MENTAL RETARDATION: Nursing approaches to care

MENTAL RETARDATION
Nursing approaches to care

Edited by

JUDITH BICKLEY CURRY, R.N., M.S.

Regional Health Consultant,
Chicago, Illinois

KATHRYN KLUSS PEPPE, R.N., M.S.

Assistant Nursing Director,
Division of Maternal and Child Health,
Ohio Department of Health,
Columbus, Ohio

with 45 illustrations

THE C. V. MOSBY COMPANY

Saint Louis   1978

The C. V. Mosby Company
11830 Westline Industrial Drive, St. Louis, Missouri 63141

Library of Congress Cataloging in Publication Data

Main entry under title:

Mental retardation.

  Bibliography: p.
  1. Mentally handicapped—Care and treatment.
2. Nursing. I. Curry, Judith Bickley, 1939-
II. Peppe, Kathryn Kluss, 1947-   [DNLM: 1. Mental
retardation—Nursing. 2. Psychiatric nursing. WY160
M551]
RC570.M419   610.73'68   77-26307
ISBN 0-8016-1196-2

C/M/M 9 8 7 6 5 4 3 2 1

Contributors

F. BRUCE ANDERSON, B.A.

School Social Worker, Suburban Community Training and Services Center, Englewood, Colorado

SUSAN BLACKBURN, R.N., M.N.

Research Instructor, Program Coordinator, Perinatal Nurse Clinician Program, Department of Maternal-child Nursing, University of Washington, Seattle, Washington

EDE MARIE BUERGER, R.N., M.S.

Clinical Nurse Specialist, Developmental Neurophysiology and Neonatology, Loma Linda University Medical Center, Loma Linda, California

JUDITH A. BUMBALO, R.N., M.S.

Assistant Professor of Nursing, Department of Maternal-child Nursing, University of Washington; Clinical Nurse Specialist, Child Development and Mental Retardation Center, University of Washington, Seattle, Washington

WILLIAM JOSEPH BURNS, Ph.D.

Associate in Psychiatry and Pediatrics, Northwestern University; Staff Psychologist, Children's Memorial Hospital, Chicago, Illinois

MARY SCAHILL CHALLELA, R.N., M.S.

Chief Nursing Consultant, Eunice Kennedy Shriver Center for Mental Retardation, Inc., Waltham, Massachusetts; doctoral candidate, Boston University School of Nursing, Boston, Massachusetts

JUDITH BICKLEY CURRY, R.N., M.S.

Regional Health Consultant, Chicago, Illinois; formerly Chief of Nursing, The Ohio State University Nisonger Center for Mental Retardation and Developmental Disabilities, and Assistant Professor, The Ohio State University School of Nursing, Columbus, Ohio

CAROL DOWLER, R.N., M.S.

Clinical Specialist, High Risk Perinatal Project, The Ohio State University, Columbus, Ohio

KAY F. ENGELHARDT, R.N., Ph.D.

Associate Professor, University of Wisconsin–Madison School of Nursing; Nursing Section Head, Diagnostic and Treatment Unit, Waisman Center on Mental Retardation and Human Development, University of Wisconsin–Madison, Wisconsin

MARCENE POWELL ERICKSON, R.N., M.N.

Associate Professor of Nursing, University of Washington School of Nursing; associated with the Child Development and Mental Retardation Center, University of Washington, Seattle, Washington

DOROTHY J. HUTCHISON, R.N., M.A.

Professor, University of Wisconsin–Madison, School of Nursing, Madison, Wisconsin

v

MARILYN KRAJICEK, R.N., M.S.

Chief Nurse, John F. Kennedy Child Development Center; Assistant Clinical Professor, School of Nursing, and Instructor, Department of Pediatrics, University of Colorado Medical Center, Denver, Colorado

WILMA LUTZ, R.N., M.S.

Assistant Professor, Capital University School of Nursing, Columbus, Ohio

BARBARA NEWCOMER McLAUGHLIN, R.N., M.N.

Assistant Professor, Child Health, Nell Hodgson Woodruff School of Nursing, Emory University, Atlanta, Georgia; formerly Assistant Professor, Department of Maternal and Child Nursing, and Clinical Nurse Specialist, Child Development and Mental Retardation Center, University of Washington, Seattle, Washington

PATRICIA McNELLY, R.N., B.S.N.

Director of Nursing Services, Central Wisconsin Center for the Developmentally Disabled; graduate student in Pediatric Nursing, University of Wisconsin–Madison, Madison, Wisconsin

SANDRA ERICKSON OEHRTMAN, R.N., M.S.

Clinical Specialist, Active Baby Care Infant Stimulation Project for High Risk and Handicapped Children, Springfield, Ohio; formerly Clinical Specialist, St. Vincent's Children's Center, Columbus, Ohio

ROSE ANN M. PARRISH, R.N., M.S.N.

Field Service Assistant Professor of Nursing, University of Cincinnati College of Nursing and Health; Nursing Educational Coordinator, University-affiliated Cincinnati Center for Developmental Disorders, University of Cincinnati, Cincinnati, Ohio

NANCY J. PATTERSON, R.N., M.S.

Mental Retardation Specialist, Human Rights Committee, Partlow State School, Tuscaloosa, Alabama

ANN WIZINSKY PATTULLO, R.N., M.N.

Program Director for Nursing, Institute for the Study of Mental Retardation and Related Disabilities; Associate Professor, School of Nursing, University of Michigan, Ann Arbor, Michigan

KATHRYN KLUSS PEPPE, R.N., M.S.

Assistant Nursing Director, Division of Maternal and Child Health, Ohio Department of Health; formerly Instructor, The Ohio State University Nisonger Center for Mental Retardation and Developmental Disabilities and The Ohio State University School of Nursing, Columbus, Ohio

MARY PATRICIA RYAN, R.N., Ph.D.

Associate Professor, Loyola University School of Nursing, Chicago, Illinois

ROBERTA G. SHERMAN, R.N., M.S.

Clinical Nurse Specialist for multiply handicapped children, University-affiliated Cincinnati Center for Developmental Disorders; Field Service Instructor, University of Cincinnati College of Nursing and Health, Cincinnati, Ohio

LUELLA STEIL, R.N., B.S.N.

Graduate student, University of Wisconsin–Madison School of Nursing, Madison, Wisconsin; formerly Perinatal Nursing Consultant, Bureau of Maternal and Child Health, Ohio Department of Health, Columbus, Ohio

SARAH S. STRAUSS, R.N., M.N.

Doctoral candidate in Educational Psychology, University of Washington, Seattle, Washington; formerly Assistant Professor of Nursing, Western Carolina University, Cullowhee, North Carolina

LUCILLE F. WHALEY, R.N., M.S.

Associate Professor, San Jose State University, San Jose, California

TO

JOHN and MIKE

Preface

Nurses have been involved for many years in the provision of care and services to mentally retarded individuals and their families. Yet little has appeared in the literature to document their efforts and contributions. This fact became obvious to us while we were teaching students of nursing and other disciplines at a university-affiliated facility for the mentally retarded. Because of our acquaintance with professional nursing colleagues, we were aware of the variety of programs and activities in which they were involved. This book is an effort by some of these nurses to present their activities and interests as a necessary contribution to the professional literature.

The purpose of this book is to serve as a resource for anyone interested in learning about nursing roles, functions, and capabilities in the field of mental retardation. Because this condition is a major health problem affecting more than six million Americans and their families, all nurses should find this book beneficial to improving and expanding their practice. It may be of special interest to nurses already working with retarded individuals, as well as to students who may consider entering this field of practice. Although written primarily for nurses, the book may also be of interest to other health professionals and to parents and families of retarded persons.

The unifying theme of the book is commitment to a humanistic, family-centered approach to services. In Part one, nursing's historical involvement and educational preparation provide a perspective for the book. Part two discusses several frameworks for nursing practice that are useful in working with mentally retarded individuals and their families. Part three progresses from presentation of preventive approaches of nursing care through identification for early case finding to interventive techniques that are useful in program planning.

Some chapters refer specifically to mental retardation, whereas others use the more encompassing term, developmental disabilities. We attempted to limit the focus of the book to mental retardation but recognized that mental retardation rarely occurs as a solitary condition. Some contributors preferred to include other developmental disabilities in the context of their chapters. For the purpose of this book, we are using the definition of mental retardation as found in the American Association of Mental Deficiency's 1973 edition of *Manual on Terminology and Classifications in Mental Retardation*. This definition requires that both adaptive behavior levels and intelligence demonstrate significant deviations from the normal before the diagnosis of mental retardation can be made. Developmental disabilities include the conditions of mental retardation, cerebral palsy, autism, epilepsy, and other neurological disorders that require similar care.

We express our appreciation to the contributors, who are both our professional colleagues and, in many cases, our personal friends. Without their interest and help, this book would not have been possible. We hope that this book will stimulate more nurses in the field of mental retardation and developmental disabilities to publish the results of their efforts.

Judith Bickley Curry
Kathryn Kluss Peppe

Contents

PART ONE

Overview of nursing in mental retardation

CHAPTER 1

Nursing in mental retardation: historical perspective

KATHRYN KLUSS PEPPE and ROBERTA G. SHERMAN

There are certain parallels between the history of mental retardation and the history of nursing. Both have been in existence for as long as man has been present in the world. The art of nursing began with the first mother who nurtured her young children or the sick. Ancient civilizations were also aware of the retarded and regarded them as objects of derision and persecution who harbored evil spirits.[2]

Few nurses have been interested in studying the history of nursing's involvement in the care of mentally retarded persons. Likewise, few historians of mental retardation have concerned themselves with what nurses have contributed to improve treatment methods. Yet nurses have indeed been participants in the care, study, and treatment of mentally retarded persons throughout their respective histories.

This chapter is limited to a brief overview of the early histories of both nursing and mental retardation. The primary focus is to trace the development of mental retardation nursing in the United States. Consideration is given to the care of re-

tarded persons and the availability of such in the community. The historical evolution of nursing roles and the educational preparation for nursing in mental retardation are identified.

There has been relatively little documentation by nurses concerning their practice or interest in mental retardation until recent years. Credit for the accomplishments of individual nurses and of the profession of nursing in advancing knowledge about mental retardation has been long overdue. This chapter is a beginning step in recording the contribution of American nurses involved in providing care to mentally retarded persons. It is hoped that other nurses will be encouraged to study further the impact that nursing has had on this specialized field.

EARLY HISTORIES OF MENTAL RETARDATION AND NURSING

In early civilizations, nursing was not recognized as a specialized profession.[3] The treatment of mentally retarded persons was also not specialized; they were confined in institutions or almshouses with the insane and received identical treatment.[2] Nursing became a distinct profession about the same time that mental retardation became a separate diagnosis requiring specialized treatment.

Note: Terms such as "the retarded" and "retardates" appear in this chapter for the purpose of maintaining consistency with their historical use as nouns. The reader is advised that these terms are not currently used.

In early primitive tribes, female relatives provided care for the sick at home. Disease and illness were believed to be caused by evil spirits and supernatural phenomena, and thus the sick were sometimes abandoned.[3] During this period of time, there is no indication of specific or organized efforts to provide shelter, protection, or training for the retarded.[6] When healing temples developed in ancient Egypt to provide nursing care for the sick, both the Egyptians and the Greeks provided humane, remedial care for those who were epileptic and insane.[3]

Extreme degrees of retardation were recognized by some early civilizations. Obviously defective children, including the mentally retarded, were abandoned by the Spartans, Greeks, and Romans. However, some wealthy Romans kept the retarded in their homes as ''fools'' to entertain their guests.[6] Roman slaves were designated as nurses to care for the sick and insane. During this time in Greece, a scientific foundation for nursing developed.[3]

The early Christian Era brought many changes to both nursing and mental retardation. Through the concept of charity, many religious nursing orders developed, which helped bring some alleviation to the lot of the retarded.[3] For example, the Bishop of Myra (St. Nicholas) showed particular compassion for them, and the Bible offered kind words.[6]

During the Middle Ages, the retarded again became the fools or jesters of nobility and religious nursing orders.[3] The retarded were no longer viewed as being ill but instead were believed to be possessed by devils and received the usual treatment of torture and cruelty. The Sisters of Charity, founded by St. Vincent de Paul, were a major exception. They gave kindly treatment to all retarded who came under their care at Bicêtre, a hospital and asylum in Paris.[2]

The Reformation led to further persecution of the retarded. They were regarded as ''godless'' creatures by Martin Luther. Both Luther and John Calvin agreed that the retarded should be killed because they were possessed by the Devil.[6] The religious wars during this period led to the closing of many monastic hospitals where nursing care had been given to the retarded. Similarly, no one received nursing care. It was not until the reign of King Henry VIII in England that hospitals were again opened and endowed to provide nursing care for the sick and disabled.[3]

The seventeenth century was a time when the mentally ill and criminals were imprisoned. However, Bethlehem Royal Hospital in England was one of the early hospitals converted to an asylum for the purpose of separating the criminals from the insane. Conditions still remained poor; hospitals were infested with vermin, and treatment was cruel. It was during this century that the first hospital to care for the sick in the American colonies was opened on Manhattan Island. In 1678, a facility in Pennsylvania was opened to care for the insane.[3]

From the early civilizations, we have seen that both nursing and care of the mentally retarded existed. However, neither nursing nor care of the retarded was considered to be a distinct part of society. Therefore, little mention of the practices in both of these fields during early times exists although they developed in a cyclical fashion. That is, nursing developed from the undifferentiated nurturing of sick individuals into the more specific purpose of the religious nursing orders. During the Reformation, most nursing orders were persecuted and disbanded. Care of the retarded followed a similar pattern of development. They were abandoned by the ancients, received kindly treatment during the era of Christianity, and during the Reformation were either killed or persecuted. Throughout all of these early periods, however, the retarded were looked upon as objects of entertainment and derision.

TRANSITION PERIOD FOR NURSING AND MENTAL RETARDATION

During the eighteenth and nineteenth centuries, nursing and care of the retarded both developed into more specific fields. Charity again became an influential force in the movement to improve care for the retarded and also helped nursing become a distinct profession.

Public attention in the American colonies during the early eighteenth century was directed toward the need to provide care for the retarded. Public care was then provided in jails, almshouses, or insane asylums. Some retarded persons were neglected and permitted to roam the countryside without care. Others were sold as slaves. Legislation during this time created guardians for the retarded and directed the overseers of the poor to take action in providing care.[2] In 1722, Connecticut's first house of correction was opened for undesirable persons, which included the retarded.[7] Blockley Hospital in Philadelphia was opened in 1731 as a federally supported almshouse. Care was provided by the inmates. In 1793, when the Blockley Hospital was under investigation for the quality of care delivered, it was found that the untrained nurses and caretakers had been negligent in conducting their responsibilities.[3]

In the American colonies during the middle eighteenth century, some special hospitals having the philosophy of providing treatment to the mentally deranged were developed. It is unclear whether the retarded received treatment in such facilities. However, the Colony of Virginia in 1769 enacted a law providing employment of nurses to care for the sick, retarded, and mentally ill.[3] By the end of the eighteenth century, it became evident that nurses must be educated in order to properly care for patients. Dr. Valentine Seaman made the first attempt to teach nurse attendants in 1798 at the New York Hospital.[4]

The reform movement of the early nineteenth century expanded into many parts of society. The concept of charity again flourished with the consequent development of many religious nursing orders in the United States.[3] For the first time, maintenance of health was thought to be a public responsibility, and public health reformers recommended establishment of state and local health departments accompanied by wise legislation.[4]

In the first half of the nineteenth century, interest in retardation spread to the United States from France, Switzerland, and the rest of civilized Europe where movements to improve the conditions of the oppressed or neglected arose. During this time, mental retardation was thought to be a unitary condition. Itard, however, hypothesized that retardation was an acquired condition that could be remedied through education. He tested his hypothesis for 5 years with Victor, the famous "Wolf Boy of Aveyron." Itard's work represented the first scientific attempt to train the mentally retarded.[6]

Guggenbühl, who believed that all retarded were cretins, opened a homelike institution in Switzerland in 1839 to provide medical treatment and education for the retarded. The Evangelical Sisters of Mercy provided daily care. Guggenbühl thus became the originator of the colony plan for institutional care of the retarded.[6] Seguin, a Frenchman inspired by Itard's efforts with Victor, opened the first successful school for educating the mentally retarded in Paris in 1839. Seguin's scientific papers encouraged Americans to open similar training schools.

In the United States, Dr. Samuel Gridley Howe had been interested in the blind and deafmute. In 1832, he established a training school for these individuals, which was later renamed the Perkins Institute for the Blind. However, the work of Guggenbühl and Seguin influenced him, and in 1848, Howe became the first superintendent of an experimental training school for the retarded. This school, first known as the Massachusetts School for Idiotic and Feeble-Minded Youth, received $2,500 a year for 3 years from the Massachusetts legislature to train ten retarded children. Appropriations became permanent when the school proved successful. The school was later renamed the Walter E. Fernald State School.[6]

In 1848, Seguin emigrated to the United States and served as a consultant in the organization of Howe's training school for the retarded. He made a major impact on the development of institutional care for the retarded in the United States and assisted in organizing these facilities in Pennsylvania, Ohio, Connecticut, and New York. In 1876, he became the first president of the Association of Medical Officers of American Institutions for Idiotic and Feeble-Minded Persons, now known as the American Association on Mental Deficiency. The objective of this professional organization was to discuss the causes, conditions, and statistics on retardation, including management, training, and educational needs.[6]

Institutional treatment for the retarded was originally envisioned by Seguin and Guggenbühl as a way to cure the condition or to attain normalcy. It soon became apparent that cure for retardation was not achieved by placement in institutions, and the hope of curability weakened to amelioration of the problem. Howe used amelioration of retardation as his purpose in establishing American institutions. Gradually, attention shifted from amelioration of retardation to concern for the needs of society. Institutions then became focused on protecting society by isolating and segregating the retarded.[6]

During this period of institutional growth, the need to reform the type of care provided to the mentally ill and retarded in almshouses and jails became evident. Dorothea Lynde Dix, a teacher and an untrained nurse, was one of the most influential reformers. Her activities were supported by Howe and Charles Sumner. In 1841, she began investigating every almshouse and jail in Massachusetts. She kept exact records of her findings, which she later used in her testimony before the Massachusetts legislature. She accomplished extension of state care for the insane. Dix was the first person to favor a state tax base to support hospitals, successfully accomplished for the first time in New Jersey in 1845. She continued her inspections of almshouses for the next 20 years in every state in the Union and took her findings to every state legislature.[3, 6] In addition, Dix established training schools for nurses in the state hospitals. At the fed-

eral level, she advocated a bill that passed through both houses of Congress to set aside 12 million acres of public land for the endowment of institutions for the insane, blind, and other helpless persons. The bill was unexpectedly vetoed by President Franklin Pierce. During the Civil War, Dix was the first woman appointed to an administrative position by the War Department and served as Superintendent of Female Nurses for the Union Army.[3] Dix's accomplishments had far-reaching effects, both on nursing and on the improvement of care for the mentally ill and retarded. By 1875, almost every state in the Union had a mental hospital supported by public funds to care for all types of mental patients.

During the middle nineteenth century, scientific knowledge about mental retardation was expanding. Down's description of mongolism (Down's syndrome) in 1866 represented a departure from the previous notion that all retardation resulted from the same cause. Down tried to classify the mentally retarded using a system based on etiology. The system included congenital idiocy, developmental idiocy, and accidental idiocy. Accidental idiocy was further classified into the categories of traumatic, inflammatory, and epileptic. A clear distinction based on severity of handicap was made between idiots and imbeciles. Other physicians began to demonstrate that there were forms of retardation closely associated with structural anomalies of the central nervous system.[6] Howe quickly grasped the importance of classification systems to treatment programs and separated the residents of his institution into three groups according to the severity of their retardation.[7]

In the last half of the nineteenth century, changes in treatment methods used in institutions continued. Although public opinion at the time viewed the retarded as a menace to society, some institution workers believed this opinion was inhumane. They developed the colony plan of institutional care by placing retarded patients into more normal living and working situations. This plan encouraged the independence of the patients but permitted supervision when necessary.[6] The colony plan had the added benefits of providing care to the retarded more economically and generating income for the institution by utilizing patients for remunerative work on farms or as domestics.[7] The first colony was established in 1878 as part of the institution for the retarded in Syracuse, New York. The first separately organized colony was started on a farm in Fairmount, New York in 1882.[6]

For the retarded who remained in the community, few treatment opportunities existed until the late nineteenth century. The first special education class for the retarded within a public school system opened in Cleveland in 1878. By 1905, special classes in the public schools were a widely accepted practice.[6, 7] At a time when the retarded were not welcome members of the community, Walter E. Fernald State School in Massachusetts began a program of parole in the community before discharge. Even with the development of thoughtful programs such as this, it is apparent that the public was not receptive to the notion of having retarded persons in the community. In 1882, the first restrictive act on immigration was passed, prohibiting lunatics, idiots, convicts, and persons likely to become public charges from entering the United States.[10]

While the retarded received care primarily in institutions, untrained nurses were the major care providers in these facilities. However, nursing was actively evolving into a profession during the last half of the nineteenth century. The religious nursing orders continued to provide the only respected nurses until Florence Nightingale established a training school for nurses in 1871 in England.[3, 10] Many of the graduates of the Nightingale School emigrated to the United States and facilitated the beginning of an organized system of nursing in this country. Nightingale influenced the development of American training schools and nursing care by guiding her former students and the founders of training schools. She was a personal friend of Dr. Elizabeth Blackwell, who founded the hospital school

in Roxbury, Massachusetts in 1872.[3] Nightingale's writings in 1865 outlined the basis for American public health nursing.[4]

One Nightingale student, Alice Fisher, went to Blockley Hospital nearly 100 years after completion of the 1793 investigation concerning the negligence in nursing care provided to mentally ill and retarded patients there (see p. 5). Fisher was instrumental in improving the nursing care provided at Blockley.[4]

The 1860s and 1870s are depicted as a period of citizen unrest and concern about the unsanitary conditions in some of the more densely populated areas. The Citizen's Association in New York City through legislative action was successful in obtaining a board of health in 1866. Social welfare groups soon developed, and the need for nurses in the community was articulated. In 1886, the Visiting Nurse Society of Philadelphia employed nurses to care for the sick in their homes. Lillian Wald in 1893 founded the Henry Street Settlement House in New York City, the first neighborhood nursing service for the sick-poor.[4]

The 1870s were not only a period of public health reform but also a time when training schools for nurses were opening in the hospitals. In 1873, Bellevue (New York), New Haven (Connecticut), and Massachusetts General Hospitals (Massachusetts) opened training schools. Almost a decade later, it was believed that hospital-trained nurses needed additional preparation in order to care for the insane, and in 1882, the first school of nursing in the McLean Asylum (Waverly, Massachusetts) was opened. Linda Richards, thought by some to be the first trained nurse in the United States, played an impressive part in the movement for training nurses in mental hospitals.[10]

The intellectual emphasis in nursing flourished during the late 1800s. *The Nightingale,* published in 1886, became the first professional journal. This journal recorded the first attempt to form an association of nurses called the Philomena Society in 1886-1887. Clara Weeks was the first nurse to publish a professional book entitled *A*

Textbook for Nurses in 1889. During the same year, religious nursing orders began opening training schools. By the end of the nineteenth century, the American Society of Superintendents of Training Schools for Nurses was formed. In 1899, it was suggested that nurses in the United States achieve legal status from a board of examiners.[4] Nursing was well on its way to gaining professional status.

In summary of the changes that occurred during the eighteenth and nineteenth centuries, social welfare movements led to improvements for both nursing and care of the retarded. A greater need for education in nursing was first recognized during this time. Consequently, programs opened in hospitals and other institutions to provide systematic training for nurses. The nursing care provided to institutionalized retarded persons also began to improve with the education of nurses. Specialty nursing practice emerged with the provision of additional preparation for nurses caring for persons in state mental hospitals. During this time, also, the foundation of American public health nursing was laid. Nursing leaders such as Dix, Nightingale, and Wald were instrumental in changing nursing to an organized profession and improving care for the retarded.

Changes in treatment practices of the retarded can be attributed to Itard, Seguin, Howe, Guggenbühl, and Down. They began developing modern scientific knowledge about retardation by questioning old theories of etiology, developing a classification system that recognized degrees of retardation, and beginning the identification of causation. New treatment methods that emerged in the United States included the use of education and the creation of specific institutions for training the mentally retarded. Due to the pressure of reformists, the American government began to assume some responsibility for the care of retarded and mentally ill persons. However, by the end of the nineteenth century, public opinion concerning the retarded had changed from a positive desire to provide necessary

treatment to the desire for isolation of the retarded and protection of society from them.

NURSING AND MENTAL RETARDATION IN THE TWENTIETH CENTURY

The twentieth century brought numerous changes for both nursing and mental retardation. Advanced preparation for specialty areas in nursing continued to emerge as nursing education in general expanded and became organized. In the field of mental retardation, society and the government increasingly assumed responsibility for providing services for diagnosis and treatment. The philosophy of care for the retarded gradually shifted from custodial care in institutions toward care in the community utilizing resources that developed from the efforts of government, parents, and professionals. The further need for educating professionals to work with the mentally retarded was evident.

Mental retardation

The "eugenics scare" was an early twentieth century movement that spread rapidly throughout the United States. Its origin stemmed from Sir Francis Galton, who first expressed his concern for the destiny of the human race in 1865. He coined the word "eugenics" in 1883 to refer to a science dealing with factors that improve the qualities of a race.[6]

The period of the eugenics scare extended roughly from 1910 to the 1930s. The pervading issue focused on the endangerment of the race due to the large number of retarded persons who rapidly multiplied themselves.[6] The eugenics scare gained initial momentum with the publications of reports indicating that entire families were retarded, paupers, or criminals. The earliest such report was Dugdale's study of the Juke family, whose members were either criminals or retarded.[7] Although the Juke family study was originally published in 1877, it did not gain widespread attention until it was reprinted in 1910. A similar report was Goddard's study of the Kallikak family, published in 1912. It increased the public's fear that retarded individuals produced only retarded offspring.[6]

The eugenics scare was characterized by social indictment of the retarded, who were viewed as degenerates spreading evil, crime, disease, and financial hardship on society.[2, 6, 12] Even prominent leaders in the care of the retarded supported the eugenics movement. For example, Fernald stated in 1912 that the retarded were parasitic predators on society who lacked sexual morals, were likely to become criminals, and were dangerous members of the community.[7] Wald agreed with the philosophy that society should be protected from the retarded.[3]

The social indictments of the eugenics movement stimulated interest in finding remedies for the spread of retardation. In 1911, the Research Committee of the Eugenics Section of the American Breeder's Association met to recommend alternatives. Although they decided that life-long segregation and sterilization of the retarded were the best solutions, they also discussed restrictive marriage laws, public eugenic education, systems of matings to remove defective genes, improved general environment, polygamy, euthanasia, neomalthusianism, and laissez-faire. From the time that states first enacted sterilization laws until 1958, records indicate that some 31,038 retarded individuals were sterilized. There was also a concurrent upsurge in segregating the retarded from society by building more institutions in which to house them. The practice of committing the retarded to institutions as a ward of the state through court action became common, thus inhibiting the discharge of retarded persons from institutions.[6, 7, 12]

Few community services for the retarded developed during the period of the eugenics scare. However, the mental hygiene movement that was prevalent during this time encouraged the establishment of child guidance clinics for all children with problems. Retardation was not particularly viewed as worthy of receiving the full service of these clinics. The first community clinic that made an effort to integrate services and research of mental retardation with its other clinical services was started in 1930 at The Johns Hopkins Hospital.[6] Special classes for the retarded were maintained within the public education system during the eugenics scare but were seen as a means of identifying the retarded for subsequent institutionalization.[7]

As a result of the need to identify appropriate children for special education classes, Binet began his work on the development of a normative performance scale in 1904 and published his results in 1905. Binet's work in developing a test of intelligence quotient (IQ) was used in differentiating the three existing categories of mental retardation: moron, imbecile, and idiot.[6] The classification system of degrees of mental retardation has been revised several times during the twentieth century. The terminology has likewise changed to currently indicate four levels of retardation: mild, moderate, severe, and profound. However, the IQ score remains one of the criteria used today to determine the level of retardation.

With the discovery of phenylketonuria (PKU) as a metabolic disorder in 1934, the eugenics scare began to lose momentum. Because retardation could be prevented in PKU by initiating dietary control, the concept of preventing mental retardation through medical treatment became important. Society became less fearful, and family care services for the retarded were offered for the first time in New York in 1933, although family care services had been offered to mentally ill individuals since 1885.[6]

The 1940s was a period of little new activity in the care of the retarded. In 1949, however, parents of retarded children organized what is now known as the National Association for Retarded Citizens (NARC), which stressed the need to provide more research, prevention, and care for the retarded.[6] This impetus led to an emphasis on families keeping their children at home and using multiple community supports.[18] Through parents' desperation to find diagnostic, evaluation, and guidance services, NARC set up clinics that were demonstration projects.[15] In 1952, NARC presented their long-range objectives to congressional leaders in an attempt to effect change.[7] In 1956 and 1957, the Children's Bureau received Congressional appropriations to establish special projects in mental retardation, which included clinical services for young children and their families.[15] It was recognized that a team approach utilizing a variety of disciplines was needed to provide this service.

Attitudes toward the mentally retarded began to change with the introduction of the "normalization principle" in 1953.[18] In 1957, Bank-Mikkelson presented normalization as the right of the retarded to attain normal existence. The principle was later refined by Wolfensberger and Nirje to emphasize individual cultural norms and to mainstream the retarded into society. Institutions were recognized as custodial environments that were not conducive to individual growth. Day care programs, sheltered workshops, and recreational facilities and agencies to assist parents were developed in the community so that the retarded had a viable alternative to institutionalization.[7]

During the 1960s, the need for institutional reform was determined. The New York State Planning Committee on Mental Disorders recommended in 1965 that institutions should become active treatment and rehabilitation centers for total community-based care and that the client population should not exceed one thousand.[9] Others thought that institutions should revert to educational training goals.[8] It was also recommended that institutional staff have consultants and university faculty available for inservice and advice.[7] In 1963, President John F. Kennedy stimulated national awareness of retardation through many social programs, particularly a request for a national program to combat mental retardation.[6] Because of Kennedy's efforts and the public disclosure of inadequate institutional facilities and programs, the effort to maintain mentally retarded persons in the community became prominent.[7] During the early 1970s, various community-oriented services, such as citizen advocacy programs, developed to assist retarded persons. Thus, the community accepted responsibility for helping maintain the mentally retarded in society outside the institutions.

Nursing's influence

The influence of the nursing profession on the field of mental retardation can hardly be measured in small terms. One of the most influential government agencies established to deal with the problems of children was the Children's Bureau, the brainchild of a prominent nurse, Lillian Wald. The Children's Bureau set the tone for governmental involvement in providing services to all children, particularly those with handicaps and mental retardation. Nursing in institutions for the retarded became a distinct and influential entity, as did nursing in community health settings. In order to better prepare nurses for these specialized fields, nursing education responded with various curricula and training opportunities. The twentieth century has so far been a time of great interaction and influence between nursing and the field of mental retardation.

Government agencies

During the twentieth century, local, state, and federal governments have assumed increasing responsibility for providing services to the mentally retarded. The Children's Bureau was one of the most prominent government agencies in this regard. Prior to its establishment in 1912, only one state and some large cities had created bureaus of child health in their departments of health. One activity of the Children's Bureau was to assist states in the development of bureaus of maternal and child health within the state health departments. The function of these bureaus was to investigate and report on all matters pertaining to the welfare of children.[4] By 1961, bureaus of maternal and child health activities had further been refined so that nearly every state offered special services for the retarded as part of their health department plan.[17]

The Children's Bureau originated from a

request to President Theodore Roosevelt by Lillian Wald. She conceptualized such a bureau to benefit all children.[3] The First White House Conference on Children and Youth, held in 1909, also encouraged the establishment of a governmental agency to focus on care of dependent children. By an act of Congress in 1912, the Children's Bureau was officially established to investigate and report on the welfare of children and child life. The Bureau's initial concern was for the problems of mentally retarded children, and it accordingly initiated three major studies from 1912 to 1919 dealing with retardation.[4, 8, 15, 17] The findings of all three studies indicated that the mentally retarded were not receiving appropriate care. In addition, a high correlation was found between retardation and the problems of poverty, neglect, dependency, and abnormal home life. These studies helped to set the direction of the Children's Bureau for subsequent years, as did the Second White House Conference on Children and Youth, held in 1919, which stressed child welfare standards.[4, 15] International concern for children and for nursing was also formalized in 1919 with the creation of the Federation of the National Red Cross Societies by world health authorities. Within this organization, a child welfare program was created as well as a division of nursing.[4]

During the 1920s, the Children's Bureau served primarily as an information clearinghouse about mental retardation. However, the Bureau recognized the importance of early detection of retardation and established mental clinics for preschool children. With the passage of the Maternity and Infancy Act in 1921, the Bureau provided educational programs for the health promotion of mothers and babies.[4] By the end of the 1920s, the Bureau stressed improved care for the retarded through legislative action for education, residential living facilities, and sterilization.[15] The Third White House Conference on Children and Youth, held in 1930, resulted in the establishment of a section on exceptional children and youth by the U.S. Office of Education. In addi-

tion, a three-stage program for child health and protection was developed. It included the identification and registration of the mentally retarded, the provision of training for some retarded while segregating others, and the social control of the retarded through supervision.[4]

The Social Security Act of 1935 gave the Children's Bureau responsiblity for financing and regulating state-administered direct service programs for maternal and child health, crippled children's services, and child welfare services. Demonstration projects were initiated to provide better services to the retarded.[8, 10, 15, 17] From 1940 to 1950, the baby boom resulted in an increased number of mentally retarded children.[15, 17] During this time, the crippled children's services programs expanded. They offered a broader range of services to children and educational opportunities for nurses, such as stipends for training orthopedic nurses. Nursing care for mothers and children in rural areas expanded during the middle 1940s through the provision of midwifery services in such agencies as the Frontier Nursing Service.[10]

Although the Fifth White House Conference on Children and Youth in 1950 identified mental retardation as one of two major problems affecting American children, the Children's Bureau reported in 1954 that its activities in behalf of the mentally retarded were quite limited.[4, 17] In an effort to expand services to the retarded, the Children's Bureau awarded a project grant to the Children's Hospital in Los Angeles to establish a diagnostic clinic for retarded children. However, public health nurses throughout the country complained that there were few, if any, resources to which children suspected of being retarded could be referred. The Bureau of Vocational Rehabilitation was meanwhile busy funding demonstration projects to establish sheltered workshops for the vocational training of the retarded in the community.[1] By 1956, the Children's Bureau had twenty-six demonstration projects to provide services to the retarded, develop new methods of service delivery, and provide training for professional workers. A budget of one million dollars was allocated for mental retardation projects, but even so, over half of the crippled children's services programs excluded the retarded. Testimony before the House Appropriations Committee, however, indicated that the greatest service gap was to infants and preschoolers. The Children's Bureau made a great effort between 1955 and 1958 to relieve the problems of service gaps. By 1958, most states offered clinical services to retarded children living at home and to their families. Over 25,000 public health nurses and 1,200 nursing students received some training to work with the retarded. Over 25,000 retarded children received complete evaluations and follow-up care. In addition, prevention of mental retardation was a concern. The need for public health screening of newborns to detect PKU was therefore emphasized.[17]

Efforts by the Children's Bureau to continue the expansion of services for the retarded continued in the late 1950s. In 1958, the Children's Bureau formed the Technical Committee on Clinical Programs, stimulating the development of disciplinary work groups. Public health nurses established an informal national committee to develop principles and guides for public health nursing activities with the mentally retarded.[17]

The trend away from custodial care in institutions toward community education and training centers offering care to the retarded was reflected in 1960 by the Bureau's expansion of maternal and child health programs in the community through new projects, clinics and increased levels of funding. Education of professionals about retardation continued through the mechanisms of conferences, symposia, training courses and institutes. It was also recognized that the needs and rights of the retarded are the same as those of other children.[13] The Sixth White House Conference on Children and Youth, held in 1960, resulted in the establishment of physical fitness programs and well-child clinics. In addition, the need for multidisciplinary services for the physically handicapped and the need for legislation for the re-

porting of battered children were identified.[4]

In 1961, the President's Panel on Mental Retardation was established, resulting in the increased involvement of the Children's Bureau with mental retardation. The Bureau focused on providing services for the multiply handicapped and, in collaboration with NARC, establishing group day care programs for retarded children. In 1962, the Bureau established diagnostic and evaluation clinics in medical centers to provide comprehensive interdisciplinary services for the retarded.[15] The President's Panel on Mental Retardation turned its attention to encouraging prevention of retardation through research, improved prenatal and postnatal care, education, and early intellectual stimulation and to focusing on high-risk groups. The need to expand professional education in order to improve the shortage of manpower resulted in the appropriation of federal funds to establish ten research centers concerned with mental retardation.[15]

The Maternal and Child Health and Mental Retardation Planning Amendments (PL 88-156), passed in 1963, permitted the Children's Bureau to establish Maternity and Infant Care projects. These projects were designed to prevent mental retardation by providing prenatal services to low-income mothers with high-risk conditions affecting childbearing. The President's Panel on Mental Retardation recommended that the responsibility for mental retardation should be shared by the federal, state, and local governments and that prevention of retardation should be a major concern.[8, 16] The Panel also recommended that the Public Health Service stimulate and support community services for the retarded. Funds for the construction of mental retardation facilities were provided by PL 88-164, the Mental Retardation and Community Health Centers Construction Act. In 1963, the First White House Conference on Mental Retardation was held, which focused specific attention on the problems of retardation.[16]

With the passage of PL 89-97 in 1965, the focus of the Maternity and Infant Care projects changed from the prevention of mental retardation to the problems of poverty. In addition, legislation establishing the Early Periodic Screening, Diagnosis and Treatment (EPSDT) Programs was assigned to the Department of Welfare. Medicare legislation resulted in making funds available through that program for maternal and child health and crippled children's services programs.[4] The Children's Bureau did not attempt to maintain control of programs relating to mothers and children and was subsequently eliminated in 1967 with the passage of PL 90-248, a revision of the maternal and child health legislation that strengthened the departments of health, education, and welfare and resulted in a reorganization.[8] In other activities during 1967, the President's Committee on Mental Retardation noted deplorable conditions within residential facilities for the retarded due to overcrowding, underfinancing, and understaffing.[7]

From 1968 to 1976, the executive branch was involved in governmental reorganization designed to decrease the federal government's responsibility for all social and health programs.[8] The concern of the federal government for the problems of mental retardation reached its peak during the early and middle 1960s and began its decline in the late 1960s and 1970s with the dismantling of agencies such as the Children's Bureau.

Throughout the twentieth century, nursing was involved in both the initiation and implementation of governmental programs that benefited mentally retarded persons. However, nursing was involved in other arenas for provision of care to the retarded, such as institutional treatment.

Nursing in institutions

In the first two decades of the twentieth century, the quality of nursing care in institutions and almshouses was questioned. As a result of matrons binding and beating retarded women entrusted to their care, a need for money to hire trained nurses in almshouses was expressed. It was thought that conscientious nurses who could create a homelike environment for the patients were desirable. One of the prominent nursing leaders during this time suggested that nurses investigate all of the almshouses and identify problems. Institutions were not for punishment but for the care, education, and training of the retarded; hence, institutional staff should provide activities to enhance the growth and learning of the mentally retarded. It was thought that well-prepared graduates from hospital schools of nursing should staff these institutions.

Little was written about the role of the nurse in institutions for the mentally retarded until the 1940s. At that time, nurses were identified as supervisors, administrators, and providers of bedside care. Nursing soon assumed the ideals of a client-centered approach to care of the mentally retarded. In 1950, the Pacific Colony in California utilized the superintendent of nurses and a trained psychiatric nursing instructor to provide orientation and evaluation of new employees who were expected to have knowledge of nursing skills and a humane attitude toward the mentally retarded.[19] During this decade, nurses promoted the goals of maximum independence and achievement within a homelike atmosphere for institution residents. Nurses advocated a team approach, acting as the team coordinator, and utilizing other disciplines as consultants in order to provide meaningful patient programs. Nurses also worked with nursing students during their clinical experiences in institutions.[15] The nurse supervisors' duties involved supervising and planning nursing care, providing a good environment for patients, providing inservice education, and arranging nursing staff time and assignments. A specific form of nursing intervention in institutions was evolving as the 1960s approached.

Many nursing staffs in the early 1960s used remotivation techniques with institution residents and obtained positive results. Remotivation is a group approach to developing human relationships through activities that bring residents in contact with the real world (such as current sports events and political happenings).[1] It was also recognized that bedridden residents needed 24-hour nursing care similar to that of patients in a general hospital.

In the middle 1960s national recognition of the plight of the mentally retarded brought pressure on institutions to provide educational training instead of custodial care.[2] Nurses were noted to begin using operant conditioning in helping residents learn daily living skills. Penny, a nurse supervisor from an institution, published a book during this time on the practical care of the mentally retarded in the institution. The book stressed the ideals of an educational environment for residents.[12] In 1967, a study on institutions for the retarded revealed that nursing personnel met minimal state requirements because most registered nurse positions were filled by licensed practical nurses. Normalization in institutions, that is, requiring the development of a normal environment for residents, was resisted for a number of reasons. One identified factor was that nurses were resistant to change.[7]

Therapeutic nursing intervention and improvement of institutional environments were the themes advocated in the early 1970s. Humanization, a recognition of the human rights and dignity of the retarded, received much attention during this time. Nursing was involved in activities that brought change in institutional care. Other chapters in this book more explicitly identify these innovative changes.

The influence of nursing on the development of governmental programs and care in institutions has been presented. Another major avenue of nursing accomplishments in providing care for the mentally retarded exists in the practice of community health services.

Community health nursing

Nursing in the settlement houses paved the way for developing nursing activities in the community during the twentieth century. In 1900, nursing in settlement houses included assessing the environments in which children lived, initiating change and reform, and developing services in the

community to meet the unmet health needs. These activities included organizing a playground in the neighborhood and establishing first-aid rooms in schools. In 1901, nurses kept daily records of the progress of children enrolled in a hospital day school for defective children. On a trial basis in 1902, Lina Rogers worked in public schools as a school nurse. By 1906, school nurses were actively involved in case finding and referral of school children in need of health care. In 1915, school nurses detected children in need of special education.[3] School nurses also obtained histories on mentally retarded children who were to be seen by an evaluation team organized by Dr. Fernald as a traveling clinic in Massachusetts. Nurses in the early 1900s also made home visits for the purpose of assessing home environments and for health teaching. Prevention and early case finding were concepts of nursing care in community health.[10]

In the 1920s, public health nurses recognized the value of the team concept. In 1922, a nurse, teacher, and social worker in the community took the responsibility of helping families with mentally retarded children find skillful diagnostic services, assisting in educational placement, and instructing parents in daily management.[10] Screening for mental retardation was made possible with the development of well-child clinics. In 1943, nurses in well-child clinics worked with physicians to help families with mentally retarded youngsters. Parents were helped to understand their children by nurses who showed sensitivity to the feelings of family members and identified resources that included more specific diagnostic work-ups. By 1948, case finding of preschool children with handicaps was a goal.[7]

In 1950, the nursing role in mental retardation in the community and in general hospitals was to serve as teacher, parent substitute, and parent advisor. In the middle 1950s, nursing's involvement on diagnostic clinic teams was delineated. Public health nurses continued some of the previously described roles and activities but became more attuned to dealing with the family's reaction to the birth of a defective child as well as follow-up home management services.[15] Public health nurses in 1954 were frustrated with the scarcity of diagnostic resources and nursing consultants.[15, 17] Nurses began to accept more responsibilities within community services for the mentally retarded. In 1956, at least one state was known to have a nurse, teacher, and psychologist involved in a home visitation program to teach parents how to manage their children at home. In addition, all children received nursing services in a community class. During the same year, there were nurses on staff for camp programs.

Mental retardation nursing consultants from maternal and child health programs were working in diagnostic clinics as early as 1956. These nurses were responsible for planning, developing, and evaluating child health programs; interpreting local and state resources to the diagnostic team; and assisting local health department nursing staff in clarifying the role and functions of public health nurses. The multiple roles and activities of nurses involved in community diagnostic and evaluation clinics were clearly delineated in the 1958 Mental Retardation Institute for Nurses. The responsibilities of public health nurses in these specialty clinics included case finding, well-child care, prevention, training for activities of daily living, family planning, identification of resources, help for families in decision making regarding health care of their children, and community organization. The activities of the nurse consultants, some pediatric nurses, and other public health nurses in the diagnostic clinics included intake evaluation, nursing assessment of children, inservice education, development of clinic policies and procedures, coordination of services, development of educational materials, liaison between clinic and health department, client referrals, community education, participation in the diagnostic team decisions, and leadership in parent group discussions.[14] By the 1960s, it was acknowledged that a multidisciplinary approach, including nursing, was the most effective way to provide service to families with mentally retarded children.

The expanded role of nurses in mental retardation programs was defined in 1960 at the Second Conference of Nurses Participating in Special Projects for the Mentally Retarded. The discussion topics for this conference focused attention on the preschool child as a target for case finding. A family-centered approach was advocated for the nurse specialist in mental retardation.[11] Educational experiences for nurses were also identified as an area of concern. Interviewing skills and tools for assessing growth and development were referred to as important areas of knowledge for nurses to gain.[13]

Interest in mental retardation grew in the 1960s. Public health nurses acknowledged their responsibility for providing professional attitudes, determining developmental readiness, and providing infant stimulation. In 1963, the Third National Conference for Nurses in Mental Retardation was held, which focused on prevention, early case finding, care of high risk maternity patients and infants, newborn assessments, day care, and needs of the multiply handicapped.[11] The realm of nursing in mental retardation became more comprehensive. With the inception of the university-affiliated centers for mental retardation, nursing specialists became nurse educators in universities and colleges. The Fourth National Conference for Nurses in Mental Retardation in 1967 focused on the clinical nurse specialist in multidisciplinary training facilities. The chief nurses in the university-affiliated centers were expert practitioners holding faculty appointments and having the responsibility for educating nursing students at the master's and baccalaureate levels. These nurses were also expected to participate in community organization, consult with community nurses, evaluate nursing programs, participate in research, and offer nursing services to children and families through evaluation and home management programs. Nurses employed in the university-affiliated centers were required to have preparation at the master's level or higher.[11]

Nurses in general hospitals also recognized a responsibility to patients with mental retardation. These nurses provided general health care and habit training and developed therapeutic relationships. During the 1970s, nurses have recognized their accountability to families in preventing institutionalization and promoting healthy parent-child interactions and community living. Guidance to families in the areas of infant care and stimulation and in parental adjustment through the techniques of crisis intervention have been major areas of concern for nurses in recent years.[7]

During the twentieth century, nursing in community health has been greatly involved with the care of mentally retarded individuals and their families. Many innovative activities and functions have been explored and defined by nurses in the community. Some of the innovations in community nursing care to the retarded are discussed in other chapters of this book.

Nursing education

Educational preparation for mental retardation nursing was identified as a specialty for those nurses who desired additional knowledge. Education for nurses in mental retardation was made available in some institutions before the turn of the century. Dr. Rogers, Superintendent of the Minnesota School for Feeble-Minded, started a 2-year training course for attendants and nurses in 1896. This course was eliminated when Dr. Rogers died in 1917. In 1901, the University of Chicago opened a training school for nurses and teachers who were working with defective children in a hospital day school. It was thought that specific training in mental retardation nursing should be a postgraduate course offered to hospital-trained graduates.

Curricula in basic nursing education in the first 5 decades of the twentieth century did not include specific courses in mental retardation nursing. However, nursing students had general knowledge and some clinical exposure to the mentally retarded in pediatric, psychiatric, and public health nursing courses.[4, 10] A pediatric nursing text published in 1936 indicates that nurses who worked with the mentally retarded needed special training. Nurses working in institutions had inservice education programs available to them in 1939. In 1945, Dr. Whitney at the Elwyn Institute offered a course on mental retardation to students in schools and colleges in the Philadelphia area. Nursing students were among those identified as participants.

In the early 1950s, it was recognized that public health nurses needed a specific knowledge base in order to work with the mentally retarded. Three levels of training were suggested: generic nursing training, interprofessional training, and specialist training in the problems of retardation. Postgraduate courses and seminars for those already in practice were considered to be sufficient.[18] With the development of clinics for the mentally retarded through maternal and child health programs, plans for providing educational preparation for public health nurse consultants evolved in 1957. This resulted in organizing regional mental retardation nursing meetings and a 2-week long training program in Tulsa, Oklahoma in 1958. Public health nurses in the field were given educational opportunities through 1-day staff education programs, inservice education, and institutes.[14]

Nursing consultants in maternal and child health and public health soon took an active part in contributing to nursing education. In 1960, Gertrude Johnson, a public health nursing consultant, acquired a faculty appointment at Boston University and began working with graduate nursing students. Many opportunities for learning about mental retardation nursing were made available to students through clinical experiences in diagnostic clinics, nursery schools, homes, and parent groups. Mental retardation nursing soon became an area for scientific study with graduate students systematically researching nursing care problems.[13]

The lack of manpower to provide

adequate services for families and their children with mental retardation was one of the forces that led to the establishment of university-affiliated centers for mental retardation (UACs). Money was appropriated for these training centers in 1966 through the Department of Health, Education, and Welfare. For nurses working with the mentally retarded, preparation at least at the baccalaureate level was considered to be a necessity. The objectives of the UACs focused on training students and professionals from the many disciplines essential to provide appropriate care for the mentally retarded and multiply handicapped. Training occurred within an interdisciplinary model, stressing diagnosis, treatment, and prevention. The activities of these centers also included research, community planning, and service. Nursing was identified as one of the disciplines essential for this educational endeavor. Graduate nursing students were the first priority for training nursing students, and undergraduate students were the second.

At the Fourth National Conference for Nurses in Mental Retardation in 1967, nurses from the UACs discussed the development of basic nursing curricula to include mental retardation nursing. Nursing concepts relevant to this specialty were identified and learning experiences explored for integration into the basic curriculum.[11] An effort to accomplish this occurred in 1968 when the University of Tennessee was funded for a 5-year project to offer elective courses in mental retardation nursing to undergraduate students. Data were also systematically collected on student knowledge and attitude change about mental retardation. The Tennessee study indicated that mental retardation nursing should be integrated into the basic curriculum of baccalaureate schools of nursing.[5] Even though specific knowledge and experience in mental retardation nursing remains on an elective course basis, nurse educators in mental retardation continue to make inroads into basic nursing curricula.

SUMMARY

This chapter has traced the development of nursing in mental retardation in the United States. A brief review of the histories of nursing and care of the retarded has been presented, placing emphasis on American developments in both fields. Through the tracing of developments in both nursing and mental retardation, it has been shown that these fields have been interactive and mutually influential. This chapter has provided a historical perspective for subsequent chapters describing current nursing theory and practice in the field of mental retardation.

REFERENCES

1. Baumeister, A., editor: Mental retardation, Chicago, 1967, Aldine Publishing Co.
2. Best, H.: Public provision for the mentally retarded in the United States, Worcester, Mass., 1965, Hefferman Press, Inc.
3. Bullough, V., and Bullough, B.: The emergence of modern nursing, ed. 2, New York, 1969, Macmillan, Inc.
4. Doland, J. A.: Nursing in society; a historical perspective, Philadelphia, 1973, W. B. Saunders Co.
5. Haynes, M.: Teaching mental retardation nursing, Am. J. Nurs. **75:**626, 1975.
6. Kanner, L.: A history of the care and study of the mentally retarded, Springfield, Ill., 1964, Charles C Thomas, Publisher.
7. Kugel, R., and Wolfensberger, W., editors: Changing patterns in residential services for the mentally retarded, Washington, D.C., 1969, President's Committee on Mental Retardation.
8. MacQueen, J.: Historical development of MCH/CC organizational structures, Biregional Conference of MCH/CC Directors, Columbus, Ohio, Jan. 27, 1976.
9. New York State Planning Committee on Mental Disorders: A plan for a comprehensive mental health and mental retardation program for New York State, report to the governor, vol. 1, July 1, 1965.
10. Nuesse, C. S., and Sellew, G.: A history of nursing, St. Louis, 1951, The C. V. Mosby Co.
11. Nursing in Mental Retardation Programs, proceedings from the Fourth Annual Workshop, April 4-7, 1967, Miami, Fla.
12. Penny, R.: Practical care of the mentally retarded and mentally ill, Springfield, Ill., 1966, Charles C Thomas, Publisher.
13. Proceedings of the second conference of nurses participating in special projects for mentally retarded children, Washington, D.C., May 25-27, 1960, Children's Bureau Conference.

14. Reports from nurses participating in special projects for mentally retarded children, Washington, D.C., June 2-3, 1958, Children's Bureau Conference.

15. U.S. Department of Health, Education, and Welfare: Historical perspective on mental retardation, 1954-1964, Washington, D.C., 1964, Welfare Administration.

16. U.S. Department of Health, Education, and Welfare: An introduction to mental retardation problems, plans, and programs, Washington, D.C., June, 1965, The Department.

17. U.S. Department of Health, Education, and Welfare, Social Security Administration, and Children's Bureau: Health services for mentally retarded children, a progress report, 1956-1960, Washington, D.C., 1961, Children's Bureau.

18. World Health Organization: The mentally subnormal child, technical report series No. 75, April, 1954, World Health Organization.

19. Wyers, R., and Tarjan, G.: The supervisor as teacher and trainer, Am. J. Ment. Defic. **54:**297, Jan. 1950.

CHAPTER 2

Nursing education in mental retardation: status and needs

NANCY J. PATTERSON

Educational preparation for a specific responsibility requires answers to the following question: Who is being prepared to do what with whom and in what location? The answers to this question will serve as a basis for setting forth certain guidelines for the educational preparation for nurses in mental retardation.

WHO IS BEING PREPARED

For purposes of this chapter, the question of who will be limited to the registered nurse. This is not to discount the value of the other members of the nursing team, such as the licensed practical or vocational nurse and the nursing assistant or aide. Indeed, the worth of the registered nurse is often dependent on the ability of these members of the team to implement the nursing plan. This brief recognition of their value is the limit of consideration in this chapter.

It is generally accepted that there are three types of registered nurses with three levels of educational preparation. The length of preparation can be as little as 2 years or as long as 5 years. The 2-year graduate, often referred to as the graduate of an associate degree nursing program, is prepared to function at beginning levels in acute care settings. The 3-year graduate, or diploma graduate, is also prepared to function in acute care settings. Many of the remaining

diploma schools are attempting to prepare graduates who can function in other health care settings at beginning levels. The third type of registered nurse is the graduate of a 4- or 5-year program, resulting in a bachelor of science degree in nursing. This graduate is also prepared to function at beginning levels and to work in a wide variety of settings, including those providing preventive services and health maintenance as well as acute care. The foregoing descriptions of the three basic levels of nursing education are perhaps open to some debate but are the operational definitions used in this chapter.

There has been considerable effort on the part of the nursing profession to more clearly delineate the levels of nursing and identify job responsibilities in keeping with the level of preparation.[1, 2, 8] The concept of "a nurse is a nurse is a nurse" is still quite prevalent, however, and is reinforced by the fact that all levels still write the same state board examinations. In addition to their basic preparation, many nurses choose to further their education in some specialty. Generally, this occurs either through further academic preparation, such as a master's degree or a doctorate, or in experiential ways through continuing education. One result of the variety of levels of nursing education is confusion for nurses, their professional colleagues, and the consumer of nursing services.

WHO IS BEING SERVED

Mental retardation is a condition that can occur in isolation but is more apt to be associated with related disabilities. Decreased intellectual capacity renders individuals less able to adapt to their environments, especially if other developmental difficulties are present. Persons who are incapacitated in such a manner are currently referred to as being developmentally disabled. The Developmentally Disabled Assistance and Bill of Rights Act of 1975 clarifies this disability as (1) attributable to mental retardation, cerebral palsy, epilepsy, autism, or dyslexia, (2) any other condition related to mental retardation by a similar impairment of general intellectual functioning or adaptive behavior, or requiring treatment and services similar to those of mentally retarded persons, (3) originating before age 18, (4) continuing or expected to continue indefinitely, and (5) constituting a substantial handicap to the person's ability to function normally in society. The U.S. Office of Education in 1970 stated that there were 7,083,000 handicapped individuals from birth to 19 years of age in the United States. If nursing services are provided for these individuals and their families, it is estimated that the population would approximate 25,000,000 people.[9]

When the definition of the population being served is discussed, prevalence of the condition should be stressed. Because of problems associated with development, there are very few linkages with ethnic background, socioeconomic levels, and other usual measures of incidence. Furthermore, because these are conditions rather than diseases, such persons often have a normal life expectancy. With recent trends toward other community alternatives to residential placement and a more rapid return to the community from a residential setting, developmentally disabled persons are becoming more visible. As efforts are increased to provide more normal life-styles,

this visibility will continue to increase. Therefore, it can be stated that mental retardation and other related disabilities are not limited to specific groups of people or particular locations but are dispersed fairly evenly throughout the overall population. Regardless of the setting in which a nurse is working or living, encounters with developmentally disabled persons will occur. It may be a trend that the educational preparation for nurses and other professionals working with the retarded will be considered less of a specialty as these individuals become more visible in the community.

WHAT NURSING SERVICES ARE NEEDED

The best treatment for a condition such as developmental disability is prevention; therefore, the role of the nurse begins with prevention. In developmental disabilities, prevention begins with the potential parents. The nurse working in a school setting has opportunities to teach (1) the importance of adequate nutrition, (2) sex education and family planning, and (3) other factors known to produce infants at risk.[4]

The role of prevention is further attended by nurses who work in labor and delivery. They can monitor the danger of oversedation of the mother and signs indicating need for surgical intervention for prolonged labor. They can also be alert to fetal distress, anoxia, or other problems.

In the nursery, nurses have a dual role of prevention and early case finding. Prevention focuses on observing for signs and symptoms of hypoglycemia, hyperbilirubinemia, and other conditions that, if not treated, could result in mental retardation and related disabilities. In addition, the staff of the newborn nursery is in a strategic position to identify the minor anomalies and soft signs of an underlying, more significant problem.

The physician's office and the public health clinic become the next focus for needs. If a developmental disability is suspected, the services needed during the first few months of the baby's life include significant contact with and support of the family. Additional data can be collected at this time, and the nurse can gather meaningful information through serial observations and careful monitoring of developmental progression. Home visits can present a better picture of how the baby is adapting to the environment and can provide an opportunity to assess family reactions, coping patterns, and their ability to deal with crisis.

If a more comprehensive diagnosis and evaluation are required, a referral to a specialized resource may be necessary. Nurses working in such settings should explore the family-child relationship in more depth and provide additional assessment of the child as a contribution to the overall team evaluation. Through collaboration with the family and other interdisciplinary team members, a plan of intervention should be developed that may require continued follow-up by the nurse. If such a plan calls for temporary placement in a residential facility, nursing services will be even more intense. The nurse functioning as an integral part of the team in a residential setting is involved in developing a plan of care designed to resolve the problems necessitating placement. Certain aspects of the implementation may be assigned by the team to the nurse. Certainly the nurse assumes responsibility for prevention of disease, maintenance of health, and nursing care during acute illness episodes. Serious illness or injury may require more specialized services in an acute care facility. The nurse in the community will then provide nursing care for the illness or disability of the individual who is also developmentally disabled.

When the individual returns to the family or to the community, the normal life cycle begins again. As the individual enrolls in a structured school setting, the nurse has the same concerns about good nutrition, sex education, and family planning. Appropriate guidance and counseling through adolescence and young adulthood are essential. The nurse sometimes assumes the role of advocate for individuals with developmental disabilities who cannot always articulate their own rights and needs. Regardless of

whether family life is a possibility or an option for them, persons with developmental disabilities do grow older. Nursing needs in the geriatric population are much the same for the developmentally disabled as the rest of the population except that they are still developmentally disabled.

The foregoing definition of the nurse, the population, the services, and to some degree the location of the services, have some implications for nursing curriculum design. It is not the intent of this chapter to develop prescriptive teaching packages but to identify the learner needs as related to services provided. Much more skill and knowledge are required to transform these learner needs into meaningful academic and practicum experiences.

The nurses identified as having a heavy responsibility for the prevention of mental retardation and related disabilities include the school nurse, public health nurse, office nurse, and labor and delivery room nurse. If such nurses are prepared at the baccalaureate level or below and are not presently receiving the information they need in the present curriculum, then either: (1) the curriculum should change to reflect factors that tend to produce mothers and infants at risk and the intervention strategies used to eliminate them, or (2) continuing education courses should be provided, preferably by the employer, to prepare nurses to provide these services.

Nurses functioning in the nursery, well-baby clinics, and physician's offices are identified as those more strategic to early case finding. The question is raised as to whether the nursing personnel presently working in such settings are provided even the basic information they need to function in this important role.

Nurses working in specialized areas, such as diagnostic and evaluation centers (or university-affiliated centers), early intervention programs, and residential settings, are those most likely to be providing follow-up services. As the need for more specialized services increases, more collaboration among other members of the team is required. The nurses providing follow-up services not only need clinical intervention skills but also opportunity to learn team roles, responsibility, and function.

The dilemma that nursing finds itself in today is at least in part centered around this very issue of inadequate preparation to assume the roles offered nurses on the job market. This may not be specific to service needs of the developmentally disabled but will be restricted to that need for this chapter. The resulting circumstances demand that the nurse be taught on the job or that the needed services not be given. For example, school nurses may not develop intensive courses in sex education and family planning, because they do not know that unwanted, out-of-wedlock pregnancy in a girl under 16 years of age can produce the risk of birth of a baby with a developmental disability.

Inadequate preparation was long ago recognized by nursing education but cannot be resolved by educators alone. The following recommendations are made in the interest of the nursing needs of persons with mental retardation and related disabilities. The suggestions for consideration are directed to nurse educators, employers, and the individual nurse.

Nursing educators

It is time to consider the nursing needs of individuals with developmental disabilities and teach those needs to nursing students. As has been identified, at least the following nurses require such skills: school, public health, office, labor and delivery, nursery, and those working in acute care settings, nursing homes, diagnostic and evaluation centers, and community and residential centers. Nursing needs for persons with developmental disabilities should no longer be considered a specialty to be learned outside the basic nursing curriculum.

Ongoing exchange between the nurse educator and the potential employer must occur, particularly when the employer is not a nurse. A greater understanding of the potential a nurse has to offer will more fully in-

form the employer of additional learning needs of the employee. Thus, the beginning levels of competence of the new graduate can be expanded through continuing education and on-the-job teaching. Through such a meaningful exchange, the nurse educator can keep abreast of additional or changing nursing needs and adjust the curriculum accordingly.

Nursing schools should fully inform the student of all potential work settings and skills needed to fill such positions. This will enable the nurse to identify individual learning needs.

Employers

Employers should be aware of the skills necessary for their agency. There are standards and guidelines for agencies serving individuals with developmental disabilities to provide the employer with this information. If the nurses hired to fill needed positions do not have those skills, it becomes the responsibility of the employer to provide learning experiences as necessary to achieve that skill level.

The employer has a responsibility to nursing educators to keep them fully informed of gaps between education and practice needs. An honest exchange between these persons will result in learning experiences for the nursing student that is specific to the needs of developmentally disabled persons.

The nurse

Nurses have the responsibility to ascertain the skills they will need to function in a specific role. If neither the nurse nor the employer has a clear idea of those functions, they should jointly consult with someone who is knowledgeable. For example, consultation should be sought from nursing educators, consultants, or agencies who have nurses functioning successfully in similar roles.

It is also the nurse's responsibility to determine additional educational needs, preferably jointly with the employer. An agency serving the developmentally disabled that does not provide ongoing educational opportunities for all professional staff is not meeting the needs of the individuals being served by that agency.

• • •

It would seem that meaningful collaboration among these three groups, the employer, the nurse, and the nurse educator, would assist in determining the academic preparation that the employee should have. On the basis of skills that are needed, it is suggested that a minimum of baccalaureate preparation be required for school nurses, public health nurses, office nurses, labor and delivery nurses, and high-risk newborn nursery nurses. In specialized care settings, such as a university-affiliated center, where a significant teaching responsibility exists, nurses should be prepared at least at the master's degree level. Some universities insist on doctoral preparation. In residential settings, all nurses required to function in a collaborative relationship with other team members should have a master's degree. These suggestions are based on the skills required of the nurse in these settings.

SUMMARY

The recommendation is made to nursing school faculties to provide learning experiences that would prepare students to work effectively with developmentally disabled persons. This recommendation does not dictate methodology. There are programs in the United States that have successfully prepared students in varying ways. Some schools are integrating concepts of mental retardation and related disabilities into the basic curriculum. Others are offering a specific clinical course. Still others are teaching nursing as process so that the nurses can apply their skills in any setting. Several schools offer continuing education courses in developmental disabilities. Some master's degree programs have clinical specialty offerings in developmental disabilities, and at least one university offers a postmaster's course for nurses interested in this field. As soon as mental retardation is no longer considered a narrow specialty, more schools will provide the education and clinical experience needed for nurses to function effectively as professionals.[3, 5, 6, 8]

REFERENCES

1. Haase, P. T. and Smith, M. H.: Nursing education in the South, 1973. Pathways to practice, vol. 1, Atlanta, 1973, Southern Regional Educational Board.
2. Haase, P. T., and others: A workbook on the environments of nursing. Pathways to practice, vol. 3, Atlanta, 1974, Southern Regional Educational Board.
3. Haynes, M.: Training in mental retardation for a baccalaureate nursing program, Memphis, 1971, University of Tennessee Press.
4. Haynes, U.: A developmental approach to case-finding, Washington, D.C., 1967, U.S. Government Printing Office.
5. Hiltz, B.: Mental retardation and delivery of health care services; implications for professional nursing education, Washington, D.C., 1970, Catholic University of America, unpublished paper.
6. Patterson, N. J.: A guide for integrating mental retardation content into the basic nursing curriculum, Seattle, 1968, University of Washington, unpublished paper.
7. Rieke, E.: An exploration in the integration of mental retardation content in the curriculum of collegiate schools of nursing, Boston, 1968, Boston University, unpublished paper.
8. Reitt, B., editor: To serve the future hour. Pathways to practice, vol. II, Atlanta, 1974, Southern Regional Educational Board.
9. Seidel, M. A.: Career development in the health professions, Seattle, 1976, University of Washington School of Nursing and Child Development and Mental Retardation Center.

ADDITIONAL READINGS

Barnard, K. E.: Planning for learning experiences in the university affiliated centers, Nursing in Mental Retardation Programs, proceedings from the Fourth Annual Workshop, April 4-7, 1967, Miami, Fla.
Barnard, K. E., and Erickson, M.: Teaching children with developmental problems, St. Louis, 1976, The C. V. Mosby Co.
Cook, C.: Nursing services. In Koch, R. M., and Dobson, J. C., editor: The mentally retarded child and his family, New York, 1971, Brunner/Mazel, Inc.
Wise, B.: Nursing in mental retardation; the taxonomy approach, Houston, 1971, paper presented at American Association on Mental Deficiency meeting.
Worthy, E., editor: Symposium on the child with developmental disabilities, Nurs. Clin. North Am. **10:**307, 1975.

PART TWO

Concepts in mental retardation nursing

CHAPTER 3

The family approach

MARY PATRICIA RYAN

Families can either facilitate or inhibit plans that professionals have made for retarded individuals. If one accepts the premise put forth by Ackerman that the family is the basic unit of society,[1] then it makes sense that the nurse should work with this total unit in assessing, planning, and implementing anything that goes on with a retarded individual who is a member of a family.

Few nurses would disagree with the above statements. The difficulty lies in the following areas: (1) who is the family, (2) how does one assess the needs of the family, and (3) how can one intervene in the family (given the need for such intervention)?

WHO THE FAMILY IS

For many years in writings about the family, emphasis was on the nuclear family—the husband, the wife, and their immediate children. It was thought that this unit reflected society's family unit. In the last decade as more has been learned and written about families, society's concept of family has broadened to include two or more people who live under the same roof and eat regularly at the same table.[5] Somewhere along the continuum of all families are those who have a retarded member.

Duvall says that the family is, ". . . two or more persons related by marriage, blood, birth, or adoption whose central purpose is to create and maintain a common culture which promotes the physical, mental, emotional, and social development of each of its members."* She maintains that one may belong to one or more families:

Family of orientation: the family into which one is born and from which the most basic association is acquired.

Family of procreation: the family one establishes through marriage or reproduction.

Nuclear family: the family of husband, wife, and their immediate children.

Extended family: any grouping related by descent, marriage, or adoption that is broader than the nuclear family.[2]

Ackerman thinks of the family as an organism—the basic unit of health.[1] Although he conceives of the family as consisting of a father, a mother, and their children, Ackerman agrees that the family sometimes represents a complicated household functioning as a unit composed of all those living under one roof and submitting to the authority of one supreme head. Ackerman contends that the family, as the basic social unit of society, has four functions: biological, psychological, social, and economic. The biological function is for the purpose of producing offspring to carry on the family and the society. The psychological function is to meet the individual family member's respective af-

---

*Duvall, E. M.: Family development, Philadelphia, 1971, J. B. Lippincott Co., p. 5.

fectional needs by mutual interdependence. The social function is the response that the family generates to the forces of society. It is through the social function that the family teaches its young members the many roles that they must play in the present and the future. The economic function is the provision of the family's material needs through mutual interdependence.[1] One can see that the biological function may or may not be carried out in the family that does not fit a narrow concept of family. Single-parent families, older nuclear families, and families in and from other cultures are but a few who would not fulfill the biological function defined by Ackerman or the narrow confines of the nuclear family as defined by Duvall.

After an extensive review of the family literature, a broad definition of family might be conceived of as a *holistic configuration of interacting individuals, interdependent in a social set of reciprocal relationships and cooperating toward the development and actualization of its members physically, socially, emotionally, spiritually, and politically.* The family members share a commitment to one another; that is, each has a form of investment in the operation of the family unit. Furthermore, the bonds of this commitment may be legal, consanguine, emotional, religious, economic, or any combination of these. More than a mere collection of unique personalities, then, the family possesses a character, organization, and function of its own beyond the sum of its diverse parts.

It is important for nurses who are working with a retarded individual to identify the family of that individual. There are several reasons for this. Nurses can recognize the strengths and weaknesses of a family only if they have identified that total family unit. Retarded individuals can grow and develop to their fullest potential only with the support and cooperation of each family member. This is not to say that the retarded individual needs all of the focus of the family's efforts but that each member has a role in meeting the other's needs. The program that

is planned for the retarded individual might succeed at the expense of other family members' needs if each is not identified and included in an initial family assessment.

HOW ONE ASSESSES THE FAMILY

One problem in assessing families is to ensure that the assessment tool is broad enough to include all the information that might be collected. Yet, it should not be so broad that the assessors get lost in the complexity of it. Nurses need a simple model that provides a means of organizing information about a family in a meaningful way and that will also lead either to further questions or to planning and intervention.

There are many available assessment models that are useful in organizing material about a family in a meaningful way. However, Howells conceptualized a model that has proved useful to many nurses working with families.[3, 4] The families with which these nurses worked covered a broad spectrum. They ranged from the beginning family, preparing for and getting to know their firstborn child, to the elderly family living in a retirement home. The problems presented included learning new roles of parenting, accepting and living with a retarded or mentally ill member, and aging.

Howells has proposed a model for assessing families that has fifteen dimensions. Five dimensions are each described in three consecutive time periods: past, present, and future. The dimensions are: (1) the dimension of individuals, (2) the dimension of internal communications, (3) the dimension of general psychic properties, (4) the dimension of external communications, and (5) the dimension of physical properties.[4]

Dimension of individuals

Individual members are identified and described as completely as possible in their physical and psychological components. It is important to record how the information was obtained: direct observation and interaction with the individual, information given by another family member or health professional, or, from a written record.

Nurses may find that they have uneven amounts of information about the family members. Illnesses and disabilities will generally yield much information about one family member. It is not necessary to pry the information out of the family. Through a continuing relationship with the family, the nurse will be able to slowly gather information about each member.

Dimension of internal communication

How does each of the family members relate to each other? How does each of these members relate with other parts of the family? The child relates with the mother, the mother with the child; child with father, father with child; child with parents, parents with child. The child also relates with each of the siblings individually and with the siblings collectively. This is a complex and important dimension to assess if the nurse is to determine which family members will be able to help in working with their retarded member. For example, if the mother is the person most available to work directly with the retarded individual, the nurse must know from whom the mother will get her support—her husband, her parents, or her grown children.

Dimension of general psychic properties

Every family has characteristics that are similar to those of all other small groups but that are particular to this family. What are the conflicts that a particular family encounters in its everyday living? How does it go about resolving these conflicts? How does it assign tasks? Who is the task leader? Who is the emotional leader? How does it communicate feelings? Can the family problems be identified? In contrast, what are its harmonies? What enjoyable things do they do together? What gives it satisfaction? What does it do as a group? How does it reward its members? How does it punish them? How does it treat ill or disabled members? These are a few of the many questions one could ask of the family as a small group in this dimension.

Dimension of external communication

Each family member interacts with some level of society, and each family interacts as a group with society. A myriad of relationships is set up between the family and the community. In many instances, the head of the family is working in the community. The children are usually enrolled in public or private schools and usually play in the neighborhood or join clubs. The adults in the family have friends with whom they interact. In many instances, special services are needed by the family for assistance in caring for their retarded member. With these services come interaction with health care or welfare systems. An important community agency with which many families interact is their church or synagogue. The family is expected to subject itself to the dictates of society; how well the family conforms is an important part of the assessment process. The nurse who works with retarded individuals and their families encounters many families who have given up on society. The family more or less shuts the door to the outside world and has as few contacts as possible with their community. Trying to get the door reopened by establishing a trust relationship is a slow and arduous task. Helping a family to reestablish ties with its community is an important function of the nurse. Many of these family members have had painful experiences with their communities. Dictates, disappointment, scorn, and ridicule are some of the negative experiences that these isolated families have. Honest answers, support, facilitation, and problem solving are some of the positive experiences that must be provided before effective links are reestablished between these families and their communities.

Dimension of physical properties

This dimension focuses on the physical properties of the family. Each family owns or rents a house or an apartment of a certain size in a neighborhood. It has an income of a certain amount that permits it to purchase food, buy clothing, buy or replace furniture,

Dimensions of:	Past	Present	Future
Individuals			
Internal communication			
General psychic properties			
External communication			
Physical properties			

Fig. 3-1. Representation of Howell's fifteen dimensions.

or pay for health services. The family has a diet that is particular to its ethnic origin and social class level. This dimension includes all the physical items with which a family surrounds itself as it grows and develops. Some families maintain themselves fairly well with a minimum of physical items, whereas others need numerous such items to survive. It is helpful to gather information on these properties in order to understand the economic needs of the family and the flow of money in and out of the family. A family may seem to have an adequate income to take care of its members, but the nurse may discover that much of the income is spent on food or recreation with little left over for long-term problems, such as health care or education of a retarded member. Help with budgeting may be one of the primary services in helping a family adjust to its optimum development.

In summary, Howells' model for assessing families contains five dimensions that are to be conceived in the past, present, and future time periods. Some nurses who have used this model have started in the present time perspective, using the past to understand the present, and including each of

them to help the family anticipate the future (Fig. 3-1).

HOW THE NURSE CAN INTERVENE IN FAMILIES

Numerous interventions can be used with the family of a retarded person. It is only after careful assessment that appropriate ones can be identified as possibly useful to a particular family. If the nurse goes into a home and begins to intervene before the needs of the family have been assessed, the family may perceive the interventions as intrusions and may fail to change and grow in the desired direction. Beyond this, it may be perceived as another invasion from the community.

Support

Support is one of the most important interventions that the nurse can provide the family who is experiencing the acceptance of a diagnosis of retardation for one of its members. The availability of the nurse as a listener of the family as it identifies and works through feelings about the diagnosis is an important function. Most families have aspirations for each of its members. Some families must face the loss of fulfillment of these plans. Grieving is a process that must take place before the family members can mobilize their energies to solve present problems and to plan for the future of their family unit. The nurse who encounters a family who has just learned that one of their members is retarded may be confronted many times with the disbelief, anger, or depression of some of the individuals. If the nurse is not aware that loss could be experienced and that grieving is in process, attempts to help may not be effective. Nurses are aware of the possiblity of grieving during the period when a newborn is diagnosed as retarded, but they may forget that this same process may occur at other stages during the family cycle. For example, the middle-aged wife who is confronted with the fact that her husband will probably never function "normally" again due to a head injury needs support in grieving over the loss of her "ideal" husband and of her plans and aspirations for their future. Each of their children also needs support to ensure that there will be some alternate plans since the husband-father will be unable to fulfill his roles effectively.

For some families, support is needed as a validation that they are doing their own problem solving. Many nurses have found that families can be very creative in finding solutions to their problems of care for a retarded member. They need a valued and trusted community worker to recognize and praise their efforts. The nurse certainly has the opportunity to fulfill this need. One must consider the fact that many families will need much support at certain times in their development and then apparently function quite well at other times without much support. Through use of the dimensional approach in assessing families, such critical periods will be identified if one keeps in mind the three time perspectives. Some parents of young retarded individuals often worry about what will happen to their children when they reach puberty and begin to be interested in members of the opposite sex. Other families worry about who will take

care of their children when the parents are gone. Many do not want their other children to be burdened with the care of a retarded sibling. The more often that a family has the opportunity to discuss such fears, the better able they will be to plan for these events.

Information giving and health teaching

Information giving and health teaching are important interventions in working with families who have a retarded member. A family that has been confronted with the fact that one of its members is retarded usually has many questions. Some of these questions are easily answered. Others are very complex. An attempt should be made to answer all of the questions that a family has raised. To do this, the nurse must know where the answers may be obtained. The nurse needs knowledge of how to get to the source of information or where the family might be referred for answers. The nurse needs patience in answering questions that arise during the grieving process because some answers might not be heard. The nurse must be prepared to answer the same questions again and again until they are heard or until the family clarifies what it really wants to know.

Although the family is a unit, some individual family members may be more ready than others to learn about its retarded member. The nurse should have identified these members in the ongoing assessment and should begin to work with these members so that they can effectively care for their retarded member.

Crisis intervention

Most families are confronted with events that are so overwhelming that problem solving breaks down and a crisis is precipitated. The nurse who is working with a family during this time should help the family members identify the crisis so that the family can be assisted in appropriate methods of coping. Once the crisis or potential crisis is identified, the nurse can help the family decide how it will resolve it. If the family's past experiences with problem solving have been successful, the nurse has only to act as a catalyst for the present crisis resolution to begin. But, if the family is already burdened with unresolved crises, more active intervention may be necessary. If the crisis is directly related to care of the retarded individual or is compounded by care of this individual, temporary placement of the retarded member in a health care facility may be necessary. There are few temporary care facilities available, but organized parent groups have begun to verbalize the need for such programs. Professional counseling may be needed before crisis can be resolved. Because of the great amount of care needed by some retarded individuals, special problems can arise between the parents, between the parents and siblings of the retarded individual, among the siblings in the family unit, or with one individual or more in this unit. Special care should be exercised in the assessment process in order to be alerted to such potential crises.

SUMMARY

It is extremely important for the nurses who work with retarded individuals and their families to have answers to the following questions. Who is the family? How does one assess the needs of the family? How can the nurse intervene in the family? It is only when nurses have answers to these questions that they will be effective in working with families.

REFERENCES

1. Ackerman, N. W.: The psychodynamics of family life, New York, 1958, Basic Books, Inc., Publishers.
2. Duvall, E. M.: Family development, Philadelphia, 1971, J. B. Lippincott Co.
3. Howells, J. G.: Theory and practice of family psychiatry, New York, 1968, Brunner/Mazel, Inc.
4. Howells, J. G.: Principles of family psychiatry, New York, 1975, Brunner/Mazel, Inc.
5. Hunger, U.S.A.; a report by the Citizen's Board of Inquiry into hunger and malnutrition in the United States, Boston, 1968, Beacon Press.

CHAPTER 4

Principles of normalization

KAY F. ENGELHARDT

The purpose of this chapter is to encourage nurses to promote an average life-style for individuals who are mentally retarded and for their families. The concept of normalization provides direction for parents and other persons working with mentally retarded individuals. Use of normalization assists retarded persons to become integrated into their communities by developing life-styles similar to their peers who are not retarded.

In the field of developmental disabilities, nursing considers both the child and the family as clients. Traditionally, the nurse has assisted the family to relate to its health care needs considering the variables that affect health. Since health includes both mental and physical well-being, the range of concerns is broad and often includes home, school, health, and work problems. The nurse should assist the family of a mentally retarded member in understanding the principle of normalization: its meaning, questions of how to apply the principle, and the long-term consequences of the principle. Parents, the primary decision makers in dealing with the health system, need to have an understanding of normalization in order to make appropriate and effective decisions.

Before promoting normalization to parents as a guide, the nurse must understand the concept. Originally defined in 1957 by Bank-Mikkelson, normalization was a state-ment of the mentally retarded individual's rights to obtain a more normal existence. The individual should have a normal life similar to that of peers who are not mentally retarded.[1] Nirje further emphasized the "normal" impact of the concept and the means by which normalization would be achieved. He proposed that mentally retarded persons have life-styles patterned after those of general society.[7] Wolfensberger refined the concept by placing the goal and means in the context of the individual's culture, that is, general social environment, including ethnic, age-peer, rural-urban, and other influences. Wolfensberger defined the goal of normalization as the development of behaviors and characteristics by the mentally retarded person that are average or normal for the individual's culture. The techniques and environments used to attain the goal were also to be the usual or accepted methods for the general culture.[9]

Wolfensberger further expanded the concept of normalization to include any group of individuals who could be identified as deviant and directed normalization toward improving services for persons viewed as different from the statistical average of the population. He defined deviancy as a significant difference from other people in a negative direction.[9] Deviancy is recognized by behavior and appearance, is of low status, and results in social segregation and isolation. In order to be considered deviant, individuals or populations must demonstrate a characteristic that is visible and negatively valued. For society to have valuing impact, the population of individuals demonstrating that characteristic must be in the minority. Examples of populations that could be considered deviant are people who are aged, obese, mentally ill, or mentally retarded. Obviously, not all members of these populations would be considered or treated as deviant at all times, in all situations, in all places, or by all people. Average behavior and average treatment of individuals in society are the basis for comparison of populations recognized and treated as different.

Social segregation or isolation is the result of being viewed as deviant by societies. For mentally retarded persons, this has taken the form of labeling, institutionalization, and separate community social and health services. Contact and interaction with people other than family, caretakers, or other individuals with the same condition are limited.

Another major problem of being a member of a deviant group is the loss of individuality. The characteristics of the most severely affected members of the group become attributed to every member of the group. As a result, self-respect, assertiveness, and opportunities for risk taking are not included as a part of life for the mentally retarded.

Normalization is promoted as a principle to improve behavior and life-style because mentally retarded individuals are often following patterns of living that deviate objectionably from the stereotyped normal lifestyle. Differences in behavior have often resulted from factors other than the condition of mental retardation, such as efficiency and economy in caretaking. With institutionalization as a major mode of care, mentally retarded persons lost their individuality, had limited contact with other persons, and learned socially unacceptable behaviors that were positively reinforced in the institution.

Behaviors that were acceptable in institutions but unacceptable to society were then attributed to the condition of mental retardation.

Wolfensberger has described how individuals of a negatively valued group assume the most deviant characteristics demonstrated in the group.[9] For example, it was believed that large numbers of individuals could be served efficiently and economically if planning could be based on assumptions about group needs. With this concept, consideration of each individual would not provide effective guidelines for long-term group planning. An institution attendant may therefore give complete care to all patients regardless of their needs. In a nursery school, all children may be assisted in drinking milk because one child may have difficulty. In the community, every person who is overweight may be viewed to have the same overeating problem. These examples demonstrate that long-term group planning is not always consistent with the consideration of individuality.

The normalization principle is directed toward the public as well as toward the deviant population. Lack of knowledge about, and contact with, mentally retarded individuals has resulted in their limited acceptance in society. People often feel inadequate in dealing with a mentally retarded individual. They have an expectation that the mentally retarded person will not respond in predictable ways to social interaction. They may also doubt their own ability to cope with the anticipated situation and thus feel vulnerable.

The normalization principle provides guidelines for the public and helps the retarded individual develop acceptable behaviors. With the application of this principle, the public would regard mentally retarded persons as people who could interact socially with their normal peers. Mentally retarded persons would learn that inappropriate behaviors, such as kissing and hugging strangers, would not be tolerated or rewarded. Negative behaviors would be rejected and an appropriate response, such as a handshake, would be substituted. Through repetition, the appropriate social behavior would become habit. Both parties could then participate more comfortably in further social interaction. As retarded persons gain a repertoire of social skills and increase the number of interaction encounters, the risk factor of social discomfort decreases. The general public must learn that appropriate responses from a mentally retarded person are the same as those used by any other person. When the general public becomes normalized, retarded individuals and their families will have less difficulty in attaining normal life-styles.

The concept of normalization is particularly relevant for mentally retarded persons who have lived in institutions and are not adjusting to community living. In addition, the principle is appropriately applied for mentally retarded persons who can be identified as living a life-style different from peers or who are recognizably mentally retarded by their behavior, that is, are deviant. The nurse can use the principle of normalization with all mentally retarded persons and their families to identify those persons who are in need of normalizing interventions.

Before assisting individuals and families in making decisions relating to normalization, nurses must be able to interpret the principle in a variety of situations. In addition, nurses should consider the implications for service delivery in their individual practice settings. Services often become traditionalized, in other words, presented in a format that previously had a rationale. In current situations, that rationale may or may not exist, and often the service is perpetuated without review of the rationale.

Individual practitioners can demonstrate creativity and relevance by reviewing their practice and adapting it to meet client needs. The normalization principle can be used to examine whether their practice relates to individuals or to groups identified as different. Patients, clients, individuals, and families should be responded to individually. As nurses review their practice and use of the nursing process, they should incorporate the

concept of normalization into their assessment, planning, implementation, and evaluation of the client's needs.

RECOGNITION OF NORMALITY

Professional nurses need to identify their perceptions of normality. The person who is mentally retarded has often lost individuality by being classified as belonging to a group in which the special need of mental retardation supercedes other needs. With normalization, the individual is assisted to a normal life-style that includes the right of individuality. Normalization as a focus in assisting families of retarded persons encourages nurses to recognize retarded persons as individuals who have a right to a normal life-style. With this focus, the retarded person is, in order of emphasis: (1) an individual with human rights and needs, (2) an individual according to actual chronological age, and (3) an individual with special needs. Services emphasizing normalization demonstrate consideration of *individuality, humanness, age needs,* and *special needs.* The person who is mentally retarded has more, rather than less, in common with the general public.

Normalization can be used as a practice guide with the simple criteria provided by Nirje.[7] Recognition of individuality, humanness, age needs, and special needs is incorporated in a life-style that has at least the following characteristics:
1. An average rhythm of day
2. An average rhythm of year
3. An average routine of life
4. Average developmental experiences
5. A bisexual world
6. An economic world
7. Choice
8. Average application of standards for general society

These guidelines can be used by professionals and parents to indicate whether the individual's present life-style is normal, whether available services will optimize a normal life-style, how to plan services that will facilitate a more normal life-style, and how to identify areas where consideration for normality has been ignored, neglected, or prevented.

A normal life-style incorporates average routines and general social standards. Routines include the recognizable societal activities of day, year, and life within the relevant culture of the individual. The general standards of society include risk, choice, a bisexual world, and an economic world. How the standards are applied is also important. Average routines and standards can be used as guidelines to assess the benefits or potential benefits of normalization for a retarded individual.

Without resorting to statistical methods, parents can identify normal routines by simply describing the community activities in which they participate. When a pattern has been established, the next step is to describe the routine followed by the child. The nurse then can appreciate whether that pattern: (1) is average or an extreme variation, (2) makes the child appear more like or different from age peers, (3) has a valid basis, and (4) could be made more similar to that of normal peers.

Most people follow predictable daily routines similar to those of their friends and neighbors. Predictability includes an expectation of specific behaviors during particular times of the day. In the morning people awaken, get dressed, eat breakfast, and begin the activities of the day. Adults spend the major portion of morning and afternoon in work, children in education. In Western culture, a break in daily activities occurs in the middle of the day for a meal. The characteristics of the meal vary depending on the place of the individuals involved. Activities resume for most individuals until late afternoon when people then merge into groups for different purposes from those which preceded. Socialization and recreation with friends and family then become the focus of an average, or normal, life-style. Another meal is a part of the early evening expectations of life. The daily routine consists of sleeping, eating, resting, and enjoying leisure time that occur in predictable cultural patterns.

Individuals who are mentally retarded, as well as the general population, should be able to participate in average year rhythms. Seasonal climate variations require people to adapt their recreational patterns and clothing. People usually celebrate holidays, such as Christmas and birthdays. The format of the celebration, decorations, gifts, and types of activities can be predicted to some extent by the age of the celebrants. Home decorations are another clue to determining the yearly routine.

Life for the average person includes the normal developmental experiences of infancy, childhood, adolescence, and adulthood. Predictions can be made about what individuals will be doing at several points in life, who their associates will be, where they will reside, and what community resources will be involved. An average child will usually live with a small group of adults and other children in a single-family residence. The child will be engaged in school activities in a building other than the family residence. Activities during childhood are based on dependency. With the guidance of parents, teachers, other adults, and the peer group, independence is learned. Activities include home life, school, and recreation. Adults, in contrast to children and most mentally retarded persons, usually live in relatively independent situations frequently with one or more age peers. When adults live in a family group, they are often responsible for the dependent children. The residence may be of several types, depending on the living situation and major occupational focus of the adult.

The day, year, and life experiences of retarded persons often have little similarity to those of normal age peers. For the person who is mentally retarded, days and life are often monotonous and have little relationship to what age peers might be doing in the community on that day, at that time, and at that point in life. Their ages and relationships to others often differ from that of normal peers. The adult who is mentally retarded has more difficulty achieving normalization than does the child. The discrepancy between mental ability and chronological age is most marked when the peer group assumes responsibility for mature, adult behaviors.

Identification of age peers is useful for both parents and professionals in order to recognize normal behavior and characteristics. Social behavior, activities, hair style, and dress are examples. One mother identified that her adolescent daughter's normalization goal was to "hang around the local root beer stand like the other adolescents." The daughter rejected her mother as a companion in those activities and desired a normal age peer to make her behavior acceptable.

Identifying dress and appearance standards of peers may also have adverse effects because the mentally retarded person is often criticized and ostracized for adopting the same characteristics of the general public. One young man was identified as being mentally retarded because he was in his late teens, wore wrinkled jeans and tee-shirts, was overweight, and carried a basketball. After considering this description, the observer decided that the label had actually been based on the knowledge of the presence of a nearby residential facility for the retarded. This example demonstrates that labeling occurs even when characteristics are common in the general population, such as obesity and casual dress for leisure activity.

Peers can also be used to identify normal routines of day, year, and life. The life of an average individual includes both rights and responsibilities. Each person is assisted toward ever increasing independence and responsibility for rights. Leisure and chores are examples of each. As a member of the general society, the mentally retarded person shares in these rights and responsibilities. Identification of peers provides a standard for identifying age-appropriate rights and responsibilities.

The application of society's general standards to mentally retarded individuals is inconsistent when compared with the application of those same standards to non–

mentally retarded individuals. Inherent in each person's rights is the accompanying ability to use those rights responsibly. Individuals are prepared for responsible citizenship and independent functioning in homes, schools, and other community settings. The individual is usually given an increasing amount of responsibility until independent functioning is achieved.

Rights are often withheld from mentally retarded people unless they demonstrate a standard of responsibility beyond that which is expected of the average population. Mediocrity in voting behavior, motor vehicle operation behavior, and budgeting behavior does not prevent individuals of the general population from voting, driving, and having salaries because they demonstrate minimum standards. Those same behaviors in a mentally retarded individual could result in a denial of rights. Rights may be denied in several ways. The most effective way is to assume that the person will never be capable of certain behaviors and to deny the person the opportunity to exercise rights responsibly. Another method is to apply more stringent standards when that individual's behavior is measured.

Concern for the welfare and safety of mentally retarded individuals, their families, and the general public is often a motivating factor in denying or limiting rights of retarded people. It must be recognized that the mentally retarded individual has rights, unless those rights have been legally removed. Parents and others responsible for mentally retarded adults should assume the role of adviser and leave risk, choice, and decision making to the retarded person. The need for adequate and appropriate preparation for such decision making has become increasingly evident with normalization.

Capabilities of mentally retarded persons to assume responsibility for their rights should be realistically examined. This may be accomplished by comparing retarded persons with members of the general population. For example, most voting members of our society are not fully informed about the slate of candidates. However, they have a right to vote whether or not they are informed. It is reasonable to assume that the mentally retarded person who votes is as well prepared as the average voter.

Individual practitioners should assess whether more stringent or inappropriate standards are being applied to retarded individuals. When the well-being of the individual or society is threatened, planning should be directed at reducing risk factors while maintaining the rights of the mentally retarded person. One method for providing responsible choice and risk taking is to use a continuum for planning services, increasing independency, and increasing the responsibility of the individual.

EFFECT OF NORMALIZATION ON THE FAMILY

As primary caretakers for their children, parents are presented with the problems of planning, securing, and sometimes demanding services for their children with developmental disabilities. The increasing sophistication and ever changing availability of services are factors that complicate parents' decision making. Parents need criteria and direction by which to make selections. The normalization concept provides a principle by which such choices can be made.

Normalization is not an easy process. Parents may be torn by conflicting feelings. They recognize the limitations of their children and want an average life for them but may feel that it is unattainable. Normalization may cause pain for these parents because of the impossibility of its realization. They internalize opposing arguments and may never verbalize the desire for normalization or may even consciously discard the concept. Parents may also have a fear of normalization and its consequences. Is normalization for retarded individuals in conflict with normalization for their families? It is reasonable to assume that intensive programs that benefit the retarded member result in heavy responsibilities for parents or other family members. This produces stress and abnormal life-styles for all family members.

The presence of a mentally retarded person in a family has been shown to have both positive and negative effects on siblings.[3-6] Researchers often found adverse effects, such as increased tension and antisocial behavior in siblings. They concluded that increased interaction and responsibility for the retarded sibling were the reasons. Possible abnormal aspects of family life may be an area toward which intervention should be directed. Berge and Stauder have attempted to determine preadolescent and adolescent siblings' knowledge and attitudes about mental retardation.[2, 8] Both studies demonstrate positive results when community contacts are increased. Stauder demonstrated that adolescents have relatively consistent knowledge and attitudes regardless of their geographical location, sex, age, or parental variables of income or education.[8] Berge found that previous experience appeared to be a factor that influenced the increased knowledge and approachability regarding mental retardation. Berge also reported that eight- to twelve-year-old siblings of the retarded demonstrated more knowledge and positive attitudes than their mothers perceived them to have. The presence of the mentally retarded sibling in the home affected the responses of the normal sibling. No normal sibling in this group had a self-concept or knowledge score above the median.[2]

The implementation of normalization is not assured by the mere presence of mentally retarded persons in their homes. Research that examines normal aspects of life for mentally retarded persons and their families is needed. Alternative residential placements, such as small group homes, foster placement, or apartment living, may be necessary to optimize normal life-styles for both the retarded person and the family. The effects of normalization probably will not be measurable until the general public becomes more accepting of social interactions with mentally retarded people. The family currently has to deal with internal and social stresses as their retarded member interacts with the community. When some of this dissonance is removed, the family may experience decreased levels of stress.

Because the effect of mental retardation on family members is complex, health professionals must consider the retarded individual within the context of the whole family. When services are directed by the normalization principle, the retarded member's life takes on more normal aspects. The other family members should also have more normal lives. If the family is placed in abnormal restraints, no one can benefit. Negative attitudes among family members will adversely effect the retarded member as well. The nurse who utilizes the normalization principle must demonstrate creativity and insight in relating to the unique needs of the individual and other family members. When normalization is viewed and promoted rigidly, the practitioner is looking at the structure and not at the objectives of the principle. Normalization can be utilized only when the needs of the entire family are considered in developing alternatives.

Normalization, as with any principle used as a guideline for services, can be used both negatively and positively. The purpose for using such a principle with mentally retarded individuals is to improve their status, life-style, and available services. Normal life-styles of children and adults are within the context of families. The individual in a family context interacts with other members and has interdependent needs. If the needs of the mentally retarded individual are disproportionate to those of other family members, there is difficulty for all individuals. The nurse who uses normalization constructively can assist families to maximize normal life-styles for all their members.

CONSIDERATION OF COMMUNITY SERVICES

What are the analogous agencies for normal persons and retarded persons? The answers to this question provide guidelines for structuring services for mentally retarded persons. Examples of analogies are residential home to family home, residential school to boarding school, sheltered workshop to factory, and special education program to public school. Services in community facilities for the nonretarded usually have a basic purpose and do not attempt to provide a variety of unrelated services. This is not true in many facilities for the mentally retarded. Services for the mentally retarded usually reflect conflict relating to both the normal and special needs of the clientele. A normalization focus should be evident in the stated objectives of the facility. Special needs should be considered only in relation to the agency's objectives. For example, a sheltered workshop is a work situation, and the special needs of the retarded person are considered only as they affect a work situation. These needs include work abilities, work routines, salary, and employer-employee relationships. The nurse working with a mentally retarded person emphasizes health and assesses the individual's capabilities to assume responsibility for health. The assessment includes emergency measures, safety, ability to obtain health care, and ability to maintain health.

Consideration must be given to whether services should be provided to mentally retarded persons by a generic agency or a special-needs agency. The use of generic agencies would integrate the retarded individual into the community by establishing these services as a right of the total population. Services would then develop without regard to any special characteristics of individuals seeking services. However, critics of the health care system claim that little consideration is now given to individual needs of the general population. Even less consideration is given by generic agencies to individual needs of the mentally retarded. The development of special services has emphasized the dissimilarities of the mentally retarded population. Critics of this approach question whether the services are adequate and meet the needs of the clients. Whether the condition of mental retardation requires special services needs further investigation.

The realist admits that variation of quality

exists in both types of service delivery systems. Parents decide which system will be
used. When comparable services are available, the generic system is the system of
choice in normalization. However, more
risk exists for parents who use the generic
system because of the potential rejection of
the individual as a client, the questionable
adequacy of services, and the possible labeling as a noncaring parent. Social and health
risks are concerns of parents for their children. The nurse can be instrumental in assisting parents to make knowledgeable
choices in these situations.

NORMALIZATION IN NURSING PRACTICE

Consideration of both short-term and
long-term goals is helpful in determing how
and when to use the normalization principle.
Because community placement for the mentally retarded is a recent venture, the implementation of normalization is in its infancy. The nurse working with families can
often assist by viewing the achievement of
normalization as a long-term goal and working toward normalization as a short-term
goal.

Attainment of normalization will be
achieved after the general public and professionals accept normal life-styles for mentally retarded individuals. Nurses who accept the principle in their practice can take
several steps: (1) incorporate normalization
into the diagnostic and treatment program,
(2) assist parents in understanding the concept as it relates to their child and themselves, (3) support parents in demanding,
planning, using, and evaluating services that
promote a normal life-style, and (4) influence other professionals to incorporate normalization in their practice and philosophy.

Normalization is a goal toward which services are directed. Nurses and other health
care professionals who incorporate normalization into their practice philosophy do
not expect immediate achievement of that
goal but use the goal in planning individual
services. Achievement is measured by demonstrating that movement toward normalization is occurring. Normalization pro-

vides direction for nurses in determining
what location, for what duration, and by
what means services are provided.

Nursing assessments and interventions
should direct an individual toward a more
normal life-style. Nursing evaluations and
recommendations for retarded individuals
are directed toward participation in normal
activities. When short-term and long-term
goals are established, a short-term intensive
program may be employed within the
framework of normalization. The results of
such a program will then assist the individual
to move into a normal life. It is helpful for the
nurse to consider a continuum when assisting persons toward independent functioning. The continuum starts with a protective
and less independent structure, moves toward the increasing responsibility of the individual, and ends with total independence.
A health professional assists persons to assume responsibilities for which they are
capable. Traditional health practice has kept
the mentally retarded person more dependent than necessary. In addition, professional liability constraints may cause nurses
to hesitate in risk taking. Practitioners need
to examine their practice and determine
when their fear of risk taking has been inappropriate. Some risk taking is necessary to
prevent the fostering of continuing dependency. Nurses may experience conflict between the roles of helper and promoter of
independent functioning in clients.

Consideration given to total family needs
is not a denial of individual rights. The right
to a more normal life for the mentally retarded individual must be promoted and
maintained. However, this will be realized
only when the rights and needs of all family
members are also considered and treated as
interactive factors. The presence of a retarded child in the family home is not an assurance of normalization. Nurses can assist
children and families in using normalization
specific to their individual situation. Variations in application of the principle will exist
for each family. The nurse must be innovative and flexible, must understand the principle, and must be able to recognize the in-

teracting dynamics of all family members.

Attitudes of professionals toward the concept of normalization range from acceptance to complete rejection. Those in favor of it emphasize the need of retarded individuals to have social interactions in order to learn and reinforce behaviors accepted by the general society. Those against normalization emphasize that adequate and intensive special services may be ignored under normalization. As with any philosophy that may be used to direct services or practice of health professionals, the individual practitioner must understand the concept in order to use normalization for positive enhancement of practice. Normalization is an ideological viewpoint that can be used negatively or positively. The individual practitioner is responsible for interpreting the concept and promoting adequate and effective services by other practitioners who use the concept.

SUMMARY

Parents are looking for direction in improving the life-style of their child who is mentally retarded. Nurses who function as family and child health consultants may be instrumental in providing that assistance. The concept of normalization when interpreted in a knowledgeable and constructive manner can assist parents to consider and obtain rights for the entire family. The use of normalization as a practice principle by nurses is based on the assumptions that mentally retarded individuals have a right to a normal life-style and that their families have a right to a normal life-style. Concern for the rights of children is an essential component in the health care delivery system. When parents are ignored or made martyrs as a result of a child's needs, the family as an interacting system is neglected. Consideration given to both children and parents is the only possible way for the mentally retarded individual to realize a normal life-style.

REFERENCES

1. Bank-Mikkelson, N. E.: A metropolitan area in Denmark; Copenhagen. In Kugel, R., and Wolfensberger, W., editors: Changing patterns in residential services for the mentally retarded, Washington, D.C., 1969, President's Committee on Mental Retardation.
2. Berge, J.: Perceptions of mental retardation by mothers and siblings in a family with one retarded member, Madison, Wisc., 1976, University of Wisconsin at Madison, unpublished master's thesis.
3. Farber, B.: Effects of a severely retarded child on family integration, Monogr. Soc. Res. Child Dev. **24:**112, 1959.
4. Fowle, C. M.: The effect of the severely retarded child on his family, Am. J. Ment. Defic. **73:**468, 1968.
5. Gath, A.: The school-age siblings of mongol children, Br. J. Psychiatry **123:**161, 1973.
6. Grossman, F. K.: Brothers and sisters of retarded children, Syracuse, 1972, Syracuse University Press.
7. Nirje, B.: The normalization principle and its human management implications. In Kugel, R., and Wolfensberger, W., editors: Changing patterns in residential services for the mentally retarded, Washington, D.C., 1969, President's Committee on Mental Retardation.
8. Stauder, C.: Knowledge and attitudes of adolescents about mental retardation, Madison, Wisc., 1976, University of Wisconsin at Madison, unpublished master's thesis.
9. Wolfensberger, W.: The principle of normalization in human services, Toronto, 1972, National Institute on Mental Retardation.

CHAPTER 5

Constructs of self-image

ROSE ANN M. PARRISH

Body schema, body image, and self-concept are terms that are being used with greater frequency by professionals interested in assisting children with mental retardation or other developmental disabilities to reach their maximum physical, intellectual, social, and emotional potential. Frames of reference differ among professionals. For some professionals these terms can be used interchangeably. For other professionals the terms have different meanings. There is general agreement, however, that children with mental retardation and other developmental disabilities are potentially at high risk to develop what may be termed a "disorganized body schema," an "unrealistic body image," or a "negative self-concept" as a result of internal or external factors. Internal factors may include the nature and degree of the disability, what the children know and understand about their bodies and disabilities, and how they feel about themselves as persons. External factors may include the opportunities the children have had to learn about their bodies and

Note: This project was supported in part by Grant No. MCT-000912-10-0, awarded by the Bureau of Community Health Services, Health Services Administration, Public Health Service, U.S. Department of Health, Education, and Welfare and Grant No. 59-P-25297/5.05, awarded by Region V, Social and Rehabilitation Service, U.S. Department of Health, Education, and Welfare.

disabilities, the availability of resources to enable children to develop to their maximum potential, and the reactions the children experience from the people with whom they come in contact.

Each of these three constructs—body schema, body image, and self-concept—can provide nurses who work in the field of mental retardation with an important theoretical framework that can be incorporated into their nursing care. These constructs can be as important to nurses who work in residential settings and in hospitals as they are to nurses who work in the community. Through an understanding of the normal development of each of these constructs, the methods that have been utilized in an attempt to assess children in relation to each of them, and the interventions that have been utilized in different situations, nurses can more effectively intervene to promote the development of an organized body schema, realistic body image, and positive self-concept.

CONSTRUCTS OF SELF

These constructs can be approached from the point of view that they are somewhat separate but overlapping and interdependent. Body schema can be defined as the awareness an individual has of body parts, their relationship to each other, and their relationship in space. This definition of body

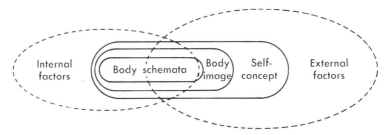

Fig. 5-1

schema has frequently been referred to as the "postural" model of body image. The posture (location in space) of the body, including the sensory impulses involved in changing posture, is viewed as a reference point against which incoming perceptions are measured. The body schema can be considered to be the foundation on which the body image and the larger self-concept are built. As Fig. 5-1 indicates, internal factors greatly influence the organization and development of the body schema. These internal factors can be considered to be the sensations that children are able to perceive from their bodies and their ability to differentiate and integrate them. Although internal factors play a major role, external factors, such as the degree and frequency of stimulation of the sensations provided by the child's environment and the people in it, also play a role in the organization and development of the body schema.

Body image can be defined as the mental impression or mental image that children have of their bodies as a whole and the parts that comprise that whole. Before children can develop a mental image of the body or a body part, they must have an awareness of the existence of the whole and its parts. Body image is thus based on the body schema. Individuals thus not only have an image or impression of their exterior physical appearances but also have an interior body image that is an image of the contents of the body and their function. The exterior and interior body images reflect both an objective and subjective component. The objective component is what individuals actually see when they look at themselves in a mirror or photograph, or what concrete,

realistic knowledge they have about their bodies. The subjective component is how individuals feel about what they see, how they interpret other people's images of them, and the frame of reference into which they integrate the concrete knowledge. For example, individuals can look at themselves in a mirror, see objectively that they are not overweight, and can intellectually know that their weight fits into an acceptable range for their height. Yet, one can still *feel* that the image seen is the image of someone who is overweight, and can *feel* that the weight is too much on the basis of what has been established as an acceptable weight by the individual. As Fig. 5-1 indicates, external factors have a greater influence on the mental image persons have of their bodies, although internal factors still play a significant role.

The self-concept can be defined as the whole gamut of attitudes, feelings, and impressions that individuals have about themselves as persons. Coopersmith points out that this concept of self consists of abstractions, and "the bases for the abstractions are the individual's observations of his own behavior and the way other individuals respond to his attitudes, appearances, and performance."[7] As Fig. 5-1 indicates, the self-concept is greatly influenced by factors external to the individual, but internal factors, such as individuals' abilities to perceive their behavior and the reactions of other individuals, also play a role. The self-concept is thus a construction that implies a great deal of complexity and subjective abstraction.

Body schema, body image, and self-concept are all dynamic constructs that are continually undergoing change as a result of the physical, intellectual, social, and emotional experiences encountered by the individual. At times, experiences influenced by internal factors may play a major role, whereas at other times experiences influenced by external factors may play a major role in either maintaining or changing aspects of the constructs. It is difficult, moreover, to deal with one construct in total isolation from the others because they are overlapping and interdependent. If, for example, the focus of intervention with a child is to promote the development of the body schema by increasing sensory experiences that will enhance awareness of a body part, there is also apt to be some effect on the child's rudimentary body image and self-concept. As the awareness of the body part develops, the child also begins to develop an image of that part that can be slowly incorporated into the total body image. The manner in which children perceive people approaching and reacting to the body part in the process of providing the sensory experiences will also influence how they effectively view themselves as people; thus, there is a potential influence on self-concept.

Theories related to child development have provided hypotheses about the manner in which body schema, body image, and self-concept develop in "normal" children. Although an attempt will be made to discuss the development of each of these constructs individually, it must be remembered that they do not develop in isolation. As body schema is developing, body image and self-concept are also developing in an overlapping and interdependent manner.

Body schema

Sensory experiences are seen as vital in the development of body schema. Newborn infants initially experience their bodies through sensations that originate from within, such as hunger, and that originate from without, such as being touched. However, there is not an awareness of a within and a without, since there is not a differentiation between a self and a nonself. Neither is there the ability to localize and respond to

many of the sensations in anything but a global manner. In respect to tactile sensation, it is felt that the newborn infant is unable to localize the source of the sensation or respond to it in a specific manner. A reflex action, such as when a tactile sensation on the cheek results in the rooting reflex, may be an exception. Gradually the infant develops the ability to localize the source of the sensation and begins to react to it in a less global manner. It has been demonstrated that at 7 to 9 months of age, a child demonstrates a generalized localization of a painful sensation, such as a pinprick, and responds with movements that are directed away from the general location of the sensation. At 12 to 16 months of age, the response is one of bringing the hand to the source of the sensation and either rubbing the area or attempting to push away the source of the sensation.[15] A similar developmental pattern can be seen in a child's response to being tickled. Initially, the child responds with a global bodily response that, as the ability to generally localize the sensation develops, results in bodily moving away from the source of the sensation. Finally, when able to more accurately localize the source of the sensation, the child moves toward it in order to inhibit the sensation.

Initially, children have very limited control over the sensory experiences they receive. As they acquire new motor abilities, they have increased opportunities for self-initiated sensory experiences. The funny objects that would go flying in and out of the line of vision and would be later known as hands can now be maintained in the visual field for longer periods and cause new sensations as they come in contact at the midline. Eventually, they can be intentionally brought to what will be known as the mouth for even new types of sensory experiences. Through exploring their own bodies and the environment immediate to them and by beginning to further differentiate and integrate the sensations involved, children begin to learn where the boundaries of their own bodies begin and end. From the viewpoint of ego development, it is felt the child differentiates a self from a nonself at about 7 to 9 months of age. This would appear to be supported by the data regarding a child's response to a painful sensation, such as a pinprick. It would appear that to have generalized movements away from the sensation, there must be a rudimentary knowledge that there is a "me" and an "out there" that makes "me" hurt.

As a sense of self and motor development continue to mature, children begin to develop a greater interest in the parts that comprise their bodies. They are no longer concerned primarily with the sensations given but are now also interested in what they can or cannot do with the sensations. They do not yet know the body parts by name but are interested in exploring if what will be called a foot can grasp a toy like the body part that will be later known as a hand. Mobility also gives children experience with their bodies in space, and they learn that there are certain laws of gravity with which to contend. They learn early that if they move full steam in an upright position from mother's arms to father's outstretched arms they have a better chance of making it than if they slow down before they reach father. At this stage, children are not only unaware of the names of body parts but also do not necessarily know that they even have a body as we think of it in adult terms. The me is still vague and composed of parts that have not been integrated into a whole.

Development of the body schema is an ongoing process that extends beyond infancy and toddlerhood. Sensory experiences resulting from continually experimenting directly with the body as an object and as an object in space further develop children's awareness of body parts, their relationship to each other, and their relationship in space. The ability to distinguish the right and left side of the body, for example, is considered an aspect of the body schema. It is often only after 6 years of age that many children can identify the right and left of the different parts of their own bodies and have developed this aspect of their body schema.

Body image

The development of body image is based on but also overlaps with the development of body schema. To develop a mental image of the body, children must have an awareness of the parts, their relationship to each other, and their relationship in space. Once an awareness has developed, tactile and visual experiences also play an important part in the development of an image. The visual experience may involve looking directly at the body part or at a reflection of the body part, such as in a mirror. One of the first images to develop is that of the face. In early infancy, children will show attentiveness to the human face and appear to be visually exploring it. When motor development occurs to the point that children can reach out with their hands, it is often the faces of the persons holding them that they reach out to explore when in close proximity. As children develop, they demonstrate interest in their own reflection in a mirror, although there is not initially a recognition that the faces are their own. Later, as children develop more of a sense of self and a mental image of that self, they are able to identify the reflections as themselves. The importance of the image of the face is seen even in the preschool years, when children will often rely on the face in a photograph to identify themselves from someone else.

As children receive verbal input from the environment, they learn that there is a name that goes with the me and then begin to learn that there are names for different parts of the me. Children are often able to associate the verbal input from the environment about the name of a body part with the body part before they are able to reproduce the word itself. It is felt that children can sometimes indicate at least one named body part by 18 to 21 months of age. Most frequently, the body parts will be those relating to the head or face, such as nose or hair. The indication may occur through actions, such as opening or closing the mouth in response to the word mouth rather than through pointing. Often it is easier for very young children to indicate the body part on a doll or a picture of a person rather than on their own bodies. This would seem to indicate that a knowledge of what the body part is and where it is located in a mirror image with visual cues occurs before the ability to localize that part on the me and before the development of a mental image of the me that includes that body part.

Berges and Lezine found that even children of 3 years of age responded more readily to indicating and naming body parts on the drawing of a doll than on their own bodies. For the most part, the children could easily indicate and name hair, hands, feet, mouth, ears, eyes, nose, back, stomach, arms, legs, and head. They also found that the body parts that were not well recognized by the children were indicated on their own bodies by a general direction, such as extending the arms toward the lower part of the body to indicate the knees. The extremities were more accurately indicated than body parts near the trunk.[3] One would wonder if the latter finding is a result of the extremities, such as hands and feet, being in most direct contact with the environment and more within the visual field when most actions are undertaken.

As an example of the influence of contact and visual field, place a pencil on a surface directly in front of you and look at the pencil with your hands out of your immediate vision. There is a vivid object "out there," but a somewhat vague and diffuse "me." Now, grasp the pencil in your hand and maintain your vision on the pencil. Not only is there now a vivid object out there, but there is also a vivid part of the me because of both being within the visual field and because of the sensations that result from grasping the pencil. That part of me holding the pencil, however, is still only vaguely connected to the rest of the me. If you lift the pencil up and down vertically from the surface to above head level while maintaining the pencil in your vision, the part out there is still most vivid. But there is somewhat greater awareness of a connection with the me as a result of the sensations arising from the movement of the arm. The arm, however, becomes

only a vivid part of the me when vision is shifted from the pencil to the moving arm.

Self-concept

The development of the self-concept also begins in infancy. When children feel discomfort, they learn that a person can bring them pleasure. This person is usually the mother, although she is not differentiated from anyone else. The manner in which the child is touched, fed, and held conveys attitudes toward the infant. It is frequently stated that children see themselves in their mothers' faces. If the face reflects acceptance and love, children will feel good about themselves as persons. If the face reflects rejection or disappointment, children will feel bad about themselves. Not only are attitudes conveyed about the whole of the children but are also conveyed about body parts. If children feel pleasure as their mothers play with or touch a body part, and this pleasure is reflected in the mothers' faces, they associate that body part with pleasure or a positive feeling. However, if children feel pleasure but displeasure is reflected in the mothers' faces, they begin to associate that body part with a more negative feeling. As children develop further, they become aware of the approval or disapproval reflected in the tone of their mothers' voices, and they also respond to this by feeling good or bad. The same thing that was said to a child in an accepting, loving tone of voice and resulted in smiles and laughter from the child can be said in a different tone of voice and result in tears.

During infancy, the self-concept is primarily formed through interaction with the primary caretaker, who is usually the mother. As children become less egocentric and become more interested in other people in the immediate environment, they slowly become aware of the attitudes that are also conveyed. Later in childhood when the environment is expanded to include peers and other significant adults, the child's self-concept is further modified based on perceptions of how they are viewed outside the family. Children can radiate pleasure and a sense of feeling good about themselves when their best friends have told them that they really like them or when such individuals as their teachers have commented in a positive manner about something they have done well. On the other hand, many parents have also experienced the pain radiated by children who feel bad about themselves as persons because their best friends have called them a name or their teachers have commented on something they have not done well.

DEVELOPMENT AND CONSTRUCTS OF SELF

Much of the information available about the development of the constructs of body schemata, body image, and self-concept is based on empirical data. However, emphasis has not been placed on documenting the development of these constructs over time with a large number of children to provide a frame of reference as to what can be considered normal and abnormal at a given developmental level. Various studies have concluded that children with mental retardation or other developmental disabilities differ from normal children in relation to aspects of the body schema, body image, or self-concept. However, it is often difficult to determine if they indeed differ in these constructs from what could be considered the norm for children of their developmental levels, or if they simply differ from the children with whom they were compared because of a difference in their developmental levels. There is very limited normative data available as to the sequence and exact manner in which the body schema develops, although the construct has provided a base for certain theories regarding perceptual-motor development. Both Kephart and Ayres view the body schema as the focal point for an individual's knowledge of the world.[2, 12] Visual-space perception is seen as beginning with an understanding that there is a front and a back to our bodies as well as an up and a down before these conceptions can be generalized to objects outside of the body. Early number concepts are also viewed as having a reference to the body schema.

Children learn that they have one of certain body parts, such as the mouth, two of certain other body parts, such as feet, and many of certain other body parts, such as fingers. The reference point of the body in relation to early number concepts can also be seen when children use fingers to indicate how old they are or to count.

Body schema

Within these theories of perceptual-motor development, movement is seen as essential to the development of the body schema. According to Ayres, "purposeful movement is the 'sine qua non' in the development of body scheme, for it provides the opportunity to synthesize and derive meaning about the body from many sources of information, especially vision, touch, and proprioception."*Kephart also stresses that only when children have achieved purposeful movement in a well-integrated pattern are they free to explore their environment since they no longer have to concentrate attention on the movement itself and can concentrate on the purpose of the movement, which is exploration.[12] To execute a purposeful movement, children must be aware of the body parts involved, their relationship to each other, and their relationship in space.

Ayres identified methods that could be utilized by the occupational therapist in promoting development of the body schema. The focus of the training methods involves techniques such as (1) increasing the flow of sensory impulses in body parts by brush stroking a body part while calling the individual's attention to the body part and naming the area being stimulated, (2) using heavy objects attached to an arm or leg to increase proprioceptive impulses, (3) engaging the individual in gross motor activities, such as rolling or jumping, to promote an awareness of how various body parts relate to one another, and (4) constructing body parts through activities such as tracing or

---

*Ayres, A. J.: Development of the body scheme in children, Am. J. Occup. Ther. **15**:99, 1961. Copyrighted by the American Occupational Therapy Association, Inc.

modeling with clay.[2] Very few studies have documented the effectiveness or ineffectiveness of these techniques in promoting the body schema of either very young normal children or children who are mentally retarded. One of the difficulties may be that an awareness is difficult to measure without relying on verbal and nonverbal techniques that involve a higher level of concept development.

Kephart also developed a sensory-motor treatment program to be utilized in educational settings with children who were considered brain injured. The treatment program emphasizes the sequential development of the motor generalizations and the body schema through activities on a walking board, a balance board, and a trampoline as well as rhythm activities, angels-in-the-snow, and stunts and games.[12] The results of a study by Maloney, Ball, and Edgar indicated that sensory-motor training can result in a significant increase in aspects of the body schema of adolescents who were moderately and severely retarded. It appeared that the major improvement in the body schema was in the area of laterality (awareness of the two sides of the body and their difference).[16]

Clapp studied the body schemata of children who were mentally retarded and demonstrated signs of organicity, children who were mentally retarded and did not demonstrate signs of organicity, and normal children who were matched according to mental age (approximately 4 years, 6 months). Finger localization, localization of tactile stimulation, and imitation of gestures of the arms, hands, and fingers were used as measures of body schema. The findings indicated that the children who were mentally retarded and demonstrated signs of organicity had the greatest overall body-schema deficit. It was also found that all three groups had more difficulty with finger localizations and imitations than with hand and arm localization and imitations, but the children with organic involvement had the most difficulty.[4]

What significance does the construct of the body schema have for nurses who work with children with mental retardation and other developmental disabilities? Foremost, it provides an additional aspect to the theoretical framework for nursing interventions. If it is recognized that developing an awareness of body parts, their relationship to each other, and their relationship in space is an important part of the foundation needed to learn certain skills and concepts, then interventions can be geared toward promoting this awareness. In part, this means ensuring that children have recurring opportunities for sensory experiences that are appropriate for their developmental levels and for their levels of body-schema development. A child who is mentally retarded will not develop this awareness as quickly as would be expected in a normal child. However, only through recurring opportunities for sensory experiences will this awareness develop to some degree. For a child who is moderately retarded, it would be expected that this awareness would develop sooner than for a child who is severely retarded. Specific intervention techniques will vary with the developmental level of the child and the particular developmental disability. The techniques, however, are basically the same ones as those currently being used under the category of "stimulation" techniques. Activities for a child functioning at a very young developmental level may involve touching, rocking, and passively moving body parts. For children at a somewhat higher development level, the activities may involve promoting self-initiated motor activities, such as reaching for and grasping objects or mouthing safe objects.

Body image

The construct of body image also lacks normative data to document the sequence and exact manner in which children develop images of themselves, although there has been a proliferation of studies and articles dealing with the body image of both children and adults. The methods utilized in studying the body image of children have included nondirective interviewing, the Rorschach utilizing-the-barrier concept, the forming of human figures from cutouts of body parts of various sizes, and figure drawings. Since it is often easier to graphically depict a mental image than to try to describe it verbally, one of the methods most frequently used to determine the body image of children has been figure drawing. The basis for the use of figure drawings as an indication of body image is the theory that when adults or children draw pictures of persons, they are projecting their images of themselves into the drawing.

From my experience in utilizing children's figure drawings as a projective technique in determining body image, I would emphasize two areas of caution. First, it must be realized that figure drawings of children proceed through a developmental sequence. A child's drawings at a particular developmental level are affected by such factors as visual-motor coordination and level of concept development. Anyone who uses figure drawings as a projective technique must first be able to recognize at which developmental levels certain characteristics are appropriate and at which developmental levels these same characteris-

tics may be an indication of modification or distortion of the external body image. The second area of caution is that of interpretation once a characteristic is identified as being unusual for a child of that particular developmental level. Interpretation must be based on a thorough understanding of individual children in terms of some of their past and present experiences. For a child with a developmental disability, a thorough knowledge of the disability is essential.

As an example of these two points of caution, it would be difficult to determine if Fig. 5-2 is usual or unusual for a 6-year-old child unless one knows that a 6-year-old is apt to draw a figure such as the one in Fig. 5-3. Knowing some of the normative data established for the typical figure drawn by a 6-year-old, one would expect the figure to consist of at least a head, eyes, nose, mouth, trunk, legs, arms, and perhaps hair.[13] It is obvious that Fig. 5-2 does not include two characteristics that would be expected in the figure drawing of a child this age—a trunk and legs. On the other hand, the figure drawing does contain characteristics that may appear in the drawing of a 6-year-old but would not necessarily be expected characteristics until a later age. These characteristics are the ears, neck, and hand representation with the correct number of fingers.

Now that the characteristics that could be considered usual and unusual for a child of this age have been identified, what information does this give? First of all, one could

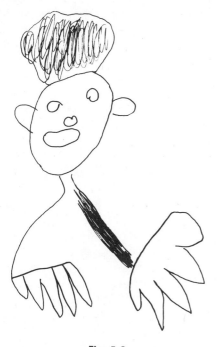

Fig. 5-2

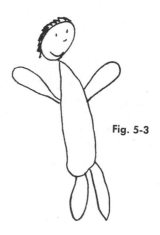

Fig. 5-3

question whether the child who drew Fig. 5-2 is mentally retarded and, therefore, not at a developmental level where the trunk and legs would be expected characteristics of the figure drawing. Among the figure drawings of younger children there is a primacy of the head, arms, and legs, although the trunk may not be present. This figure drawing does not include legs, which would be expected characteristics at a younger age, but does include characteristics that one would not necessarily expect to appear until the child is older. The presence of these characteristics would lead the professional to question if mental retardation is the primary reason for the absence of the trunk and legs. From a psychiatric point of view, the omission of certain body parts at a developmental age when they are expected characteristics in the figure drawing can be suggestive of denial of the function of the body parts and imply a degree of emotional disturbance. Thus, one might say that for some unconscious reason the child is denying the existence of the trunk and legs and only recognizes the existence of the head, neck, arms, and hands. This is a logical interpretation of the figure drawing based on what can be seen or not seen in the figure drawing. Still, however, nothing is known about the child who drew the figure except that it was drawn by a 6-year-old. What is needed at this point is some information about the child in order to validate whether the child is denying the existence of the trunk and legs because of some unconscious reason or whether there is another explanation for their absence.

The child who drew the figure was a 6-year-old girl who was born with myelomeningocele. Because of the location of the birth defect and the degree of spinal cord involvement, she lacked all sensation and movement below the umbilical area. The figure drawing was done while she was hospitalized for corrective spinal surgery and was immobile in a body cast. On the day she drew the figure, an IV that had prohibited the full use of her left hand and arm had been removed. Now that something is known about the child, what information does the

figure drawing reveal in terms of her exterior body image? Obviously, as has been discussed earlier, it reveals that at that point in time, her image of herself did not include having a trunk or legs, but why is still not known.

Exterior body image. Goodenough contends that children do not represent in a drawing all the knowledge they have about what they are drawing but represent only the particular aspects that have the most meaning to them without the power of suggestion from external sources. The drawing is seen as composed of two components. The first component is the aspects that have already been integrated into the concept of the object and appear with consistency in the child's drawing of the object. The second component is the aspects that are undergoing the process of integration and have not yet become a consistent feature.[10] Therefore, lack of a trunk and legs in Fig. 5-2 may not be so much a denial of their existence but a lack of awareness of their existence or an indication that they are body parts that are in the process of being integrated into the body image. As discussed previously in relation to the body schemata, sensory experiences play an important role in the development of a child's awareness of body parts. Without an awareness that a body part exists, a child cannot develop an image of that body part. This child had not had the same sensory experiences or, in all likelihood, the same opportunities to explore her body as had most children of this same age. Moreover, with the child's trunk hidden by a body cast and her legs out of her field of vision, she was unable to reenforce their existence through vision. If the example of the importance of contact and vision is recalled, the concrete existence of body parts is often reenforced visually even when an awareness exists.

The figure drawing also gives an indication of the body parts that are important to the child in experiencing herself as a person and her environment—eyes, ears, nose, mouth, arms, and hands. The shading of the arm that had been restrained because of the IV perhaps indicates the degree of anxiety and anger the child experienced by having one of her major means of interacting with and defending herself from the environment taken away. One of the goals of nursing intervention with this child would be aimed at promoting the integration or reintegration of these body parts into her exterior body image. Initially, intervention would be geared toward the body schemata by increasing sensory experiences related to these body parts available to the child through vision, hearing, and touch. Whenever possible, the sensory experiences should be related directly toward the child's own body. When this is not possible because of the restrictions imposed by such factors as the body cast and her supine position, these same senses can be utilized to increase the child's awareness of these body parts in relation to people in her environment, a doll, or pictures of people. Once an awareness develops, the sensory experiences available to the child can then be utilized in promoting a realistic "image" of the body parts.

Fig. 5-4 is an example of how another type of chronic, handicapping condition can possibly influence a child's exterior body image. The figure was drawn by an 11-year-old girl with juvenile arthritis who was confined to a wheelchair. The drawing is excellent for a child of her age in terms of artistic ability. Note the manner in which the figure's right elbow, right hand, and the knees are depicted. Joints, especially knee joints, are considered uncommon characteristics of figure drawings.[13] In this case, it is possible that they appear because of the girl's artistic ability in representing the human figure. It is also possible, however, that because of her juvenile arthritis, joints have become significant in her body image. The importance of sensations in the development of the body schema was discussed previously. One sensation is that of pain. Just as pain may contribute to an awareness of certain body parts, it may also contribute to an overawareness when it is recurrent in that body part. This overawareness, in turn, can influence the image that is developed of that body part. The manner in which the left arm

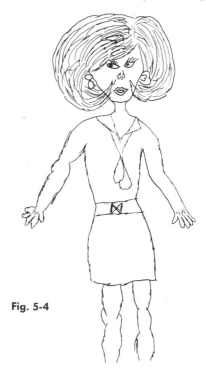

Fig. 5-4

and hand were drawn is interesting in comparison with the manner in which the right arm, right hand, and legs are drawn. The lines of the arm flow in a somewhat less broken manner, and the fingers appear less crude than they do on the right hand. This would lead one to question if the girl has had less pain and difficulty in her left arm and hand than in her other extremities.

Whether figure drawings can be used to gain information about the body image of children with developmental disabilities when there is severe involvement in the upper extremities depends on the individual child and the nature and degree of the disability. Fig. 5-5 was drawn by a 10-year-old girl who was quadriplegic as a result of an accident that occurred when she was approximately 5 years of age. Although the girl had a great deal of difficulty using her upper extremities for fine motor activities, she was able to demonstrate enough control, with a great deal of effort, to draw. The body parts depicted in the drawing are those which could be expected, according to certain normative data, to be present at approxi-

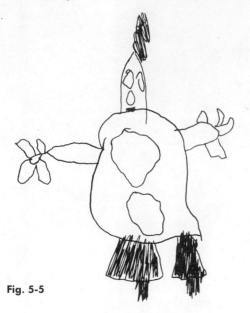

Fig. 5-5

mately 8 years of age.[13] Psychological testing had indicated she was functioning in the mildly retarded range, and it was reported that she was functioning at about a second-grade level academically. The items not depicted in the drawing that are reported to be expected at age 10 years were a representation of the neck and the arms in a downward position. The drawing would indicate that the child's body schema is grossly adequate as depicted by the image she has of the human figure. It would be difficult to draw any other conclusions, however, related to the possible effect the child's disability has had on her image of herself. One might question the significance of the shading of the lower extremities. This could be an indication of how the child feels about her lower extremities, but it could also be an attempt to indicate pants on the figure.

In discussing the drawings of children with cerebral palsy, Abercrombie and Tyson pointed out that some children have difficulties in drawing things other than a person, and characteristics that appear in their figure drawings may be more a reflection of their general weakness in drawing than an indication of a disturbance in body image. They studied the figure drawings of a group of children with cerebral palsy who were between 8 and 18 years of age.[1] A Goodenough mental age was obtained, and the drawings were compared with those of normal children of the same mental age (6 years).[10] It was found that there was as great a tendency for the normal children to draw people who might seem to be physically handicapped as there was with the children who had cerebral palsy.

Wysocki and Whitney also utilized figure drawings to study the body image of children whom they termed "crippled." The children had such conditions as polio, cerebral palsy, clubfoot, congenital dislocated hip, myelomeningocele, and scoliosis. The drawings of these children were compared with the drawings of a group of normal children of the same intelligence quotient (IQ) and age. The significant findings from the study indicated that the children who were considered crippled drew large figures, placed their figures toward the edges of the paper, and had more shading in their drawings. It was concluded that the drawings of children who were crippled contained more indicators of aggression (as determined by pressure applied to the pencil in making the figure and the amount of shading) and negative compensation (as determined by the large figure). Since 36% of the children indicated in their drawings an area of input that corresponded to their own handicapping conditions, it was felt that children who most probably had not adjusted to their physical disabilities would indicate the handicap in their drawings.[24]

When children's figure drawings are used as an indication of body image, the question often remains as to whether the drawing depicts the children's actual body images or only those aspects that their visual-motor abilities permit them to reproduce. Since children usually do not indicate dissatisfaction with what they have drawn, it is assumed that their creations are congruent with their images. Fig. 5-6, for example, was drawn by a 9-year-old boy who was considered normal intellectually, had no significant difficulties in school, and had no identified handicaps. The child was satisfied

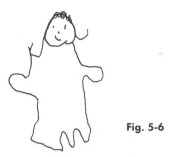

Fig. 5-6

that what he had drawn was a person. However, the drawing does not depict a figure that adults would be satisfied with as a person. There seems to be an awareness of certain body parts, such as the arms, legs, and trunk, but either the presence of an unclear image of the parts or a perceptual-visual-motor problem may be influencing a more accurate representation of the figure. If the difficulty were in reproducing the image, would the child not have tried to correct the representation by either erasing segments and attempting them again or by indicating that it was not what he wanted to do? Since he did neither of these things, it would appear that the figure approximated his current image of a person.

A recent study by Gellert has added to the understanding of the range representing adequate or normal body-image development by a method that does not rely on figure drawings. A large group of elementary school children between 5 and 12 years of age was given the task of assembling self-replicas from jigsaw pieces representing various body parts. The head was given as a starting point, and the children were requested to select and place body parts to make a figure they felt resembled their own bodies. In addition, self-drawings were obtained from the children between the ages of 5 and 7 years to use as a comparison. Emphasis was placed especially on children in the 5- to 6-year age range based on the assumption that the most marked errors and changes in performance would occur in this age group. The findings, however, indicated that more shifts in performance seemed to take place in the 6- to 7-year age range.[9]

The results of the study included the following. First, the constructions tended to improve with age, and leveled out at about 10$\frac{1}{2}$ years of age. Second, the most notably asymmetric treatment of the upper extremities occurred in relation to the size of the two hands, with 39% of the youngest children using hands that were grossly different from one another in size, and although this tendency declined with age, it did occur at all ages. Third, two members of particular pairs (that is, arms) often looked quite unequal and asymmetric on the assembled figures, although gross deviations in symmetry declined markedly after age 7 years. Finally, no child omitted some representation of paired legs.[9]

When the constructions with the figure drawings were compared, it was found that there was a tendency in both to overestimate the size of the head in proportion to the rest of the body. There was some omitting of the hands and arms or attaching of the hands directly to the trunk as occurred at times in the figure drawings. There was also a tendency, although less than occurred in drawings, to locate the legs too far apart at their juncture to the trunk. Some differences were noted between the constructions and the figure drawings. With the constructions, there was no significant relationship or consistent trend between IQ and performance. With figure drawings, however, IQ influenced performance. Only three children attached the arms to the head or neck, and only one child omitted the trunk altogether as is typical in figure drawings at an early stage.

The aspects of the representation of the human body that appeared in both the constructions and the human figure drawings appeared to indicate that: (1) the head assumes a primacy in a child's body image, (2) hands and arms do not necessarily have as major place in the body image of the young child as one would assume, and (3) the relationship of the legs to each other at the juncture to the trunk is an aspect of the body image, and probably body schema, that is not easily developed. The differences that occurred between the constructions and the figure drawings indicated that construction of a self-replica out of jigsaw pieces may be a more valid technique than figure drawings in obtaining information about the body image of children who are mentally retarded or who have severe physical handicaps. It would also seem that this technique has the advantage of obtaining information about normal children who can be considered to be in a transitionary state between body schemata and body image. They have an awareness of the body parts and the relationship to each other, but their image of these parts and the relationship to each other is still too fuzzy for reproduction through drawing. The child who drew Fig. 5-6 may be an example of a child in the transitionary stage.

Two aspects of Gellert's study are significant to the earlier discussion of the figure drawn by the child with myelomeningocele (Fig. 5-2). First, the findings that only one child omitted a trunk and no child omitted some representation of paired legs support the conclusion that the child's body image differed from what would normally be expected of a child of her age. Second, it points out a technique that could possibly have been utilized to determine if her trunk and legs were still in the process of being integrated or reintegrated into her body image, or if she still lacked the basic awareness of them as a part of her body schema.

The body image of children with myelomeningocele has been studied by Weininger, Rotenberg, and Henry utilizing a method that involved assembling the figure of a person. The purpose of the study was to determine whether there would be significant differences in body image among children with myelomeningocele who were in an institution, children with myelomeningocele who were living at home, and children who were not handicapped. All the children were within the normal range of intelligence and were between 11 and 18 years of age. To construct the human figures, the children were given oval styrofoam shapes of various sizes, a bundle of heavy, colored plastic drinking straws, a pointed wooden stylus for boring holes in the styrofoam, and a pair of scissors for cutting the straws. The completed figures were measured in terms of length of the total figure, length of the arm, length of the leg, proportion of the arm to the body, proportion of the leg to the body, and proportion of the arm and leg to the body.[23]

Results of the study indicated that children with myelomeningocele who were institutionalized consistently created smaller figures in relation to both length and proportion than did the children in the other two groups. No significant difference was found between the children with myelomeningocele who were living at home and the group of children without handicaps. It was concluded that the body image of the institutionalized children was underdeveloped, and it was hypothesized that the life experiences within an institutional setting resulted in an encapsulation and a reduction in the perception of the space occupied by the body. Other aspects of the constructions, such as the body parts actually depicted, were not specifically documented as part of the study. It was observed, however, that the children who were institutionalized omitted, or barely indicated, arms and legs in more than half of the constructions.[23] The investigators questioned whether this observation might indicate a greater tendency to perceive oneself as a deformed person when institutionalized, but it might also indicate difficulty with the basic body schema because of limited and inconsistent sensory experiences within the institutional setting.

The body image of children who are mentally retarded has been studied by Wysocki and Wysocki. Figure drawings were used with a group of institutionalized children with an IQ range of 52 to 72 and with a group of normal children of approximately the same chronological age, 9 to 13. Eight aspects of the drawings were assumed to be indicative of body image: size, erasure, environment, clothing, fingers, detail, symmetry, and arm position. The drawings of the children who were retarded contained significantly larger figures, fewer erasures with a tendency to draw over lines rather than erase them, a significantly smaller amount of clothing, less frequent representation of fingers, a tendency to draw no detail, a significant tendency to draw asymmetrical figures, and horizontal, rigid arm positions. The investigators did not make any statements about their conclusions regarding body image.[25] The results of this study would seem to indicate that the drawings of children who are mentally retarded differ in some respects from the drawings of normal children of the same chronological age. The question remains, however, as to how the human figure drawings of children who are mentally retarded differ from normal children of the same developmental age.

Spoerl studied a small group of children with an IQ range of 42 to 98 (the majority of whom had an IQ score above 70) to determine the developmental tendencies in drawings of retarded children to compare their performance with normal children of the same chronological age and to determine if there were specific items that would distinguish the drawings of the children who were mentally retarded. The results of the study indicated that the development of drawing ability in children who are mentally retarded is dependent on mental age and that children with an IQ score below 70 tended to do consistently better work (in other words, included more detail) than would be expected of their mental age.[22]

Many questions remain in an attempt to utilize figure drawings to determine the body image of children who are mentally retarded. First, documentation on a large scale is needed to determine whether the figure drawings of children who are mentally retarded do indeed differ from the drawings of normal children of the same mental age. Second, does the figure drawing of an adolescent of 16 years of age and a mental age of 8 years differ from the figure drawing of an 11-year-old with a mental age of 8 years or a normal child with the chronological and mental age of 8 years? Is there a normal developmental progression in the depiction of the human figure by children who are mentally retarded, and does this progression dif-

fer from that of normal children? These are only some of the questions that need to be answered before figure drawings can be used with any accuracy to determine if a child who is mentally retarded has a realistic body image or if there are distortions of body image that should not be explained away simply on the basis that the child is retarded.

Interior body image. Thus far, body image has been discussed solely in terms of the exterior body image. There is another aspect of the body image termed the interior body image. It can be defined as the mental image that children have of the contents of their bodies and of the body functions. The concept of interior body image should have an importance to nurses in a variety of settings. For the nurse who is caring for a child who is mentally retarded in a hospital setting, it can provide a frame of reference as to why the child may become extremely difficult during certain procedures. For the nurse in a community or residential setting who is working with a mentally retarded adolescent girl concerning the issue of sexuality, it can provide a framework to understand the girl's frame of reference regarding the inside of her body and her body functions. For the nurse who works with children who have conditions such as epilepsy or PKU, it can provide a means of determining if the condition or treatment had less than a positive influence on the manner in which the child perceives the inside of the body.

Nurses are frequently in the position to incorporate patient teaching that is related to what is happening to a child's body or how a certain treatment is helping the child's body. Yet, teaching is not just telling. Too frequently when we tell someone about something, we assume that they have the same frame of reference as our own. Children have their own interior body images to which they apply the information they receive. If nurses do not understand how children view the inside of their bodies and the body functions at their particular developmental levels, the information given to children can be distorted by the children to fit in with their existing knowledge. If a distortion exists, just being presented with accurate information will not necessarily correct it. With children who are mentally retarded, however, there may be a tendency not to even present any information on the assumption that the children lack any understanding or frame of reference.

My interest in interior body image originated from working with children with asthma. The condition and what occurs during an attack may have been explained to a child several times in what was thought to be clear and understandable terms for the child's developmental level. Yet, when feedback from the child was requested, it was striking to discover the lack of understanding and the amount of distortion that occurred. This interest led to the realization that there is very limited information available as to how children normally view the interior of their bodies. Therefore, it was difficult to determine if children with asthma were any different from other children. Thus, I became interested in attempting to approach the concept of interior body image from a developmental point of view.[19]

The literature related to how children view the inside of their bodies has focused in most instances on the children's knowledge of their bodies and bodily functions utilizing verbal techniques rather than focusing on the mental image that children have of the interior of their bodies.

A study by Gellert regarding children's conceptions of the inside of the body has been published in extensive form. Her study group consisted of 96 hospitalized children, 4 through 17 years of age. The results of the study indicated that as children develop, different systems assume different levels of importance or awareness. The circulatory and musculoskeletal systems were of primary significance until about age 13 years when the digestive system began to assume greater significance. In response to a general question as to what was inside their bodies, about 70% of the children reported bones as all, or at least part, of what they had inside their bodies. The next items mentioned most often, in order of frequency, were blood

vessels, heart, blood, brain, intestinal tract, lungs, kidneys, and stomach. When the children were asked what the most important part of their body was, the heart was most frequently mentioned, followed by the brain, eyes, head, lungs, and stomach. In response to the question as to what body part they felt they could live without, approximately 20% of the children firmly believed that they needed all parts of their body to live. All of these children were below 11 years of age. As the children became older, there was a tendency to identify a greater number of body parts that they could live without. The contents of the trunk, with the exception of the appendix, were considered needed for life by most of the children, whereas the extremities were often regarded as less crucial for life.[8]

This information related to what body parts children view as necessary for life can give an indication as to why young children may become so upset over such surgical procedures as tonsillectomy and adenoidectomy. Children may have difficulty in really believing that they are going to live without their tonsils if their frame of reference is that they need all body parts to live. It is also interesting to listen to a young child who is losing first teeth. Although the child may be happy about it because it means becoming a "big boy" or "big girl" and perhaps means that the child will be like classmates who have already lost teeth, the child will verbalize concerns as to the ability to eat and ask for reassurance that a new tooth will definitely replace the lost one. In this case, the child is not directly verbalizing a concern about dying, but one would wonder if the concern about being able to eat is not related to a basic belief that all body parts, including teeth, are needed in order to live. These concerns about body integrity may be factors that contribute to both normal children and children who are mentally retarded becoming difficult to manage during certain hospital procedures.

A more recent study of interior body image by Porter supported some of the findings of previous studies but also indicated some differences from previous findings. One-hundred forty-four elementary school children between the ages of 6 years and 11 years were studied. The findings indicated that the children depicted the heart, bones, and brain more frequently than in previous studies.[20] Children who were 6 or 7 years of age were able to name more internal body parts than those children up to 9 years of age in Gellert's study. Children who were 10 or 11 years of age usually named at least two more parts than the children who were 16 or 17 years of age in Gellert's study. As was pointed out in the discussion of Porter's study, an increased emphasis on health teaching within the schools and the influence of advertising on television could be factors that contributed to some of the differences in the findings.

The results of these studies give an indication of how children have responded to questions about the inside of their bodies. But, how do children graphically depict the mental image they have of the inside of their bodies? Fig. 5-7, which was drawn by a 7-year-old, is an example of how young children tend to depict interior body parts existing in space without any particular boundaries differentiating the inside from the outside of the body and how they tend to think

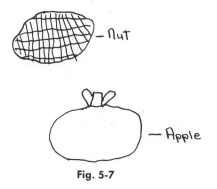

Fig. 5-7

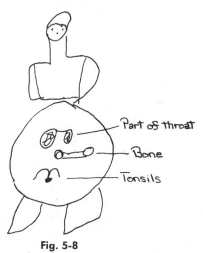

Fig. 5-8

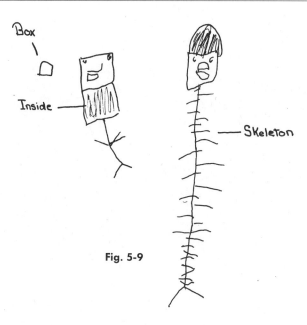

Fig. 5-9

of the contents of the body in terms of the food they put in it. Fig. 5-8, which was drawn by an 8-year-old, is an example of a child who differentiates the inside from the outside but tends to view body parts as being contained in something that resembles a large stomach. Fig. 5-9, which was drawn by a 9-year-old, is an example of the difficulty children can have in integrating different concepts. In all likelihood, the child knows he has an "inside" and bones that comprise

a skeleton, although he is either not able to depict or to understand how the two relate. Also the presence of the "box" is interesting, and may be a result of the child having heard reference to the "voice box."

The child who drew Fig. 5-9 appears to have difficulty integrating concepts. However, the 8-year-old child who drew Fig. 5-10 is more able to integrate the concepts, does not view all interior body parts as contained in the trunk or stomach area, and demonstrates a greater awareness of different body parts. Fig. 5-11, drawn by a 10-year-old, and Fig. 5-12, drawn by an 11-year-old, are additional examples of the progression that occurs in the representation of interior body image. One should not assume, however, that a child's chronological age will definitely mean a certain level of interior body image. Fig. 5-13 was drawn by a normal 11-year-old whose interior body-image concept is much different from that of the 11-year-old who drew Fig. 5-12.

Similarly, Figs. 5-14 and 5-15 were drawn by two 12-year-olds who have very different interior body-image concepts. What effect

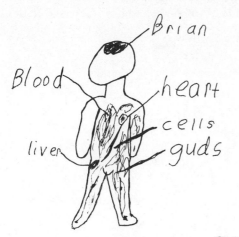

Fig. 5-10

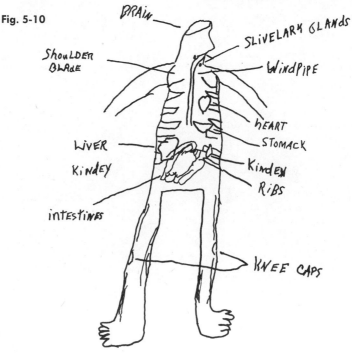

Fig. 5-11

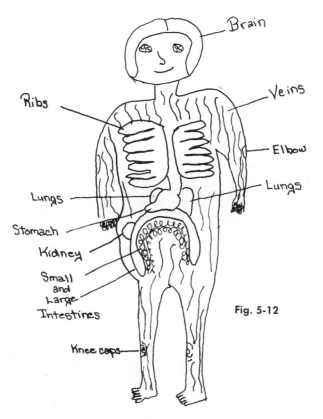

Fig. 5-12

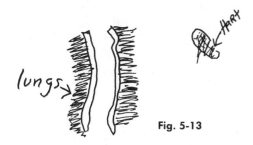

Fig. 5-13

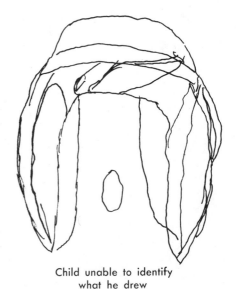

Child unable to identify
what he drew

Fig. 5-14

may a specific condition have on a child's interior body image? Figs. 5-16 and 5-17 were drawn by children with asthma. In Fig. 5-16 the only body part depicted is the lungs, and in Fig. 5-17 the lungs are represented in a very unusual manner. The child who drew Fig. 5-18 had asthma as well as a congenital heart condition. Fig. 5-19 was drawn by a 14-year-old girl with PKU who at the time of the drawing was verbalizing how restricted she felt in respect to the food she could eat because of her diet and how she always seemed to be hungry.

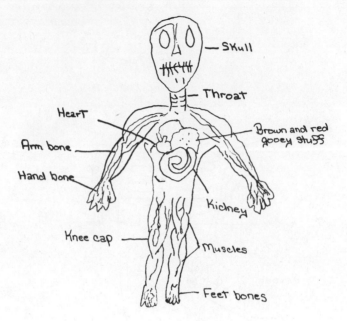

Fig. 5-15

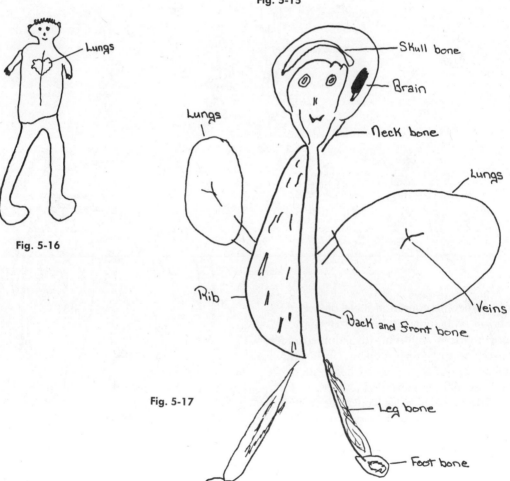

Fig. 5-16

Fig. 5-17

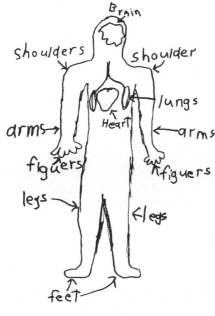

Fig. 5-18

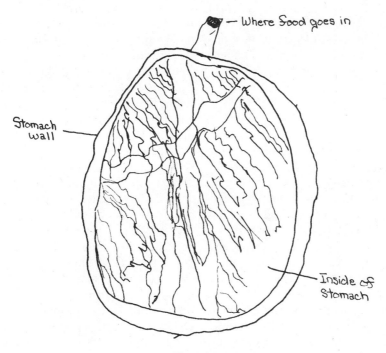

Fig. 5-19

Self-concept

The self-concept, as pointed out earlier, is a construct that implies complexity. Based on subjective abstractions, it has created controversy as to whether it can be objectively measured in individuals who are normal, not to mention individuals who are mentally retarded and thus considered to have some degree of impairment in their basic ability for abstraction. Cobb points out that although the ability for abstraction may be limited in some degree, ". . . the retarded person does develop a complex set of self-referent perceptions, attitudes, and behaviors which permeate and profoundly influence his relationship with the world around him."[5]

Interest and research in the construct of the self-concept gained momentum in the 1950s, but it was not until the 1960s that interest increased in the self-concept of individuals who are mentally retarded. A variety of scales and approaches have been utilized to determine what effect certain experiences (such as special class placement or institutionalization) have had on the self-concept, what the possible correlates of self-concept may be, and what general conclusions can be drawn regarding the self-concept of various groups of individuals who are mentally retarded.

One approach to the study of the self-concept has been to compare individuals who are mentally retarded with individuals who are considered normal. Ringness compared the reported self-concept of children who were considered to be of low (IQ 50 to 80), average (IQ 90 to 110), and high (IQ 120 or above) intelligence over a 2-year period. Measures of the children's achievement in eight areas (for example, success in learning arithmetic, acceptance by peers, and success in sports) were obtained from a standardized achievement test, a sociogram, and teachers' ratings. These measures were then compared with the children's estimates of themselves in each of the eight areas. The conclusion was that children who are mentally retarded tend to overestimate their success and thus have unrealistic self-concepts.[21] Meyerowitz studied sixty first-

grade students with an IQ range of 60 to 85 who were assigned to special classes, sixty students with the same IQ range who were in a regular first grade, and sixty first-grade students with an IQ range of 95 to 110. He concluded that the children who were retarded were more derogatory of themselves than normal children, and the children who were in special classes were more derogatory of themselves than the children who had remained in a regular first grade.[18]

Ringness concluded that children who are mentally retarded tended to overestimate their success, and Meyerowitz concluded they tended to be more derogatory of themselves than normal children, but Collins and Burger found that both adolescents with an IQ range of 50 to 78 and normal adolescents generally had a negative perception of self. In studying a group of adolescents in special class placement, they found that these students differed from normal adolescents only in self-criticism and social self. The normal adolescents had more positive concepts of their relationships with others and were more apt to self-criticize.[6] Mayer also studied adolescents with an IQ range of 50 to 75 to determine the relationship of early special class placement to self-concept. He found that the adolescents who were mentally retarded, as a group, did not differ significantly from the norms, and it could not be concluded that they had a more negative self-concept. He also was not able to conclude from his data that early placement in special classes promoted a more positive or negative self-concept.[17]

Zigler, Balla, and Watson attempted to approach the study of self-concept from a developmental viewpoint. Using two self-image disparity measures, they compared the self-image of institutionalized mentally retarded children, normal institutionalized children of the same mental age (approximately $10^1/_2$ years), and older normal institutionalized children with the self-image of three similar groups of children who were not institutionalized. Results of their study indicated that children at a higher mental age have greater disparity scores between the self-concept and ideal self-image than both children who were retarded and normal children at a lower mental age. The children who were mentally retarded were found to have a lower self-image disparity, and their ideal self-image was lower than that of normal children of the same mental age. The self-image disparity was also found to be greater among institutionalized than noninstitutionalized children.[26]

Patterns of self-attitudes of individuals who are mentally retarded have been studied by Guthrie, Butler, and Garlow utilizing the Laurelton Self-Attitudes Scale, which they developed. The data that resulted from their study of institutionalized and noninstitutionalized females with an IQ range of 50 to 80 indicated that there were seven general patterns of self-attitudes. Three of the patterns of self-attitudes ("There is nothing wrong with me, I do as well as others do, and I don't give trouble.") were considered indicative of a favorable outlook, whereas the remaining four patterns ("I act hatefully, I am shy and weak, I am useless, and nobody likes me.") were considered indicative of an unfavorable outlook.[11]

The studies that have been discussed in relation to the self-concept of individuals who are mentally retarded are only a few of those which have been done. An excellent review of the research related to the construct of the self-concept and individuals who are mentally retarded was done by Lawrence and Winschel.[14] In addition, Cobb has written a comprehensive theoretical article on the development of the self in individuals who are mentally retarded. In Cobb's article, six aspects of the development of the self (primitive differentiation, identity, self-portrait, level of aspiration, systems of control and defense, and adolescent transition) are discussed and suggestions presented as to what can be done to promote the best possible development of the self in individuals who are mentally retarded.[5]

SUMMARY

Nurses who are interested in assisting individuals with mental retardation and other developmental disabilities to reach their maximum physical, intellectual, social, and emotional potential will find that the constructs of body schema, body image, and self-concept provide them with an additional theoretical framework for nursing interventions. Hopefully, through developing an understanding of the normal development of each of these overlapping and interdependent constructs, the methods that have been utilized in an attempt to assess individuals in relation to each of these constructs, and the interventions that have been tried, nurses can more effectively intervene to promote the development of the self at all levels of development.

REFERENCES

1. Abercrombie, J. L. J. and Tyson, M. C.: Body image and draw-a-man test in cerebral palsy, Dev. Med. Child Neurol. **8:**9, 1966.
2. Ayres, A. J.: Development of the body scheme in children, Am. J. Occup. Ther. **15:**99, 1961.
3. Berges, J., and Lezine, I.: The imitation of gestures, Clin. Dev. Med., No. 18, London, 1965, The Spastics Society Medical Education and Information Unit in association with William Heinemann Medical Books, Ltd.
4. Clapp, R. K.: The body schema of normal and mentally retarded children, J. Psychol. **80:**37, 1972.
5. Cobb, H. V.: The attitude of the retarded person toward himself. In Stress on families of the mentally handicapped, Third International Conference, International League of Societies for the Mentally Handicapped, Bruxelles, Belgium, 1966, Imprimerie Hayex, S.P.R.L., 62-76.
6. Collins. H. A. and Burger, G. K.: The self concepts of adolescent retarded students, Educ. Train. Ment. Retarded **5:**23, 1970.
7. Coopersmith, S.: The antecedents of self-esteem, San Francisco, 1967, W. H. Freeman & Co. Publishers.
8. Gellert, E.: Children's conceptions of the content and functions of the human body, Genet. Psychol. Monogr. **65:**293, 1962.
9. Gellert, E.: Children's constructions of their self-images, Percept. Mot. Skills **40:**307, 1975.
10. Goodenough, F. L.: Measurement of intelligence by drawings, New York, 1926, Harcourt Brace Jovanovich, Inc.
11. Guthrie, G., Butler, A., and Garlow, L.: Patterns of self-attitudes of retardates, Am. J. Ment. Defic. **66:**222, 1961.
12. Kephart, N. C.: The slow learner in the classroom, Columbus, Ohio, 1960, Charles E. Merrill Publishing Co.

13. Koppitz, E. M.: Expected and exceptional items on human figure drawings and IQ scores of children, J. Clin. Psychol. **23**:81, 1967.
14. Lawrence, E. A. and Winschel, J. F.: Self concept and the retarded; research and issues, Except. Child. **39**:310, 1973.
15. Lowery, G. H.: Growth and development of children, ed. 6, Chicago, 1973, Year Book Medical Publishers, Inc.
16. Maloney, M. P., Ball, T. S., and Edgar, C. L.: Analysis of the generalizability of sensory-motor training, Am. J. Ment. Defic. **74**:458, 1970.
17. Mayer, C. L.: The relationship of early special class placement and the self-concepts of mentally handicapped children, Except. Child. **33**: 77, 1966.
18. Meyerowitz, J.: Self-derogations in young retardates and special class placement, Child Dev. **33**:443, 1962.
19. Parrish, R. A.: Exterior and interior body-image. In Social Systems and UAC Nursing, proceedings of Sixth National Workshop for Nurses in Mental Retardation, Cincinnati, Ohio, 1976, pp. 100-136.
20. Porter, C. S.: Grade school children's perceptions of their internal body parts, Nurs. Res. **23**:384, 1974.
21. Ringness, T. A.: Self-concept of children of low, average, and high intelligence, Am. J. Ment. Defic. **65**:453, 1961.
22. Spoerl, D. T.: The drawing ability of mentally retarded children, J. Genet. Psychol. **57**:259, 1940.
23. Weininger, O., Rotenberg. G., and Henry, A.: Body image of handicapped children, J. Pers. Assess. **36**:248, 1972.
24. Wysocki, B. A. and Whitney, E.: Body image of crippled children as seen in draw-a-person test behavior, Percept. Mo. Skills **21**:499, 1965.
25. Wysocki, B. A., and Wysocki, A. C.: The body image of normal and retarded children, J. Clin. Psychol. **29**:7, 1973.
26. Zigler, E., Balla, D., and Watson, N.: Developmental and experimental determinants of self-image disparity in institutionalized and noninstitutionalized retarded and normal children, J. Pers. Soc. Psychol. **23**:81, 1972.

ADDITIONAL READINGS

Bender, L., and Faretra, G.: Body image problems of children. In Lief, J., and others, editors: The psychological basis of medical practice, New York, 1963, Harper & Row, Publishers, Inc.
Caplan, H.: Some considerations of the body image concept in child development, Q. J. Child Behav. **4**:382, 1952.
Corbeil, M.: Nursing process for a patient with a body image disturbance, Nurs. Clin. North Am. **7**:155, 1971.
Easson, W. M.: Psychopathological environmental reaction to congenital defect, J. Nerv. Ment. Dis. **142**:453, 1966.
Fisher, S., and Cleveland, S.: Body image and personality, New York, 1968, Dover Publications, Inc.
Grossman, B. D.: Enhancing the self, Except. Child. **38**:248, 1971.
Horowitz, M. J.: Body image, Arch. Gen. Psychiatry **14**:456, 1966.
Mosey, A. C.: Treatment of pathological distortion of body image, Am. J. Occup. Ther. **23**:413, 1969.
Nagy, M.: Children's conceptions of some bodily functions, J. Genet. Psychol. **83**:199, 1953.
Schilder, P.: Image and appearance of the human body, New York, 1950, International Universities Press.
Schilder, P., and Weshsler, D.: What do children know about the interior of the body? Int. J. Psychoanal. **16**:345, 1935.
Shontz, T. C.: Perceptual and cognitive aspects of body experience, New York, 1969, Academic Press, Inc.
Shontz, T. C.: Body image and its disorders, Int. J. Psychiatry Med. **5**:461, 1974.
Simon, J. I.: Emotional aspects of physical disability, Am. J. Occup. Ther. **25**:408, 1971.
Tait, C. D., and Ascher, R. C.: Inside-of-the-body test; a preliminary report, Psychosom. Med. **17**:139, 1955.

CHAPTER **6**

The transdisciplinary approach

DOROTHY J. HUTCHISON

From
> **trans-** *prefix* [L *trans-*, *tra-* across, beyond, through, so as to change, . . . or transfer]
> **discipline** *n* [L *disciplina* teaching, learning] a subject that is taught, a field of study.

> **transdisciplinary** *adj* relating to a transfer of information, knowledge, and skills across disciplinary boundaries.

Transdisciplinary is a new word for a new approach to the delivery of services to individuals at risk or known to have multisensorimotor handicaps or mental retardation. Drawing on the pooled resources of an interdisciplinary team, the members embark on a conscious, deliberate, systematic sharing of information, knowledge, and skills across traditional disciplinary boundaries. Thus evolved the unique teaching/learning/working triad, hallmark of the transdisciplinary approach.

Tested in a variety of settings since 1969, the transdisciplinary approach ensures effective utilization of professional manpower, reduces compartmentalization and fragmentation, and enables an individualized developmental program for the client. Through role release and expansion, it enhances the competencies of the providers of services and fosters the coping abilities of parents and those who care for the retarded individual. Although designed for a special clientele, the approach has ap-

plication to other populations where the complexity of needs, the magnitude of problems, and the life-span nature of the disability demand the most skillful utilization of manpower.

Throughout this chapter, transdisciplinary is used to designate a particular approach to the delivery of services to individuals at risk and those who are multiply handicapped or mentally retarded. It is used also to designate the continuing education preliminary to, and concurrent with, the delivery of such services.

NURSING INVOLVEMENT

The transdisciplinary concept was originated by nurses. Ackerman has described this approach as a "high yield, moderate cost investment that represents a viable, national change model for the delivery of services to handicapped infants and their families."[1] The transdisciplinary approach has also been cited by Lynch as one of three efforts in this decade having a great impact on care of the developmentally disabled. He identified the other efforts as legislation for the developmentally disabled and the standards developed by the Accreditation Council for Services for the Mentally Retarded and other Developmentally Disabled Persons.[3] The involvement of many of the same people in each of these three efforts has resulted in a common philosophical resolve leading to improved services along a broad front.

The visible outcome of efforts to improve services was two projects administered by the United Cerebral Palsy Associations, Inc. (UCPA). Both were directed by Una Haynes, Associate Director of UCPA's Professional Program Services Department and Nurse Consultant. One project was the development of miniteams working with multiply handicapped clients in institutions.* The other was a collaborative attempt to provide comprehensive services to infants and families.†

Joining Mrs. Haynes in her concern were Ida Axelrod‡ and Doris Haar.§ The nature of their work took these nurses into facilities and service agencies for the retarded. They were deeply moved by the neglected and warehoused multihandicapped and by the preventable secondary disabilities that developed when care was custodial rather than habilitative. Their goal of improving services led to the involvement of additional nurses.‖ Nurses have provided a continuing

---

*A service approach toward the improvement of programs for individuals with neuro-motor and sensory handicaps in addition to mental retardation, made possible in part by grants from the Division of Developmental Disabilities, Social Rehabilitation Services, U.S. Department of Health, Education and Welfare.
†A nationally organized collaborative project to provide comprehensive services to handicapped infants and their families, supported in part by grants from the Bureau of Education for the Handicapped, Office of Education, U.S. Department of Health, Education and Welfare.
‡Ida Axelrod, Consultant in Public Health for the National Association for Retarded Children (NARC), was succeeded after her death by Gene Patterson, Program Consultant for NARC (now National Association for Retarded Citizens).
§Doris Haar, Chief, Division of Research and Development, Office of Developmental Disabilities, Office of Human Development, U.S. Department of Health, Education, and Welfare.
‖Later to be involved were Frances Orgain of Indiana University School of Nursing; Patricia McNelly, Violet Moran, and Helen Lovell of Central Wisconsin Colony and Training School, Madison, Wisconsin, who spearheaded an institutional involvement and a commitment that still persists; and Kathryn Barnard and Anita L. Spietz of the University of Washington.

force throughout the development and implementation of the transdisciplinary approach. They have been members of planning, advisory, and technical groups and have served as consultants, faculty, and members of action level teams.

Many nurses have long been aware of the significant contribution they can make in the area of mental retardation. They are also aware that nursing expertise alone is not enough. The nature of developmental disabilities requires the input of many disciplines.

The number of professionals prepared to work with the handicapped has increased. However, problems of manpower distribution and the lack of funds to secure their services continue to plague the field. Such scarcities are a major concern for voluntary agencies developed around selected clientele groups and for governmental agencies that are expected to serve all people. It is paradoxical that although more specialists are being prepared, the handicapped do not receive the special services they require. Education has produced an expert society, yet expertise has not been channeled to all segments of the population. There is urgent need for providers of services to learn to work more effectively together in behalf of the client.

A UNIFYING PHILOSOPHY

The first challenge to the transdisciplinary approach was the identification and collaboration of professionals from many fields. Their shared concerns and experiences in working with the multiply handicapped were a common bond. They met to pool their knowledge, information, special strategies, and techniques as well as educated guesses and feelings. They believed that severely involved individuals could be helped. Although there was disagreement as to theoretical framework and approaches, they began with a basic premise:

The Transdisciplinary Approach grows out of the belief that each member of the family of man is a unique being; a whole person with potential to achieve and a life to be lived. The quality of life is of importance to the individual, the family, the community and society as a whole. Therefore, effective ways must be found and used to prevent developmental disabilities and to intervene effectively to prevent secondary disabilities and to habilitate or rehabilitate those so affected.*

Doris Haar offers a retrospect on how the transdisciplinary approach came about:

In 1969, a few people with vision put their heads together and began working on developing a curriculum that would assemble the best materials of all disciplines in the field.

The representation in this working group was unique for its time. It brought together UCPA, Inc., NARC, Central Wisconsin Colony and Training School, the University of Wisconsin-Extension, and a "Fed."

By pooling really meagre resources we were able to bring to one place the few leading proponents of a wide variety of disciplines. They pooled their philosophies, they contributed their resources of information, skills, techniques, and pointed out their gaps in knowledge, their weaknesses, and their frustrations.

Their combined biographies were staggering. Their techniques at first blush seemed to be at odds with one another, while seemingly duplicating one another at other points.†

These discussions resulted in a planning effort and the identification of essential content areas for a curriculum to be used in the preparation of teams. An ad hoc interdisciplinary teaching faculty and a number of consultants were recruited.

After intensive training coordinated by Hutchison, professional teams adapted the content and offered it in an on-the-ward training program for aides. This preparation enabled them as principal caregivers to take their places with therapists and nurses as full-fledged members of the transdisciplinary team. Thus began the attempt to improve services to habilitate and prevent secondary disabilities among severely involved residents in institutions and to enrich the living environment through transdisciplinary action.

TOWARD A TRANSDISCIPLINARY FOCUS

Human services usually develop in response to human need. The transdisciplinary approach is an example where the focus is on the individual who is handicapped or at risk. The needs of the clients generate multidimensional needs in their parents or substitute family. Similarly, the needs of the clients and their families (or substitute families) engender learning needs in the providers of service as well as new patterns for the delivery of required services (Fig. 6-1).

The primary concern centers on the individual who is handicapped. Such a focus is not unique to the transdisciplinary approach since most other service approaches share this concept. However, the significant difference between the transdisciplinary approach and other service approaches is the expanded focus of the transdisciplinary model. It includes parents/surrogates, providers of services, and the caring community as well as the handicapped individual (Fig. 6-2).

A transdisciplinary stance is not easily achieved. It is made possible by the deliberate pooling of information, knowledge, and skills across disciplinary boundaries. Moving toward a transdisciplinary stance takes time. It occurs as a series of steps toward

*From Hutchison, D.: Instructional Foundation Document No. 1, Basic Premise, Rev. 1971, Madison, University of Wisconsin—Extension at Madison, Wis.

†From Haar, D.: Excerpt from telelecture to conference group, Madison, University of Wisconsin—Extension at Madison, Wis., undated.

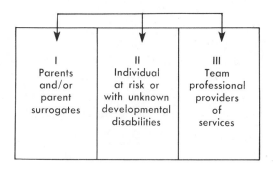

I Parents and/or parent surrogates	II Individual at risk or with unknown developmental disabilities	III Team professional providers of services

Fig. 6-1. Transdisciplinary focus on needs.

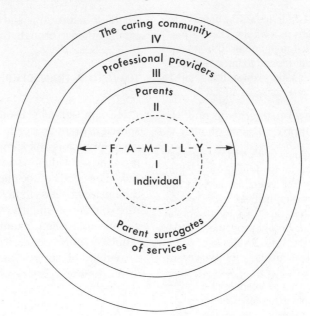

Fig. 6-2. The expanded focus.

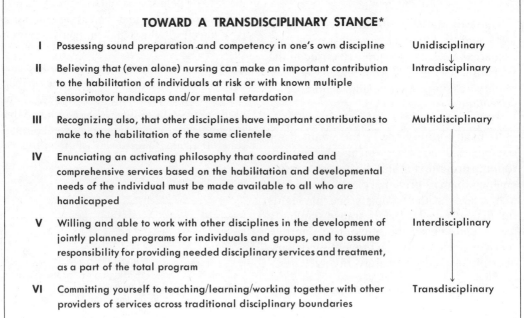

TOWARD A TRANSDISCIPLINARY STANCE*

I	Possessing sound preparation and competency in one's own discipline	Unidisciplinary
II	Believing that (even alone) nursing can make an important contribution to the habilitation of individuals at risk or with known multiple sensorimotor handicaps and/or mental retardation	Intradisciplinary
III	Recognizing also, that other disciplines have important contributions to make to the habilitation of the same clientele	Multidisciplinary
IV	Enunciating an activating philosophy that coordinated and comprehensive services based on the habilitation and developmental needs of the individual must be made available to all who are handicapped	
V	Willing and able to work with other disciplines in the development of jointly planned programs for individuals and groups, and to assume responsibility for providing needed disciplinary services and treatment, as a part of the total program	Interdisciplinary
VI	Committing yourself to teaching/learning/working together with other providers of services across traditional disciplinary boundaries	Transdisciplinary

*From Instructional Foundation Document No. 4, Toward a transdisciplinary stance, Madison, 1971, University of Wisconsin—Extension at Madison, Wis.

fuller understanding and involves both motivation and effort.

THE TEAM: FOUNDATION OF THE APPROACH

The foundation of the transdisciplinary approach is the team. Drawn from a number of disciplines, its composition is determined by client needs. The team construct will differ from agency to agency and sometimes among multiple teams in larger agencies. The need to pool information, knowledge, and skills in the critical areas of physical, cognitive, and psychosocial development must be coupled with the in-depth clinical experience of those who have centered their professional careers on ameliorating existing disabilities and preventing secondary handicaps.

The earliest attempt was the miniteam project developed by UCPA. The first teams to be established were composed of two nurses and two therapists. One of the nurses had experience in in-service education, assisting team members to teach each other and, in turn, to transmit the essential knowledge and skills to those caring for the resident. The second nurse had an administrative position, thus providing the authority to structure change in care.

In 1970, when the miniteams were developing, many problems existed in institutions. It was difficult to find institutions that had both physical and occupational therapists on their staff. Most frequently, nurses and therapists functioned as department heads, giving little direct client service. In addition, there were problems with confusion of roles between physical therapists and occupational therapists. It was also believed that nurses could function in any setting without specialized training. Few professionals employed in institutions had special preparation to work with the mentally retarded and multiply handicapped.

From the beginning, teams were provided consultation and encouraged to seek additional assistance from other staff members in their agencies. As needs became more clearly defined, the teams were expected to be augmented with other disciplinary members. Although the team served a defined target population of the severely involved multiply handicapped, its most essential expansion occurred when natural parents or parent surrogates (aides) joined the team.[2] They participated with the professionals in assessing the needs of particular clients. They collaborated in the design of the individual program plan and were responsible for its implementation. The concept of continuity of relationship as "aide parents" to a "family" of individuals was instituted.*

Over time, expanded teams were characteristic of the transdisciplinary approach. In some settings second teams were initiated. The number of expanded teams increased as the second UCPA project developed. This project was an outgrowth of UCPA's long-standing interest in infants and their families. It was also responsive to the belief of institutional teams that there was failure in providing appropriate and early help to high-risk infants or those with known cerebral dysfunction and their families.

The concept of combining the medical model with the educational model, giving rise to a developmental model, afforded a common ground for the mix of disciplines. Special recognition was given to the role of early childhood educators who became infant educators through transdisciplinary action. The roles of community physicians and public health nurses were also strengthened because they provided the early identification and referral to programs. Increasingly, physicians were integrated as members of the team. Orthopedists, who have long been interested in cerebral palsy, were joined by pediatric neurologists and developmentalists. Specialists in communication disorders, community organization, adaptive equipment, administration, social work, psychology, and outreach, and increasing

---

*The group-parent concept was pioneered at Central Wisconsin Center for the Developmentally Disabled by Patricia McNelly, Director of Nursing, and without exception was established in every institution.

numbers of volunteers and foster grandparents joined some of the teams.

Teams recognized that they could not realize project goals unless the parents or surrogate parents were included as members of the team for each client. There was recognition of the need to teach them therapeutic handling and to help them incorporate it into the life of the individual. The team also identified the need to incorporate the daily developmental plan for the handicapped individual into the life-style of the family in a positive way.

Calling a small group of people a team does not make them so; team relationships are forged over time. As understanding of the preparation and expertise is reached, trust and confidence begin to develop. Individuals exploring the transdisciplinary approach are often surprised that no one theoretical frame is held in common guiding the actions of all teams. In a developmental model, all theories are examined and evaluated in terms of the identified needs of clients.

Since the team members represent different disciplines, the potential body of theory is enlarged. Theoretical presentations by each discipline are essential. Applications of principles to practice are thoroughly considered and become central elements in team teaching and learning. They are incorporated in teaching by the exploration, study, analysis, and decision as to when and for whom they are most useful.

Few staff have previously been involved as members in the close team interaction typical of the transdisciplinary approach. Few have been prepared for the stresses and anxieties that such a teaching/working/learning relationship engenders.

The team is essentially a small group. It is important for team members to understand that there are interpersonal as well as task dimensions in any team interaction. The pattern of interpersonal relationships constitutes the group structure. The content of the interaction is addressed to task completion.

A review of the phase movement in groups [from 1949 to the present by Hutchison] shows that many observers identify similar developmental stages. Most new groups evidence orienting behavior. In their insecurity they become dependent. After initial newness has been reduced, emotional reactions to the group and the task surface and are released. Sometimes these are sufficiently severe that the group self-destructs entirely or loses some of its early members. If the members win through the emotional stage, group identity and cohesiveness begin to develop. Early traumas are relegated to the past and they address themselves realistically to the task at hand.

Tuckman's model has special relevance for the transdisciplinary team.

Stage 1: Forming	Testing and dependence
Stage 2: Storming	Intragroup conflict
Stage 3: Norming	Development of group
Stage 4: Performing	cohesion
	Functional role relatedness and productivity

Fortunately, most teams have access to experts in the field of group process. It is sometimes useful to establish a relationship with a consultant in order first to understand better group dynamics and process, and, second, to be facilitated where conflicts develop.

It is the author's observation in working with some 23 institutional and 50 community agency teams that those enduring greatest stress emerge and achieve a high functional level of team effectiveness and productivity.*

A COMMON GROUND

The varieties of educational preparation and experience represented on a team necessitate a search for commonalities. Theoretical overlap supplies the answer. It is easily found in the shared concern for the client. The common goal is to help handicapped individuals develop to their potential. All team members have some background in human development. The pooling of what each one knows, extended and expanded by what can be learned from each other, fosters a developmental model. The model is dynamic, changing, and open to new inputs. It derives from the concept

---

*From Hutchison, D.: A model for transdisciplinary staff development, New York, 1974, United Cerebral Palsy Associations, Inc., p. 16.

that developmentally disabled persons are capable of growth, maturation, and learning within the limits of their handicaps. This process often occurs in spite of the handicaps when the client is presented with appropriate opportunities.

Developmental programming may appear to be too broad to be functional. It will not occur until team members and parents think about development as something each can influence and foster. It calls team members to understand and identify individual and shared responsibilities as they relate to developmental programming.

Some basic assumptions underlie the UCPA transdisciplinary projects. For miniteams dealing with severely involved individuals residing in institutions, the following became guiding statements:

1. Any developmentally disabled person is capable of growth, maturation, and learning within the limits of his handicap, and often in spite of it. Thus, disability must be viewed within the overall context of development.
2. Specific opportunities to learn, grow, and develop must be available to every disabled person regardless of age, type, or degree of disability if growth and development are to occur.
3. Such individuals must also receive special services directed toward the amelioration of the disabilities and prevention of secondary disabilities.*

The underlying assumptions of the second UCPA project, which dealt with infants and families, included:

1. The atypical child is first of all a child—a whole child and not a series of affected parts.
2. Infancy is a crucial period in the life of the child; for the atypical child, the period is even more crucial.

3. In the early years, parents are the most crucial factors in the life of the child.*

Members of the infant and family teams developed an individual program plan (IPP or Infant Curriculum) based on comprehensive disciplinary assessments of strengths and problems. The plans were designed collaboratively by the team and the parents and specified developmental goals and the strategies that parents and team must learn from each other. The goal of the plan was to assist clients in achieving their potential. Ongoing research and evaluation must be incorporated in the program plans to the benefit of clients. Thus, the theoretical frame is dynamic and open to new inputs.

THE TRANSDISCIPLINARY PROCESS: INTERACTION/TRANSACTION

The transdisciplinary process has two major components, interaction and transaction. In a framework of interaction, the team embarks on a conscious effort to become familiar with the purposes, education for entry into the field, role, and usual functions delegated to it by society or assumed as a professional prerogative of each of the disciplines represented. Interaction also requires that the team identify the core of attitudes, knowledge, and skills held in common by all or some of the team members. The team should specify the unique functions of each discipline. Such functions include those mandated by law or declared by the profession as its particular province. Some functions may be viewed by the team as expertise to be developed as a part of advanced education within a university or under the tutelage of acknowledged experts in the field. The team must also look at separatism of disciplines in terms of positive or negative impact on services for the multihandicapped.

---

*From Hutchison, D.: Instructional Foundation Document No. 5, Guiding Statements, Madison, 1970, University of Wisconsin—Extension at Madison, Wis.

*From the first three years; programming for atypical infants, Project Report, New York, 1974, United Cerebral Palsy Associations, Inc., pp. 2-7.

In the transaction, the team systematically seeks to enlarge the common core of knowledge and competency of each team member within the group through planned individual study, one-to-one instruction, and team teaching/learning. It provides for role release to other team members so that each may fulfill an expanded role when the ability to carry out the interventions safely, effectively, and responsibly has been demonstrated. The team makes role release possible to parents and parent surrogates through systematized instruction and supervised practice. Each may then be able to sustain the individual developmental plan and carry out specified interventions safely, effectively, and responsibly for their own child or for groups of children in an institutional setting.

Through the transaction component, the team must also develop each member's capacity to serve as program facilitator through the mechanisms of collegial instruction and role expansion. In this role, the facilitator implements the individual program for selected clients and their families as assigned by the team and maintains a continuity relationship with the client/family and with the team in relation to the changing needs of the client.

TRANSITIONS TO ROLE RELEASE

Every discipline involved in transdisciplinary teamwork experiences role release. The following discussion of nursing's role release may be helpful to any professional involved in teams:

Nursing's preoccupation with role has produced a spate of words that relate to evolution in role. Role extension, role enrichment, role expansion, and role exchange surface in the literature. Each enlarges the area of nursing function. Role enlargement, however, calls for the most discriminating judgment as to priorities for the profession and what preparation is needed to serve the client. Enlargement in particular directions may ultimately call for reduction in others. The time has come to take a long hard look at the process involved in releasing certain traditional aspects of the nursing role, as simultaneously we seek to add to its dimensions.*

Role release requires a series of transitions. The transdisciplinary team views each disciplinary member as an authority. Further, the expectation is held that each brings depth in a discipline and seeks constantly to extend it through self-directed learning.

Such *role extension* adds to the knowledge base for teaching—a forerunner to role release. It also holds before each member the challenge of keeping abreast of research, reviewing new developments in practice, and applying them as appropriate for their shared clientele.

Much serendipitous learning takes place in the work setting, and *role enrichment* follows. The planned pooling of information, knowledge, and skills leads to *role expansion*. *Role exchange* follows systematic teaching as the authoritative discipline supervises another in carrying out the newly acquired interventions. The close supervision continues until both teacher and learner are satisfied that the desired level of competency is achieved.

Role release to a team member occurs when the learner is able to carry out the interventions skillfully as *program facilitator* for a particular client or clients. It also occurs when parents as *primary programmers* learn to carry out specific interventions for their child guided by a plan they have helped to develop. Role release takes place as well after parent surrogates are taught and demonstrate their ability to function responsibly and effectively in caring for an individual or group of individuals within a personalized program plan. They, too, are known as primary programmers.

None of the foregoing transitions leading to role release are possible without continuous team support. Consultative backup is continuously available to the program facilitator and primary programmer. Further, each authoritative discipline continues to

---

*From Hutchison, D.: The evolving role, J. Cont. Educ. Nurs. **5:**5, 1974.

provide the highly complex interventions demanding extensive expertise and the functions mandated by law and to institute new interventions necessitated by the changing needs of the client. Each discipline also tests and practices interventions growing out of new information and research before transmitting them to the team. Team members remain accountable for what they teach, whom they teach, how well the learner has learned, and the resulting benefits to the client.

ADULT EDUCATION: AN INSTRUMENTALITY

In describing their multiple roles, few team members use the descriptive term "adult educator." In the early days of the UCPA projects, because of the strong therapeutic and remedial thrust the team realized that each had a teaching function for which some additional preparation was needed. When asked to examine what they were trying to do with and for their clients, the team recognized an inescapable, inherent teaching role. The expanded team recognized that the outcome of its interventions might well depend on the ability to teach adults, each other as team members, parent/surrogates, and ultimately the larger community. Although most of the community agencies had infant educators on staff who provided effective role models for other team members in teaching handicapped individuals, few were skilled in adult education.

The work setting is an exciting milieu for learning when each team member actively assumes a teaching role. In the transdisciplinary approach, the most frequently used teaching strategy is collegial instruction. When the team recognizes itself as a learning group as well as a working group, learning by choice rather than by chance becomes a team goal. The team consciously strives to become a cooperative, collaborative, teaching/learning group. The teaching is shared among members in terms of their expertise. The climate is marked by the full, participatory involvement of each

member—sometimes as teacher, sometimes as learner. Colleague review ensures effective learning toward defined criterion performance.

The term "inservice education" may evoke an image of a carefully designed program of systematic learning. An honest appraisal in many agencies finds that inservice education is actually a nonsystem. It tends to be sporadic, fragmented, and nonsequential. It develops in response to crises; planning is shaped by expediencies. In many agencies, time for staff learning is seen as depriving the client of services. Sheets has made the following observation:

> Time for the inservice education must be set aside and rigorously adhered to as an integral part of the working day, and the working responsibilities of all staff members. Specific goals and training directions need to be thoughtfully established.*

The transdisciplinary approach confers a great measure of autonomous functioning to the team. How the team will structure activities to accomplish the goals of the agency and their own contributory objectives is the decision of the members. Creating a structure for learning that will provide for maintaining and extending competencies may be the most significant decision to be made by the team.

SUMMARY

The transdisciplinary approach reduces the numbers of professional persons rendering direct service to the individual, hence reducing compartmentalization and fragmentation. Continuity of relationship and many of the direct services are provided to the individual by the program facilitator. Parents, or those who substitute for them, are helped to acquire coping skills as primary programmers for their child.

With a team as the basic unit of service delivery, members merge their concerns for

---

*From Sheets, B.: Supplemental report to the project director, New York, 1973, United Cerebral Palsy Associations, Inc.

the individual and their basic understandings of human development and offer their expertise not only directly to the client but also across disciplinary boundaries to each other.

Enhancement of professional competence is inherent in the transdisciplinary approach, but the enhancement of the quality of life for the developmentally disabled is the ultimate goal.

REFERENCES

1. Akerman, P.: Excerpt from telelecture to conference group, Madison, University of Wisconsin—Extension at Madison, Wis., undated.
2. Haynes, U.: Nursing approaches in cerebral dysfunction, Am. J. Nurs. **68:**2170, 1968.
3. Lynch, F.: Excerpt from telelecture to conference group, Madison, University of Wisconsin—Extension at Madison, Wis., undated.

CHAPTER 7

Quality assurance in residential settings

PATRICIA McNELLY

Nursing in mental retardation has been described as a function of being able to work with a child and parents or with groups of children and parents in a variety of situations.[18] Current descriptions of nursing in mental retardation should reflect the ability to work with clients of all ages as well as with parent surrogates, advocates, guardians, and a variety of other professional disciplines. Nursing contact with clients who are mentally retarded will most frequently occur in clinics or in home or school settings, since a major portion of health care services are normally provided in locations other than hospitals. Nurses are actively involved in providing primary health care in adult day services, sheltered employment situations, or in a variety of community residential settings, such as intermediate care facilities, group homes, or semi-independent living situations.

The provision of services to individuals with retardation and their families has undergone fundamental changes during the past decade. Nursing roles within the spectrum of services have changed even more dramatically. Nurses have assumed greater responsibility for physical and behavioral assessment, and they foster the development of motor skills and adaptive behaviors necessary for accomplishing activities of daily living. Nurses plan programs to modify clients' problematic behaviors and increase their coping abilities. They also provide counseling services for clients and families and often serve in a coordinating capacity to maximize the effectiveness of the involvement of many agencies. These changes in the nursing role require an expansion in the knowledge base and clinical expertise of the professional nurse in order to provide quality service.

Nurses, along with other professionals, strive to alter the effect of a variety of factors that hinder the mentally retarded individual's ability to function. Nursing efforts are directed toward assisting individuals to achieve their capabilities in terms of human potential and individual integrity and to conserve those resources essential to coping with deviations in normal growth and development.[18] It must be emphasized that development is a life-long process. The individual who is mentally retarded will require varying amounts of intervention and assistance depending on the nature and severity of the developmental disability and the availability of a supportive environment during crisis periods.

Because of the expanding role of nurses in mental retardation and because of the current service delivery systems, nursing accountability needs to be explored. Nurses are accountable to clients and families for appropriate and timely assessment and intervention, with subsequent evaluation of the nursing services rendered. Too often nurses use the excuse that they have not received adequate training to work with mentally retarded individuals. Whether employed in community, residential, governmental, academic or other settings, nurses should recognize that they have a basic foundation of knowledge and skills needed to work with mentally retarded persons as well as other clients. They can readily update and expand that knowledge and skill through continuing education, inservice programs, and formal academic programs that are increasingly available.

Another component of accountability is the application of objective standards to improve the quality of services. Nurses are becoming more aware of the importance of applying standards developed by organizations such as the American Nurses' Association and the Joint Commission on Accreditation of Hospitals (JCAH). This chapter focuses on the quality assurance program through the use of JCAH standards, with emphasis directed toward residential settings. However, the information presented should be helpful to nurses regardless of the setting in which they are employed or the origin of standards being utilized.

COMPONENTS OF QUALITY ASSURANCE

Working independently or with other members of an interdisciplinary team, nurses contribute to the development of measures that determine quality in the total program. All the available approaches to evaluation, including assessment of structure, process, and outcome, need to be examined in order to determine the quality of services provided.[5] *Structure* is defined as the material and human resources used to provide care, their properties, and the manner in which they are organized. Standards relating to those resources allow judgments to be made about the quality of the structure. This is the most commonly used approach in assessment for certification or accreditation by official and voluntary agencies. It is based on the assumption that when certain

defined conditions are present, quality services are being provided. However, what is actually being assessed is the capability for providing quality service, not the actual provision of that service.

Evaluation of *process* requires a review of the sequence of activities that have been arranged in a particular manner to accomplish defined goals of service. Here, the assumptions that particular structural characteristics are related to specific levels of performance are tested. There is very little data to either support or refute the basic assumptions relating to the usefulness of structure and process standards.

Evaluations of *outcomes* consist of measuring the end result of the service or what actually happened to the client as a result of the service provided. This type of evaluation can be used to measure achievement of desired outcomes, health status, general welfare, and satisfactions. Outcome evaluation offers the ultimate test of the assumptions employed in using either structure or process measures for assessment of quality. Outcome evaluation is considered a more precise method of measurement, but it is also more difficult to develop and implement. Often there is lack of concensus on precisely what the expected outcomes are. Other variables, such as the span of time involved, the participation of a variety of agencies, the ongoing nature of services, and the multiplicity of client problems, may also need to be considered.

Current methods for assessing quality through outcome evaluation have been designed primarily for use in acute care facilities. The use of clinical case entities for identification of groups of clients to be evaluated creates a major problem for the residential facility providing long-term care. JCAH believes that there are essential characteristics of an evaluation system that can be adapted for use by any facility providing a health care component. The characteristics defined by the JCAH retrospective outcome audit, the Performance Evaluation Procedure for Auditing and Improving Patient Care (PEP), are[21]:

1. The system must be objective, using reliable, valid measures.
2. The system must provide for measurement, and care must be defined and compared with the measurements.
3. Variation from the measures must be analyzed in terms of their justification.
4. If not justified, the deficiencies must be identified and corrective action taken.
5. The action must be evaluated for effectiveness in correcting the problem.
6. The action must be documented and reported to those persons who have final responsibility for the level of care provided to the consumer.

The JCAH system used in the evaluation of outcome in the long-term care setting has two major components, the patient care profile and the primary audit.[16] The patient care profile, which includes medical and psychosocial data, provides the basis for continual evaluation of the status and care of individuals. The profile also provides the basis for primary audit, retrospectively assessing success in goal achievement for a distinct group of clients. When there is failure in goal achievement, further analysis is employed to determine if care is appropriate. Since goal achievement represents staff efforts to establish programs that meet priority needs, the rationale is that this system will measure program effectiveness in the resolution of problems. Since diverse needs may be represented within any medical diagnostic category, such as cerebral palsy, microcephaly, or Down's syndrome, other methods may have to be employed to identify distinct groups of clients whose needs are similar.

HISTORY OF STANDARDS IN QUALITY ASSURANCE PROGRAMS

Recent developments in both the governmental and voluntary sectors have provided objective tools for assessing the quality of residential and community services for mentally retarded persons. The voluntary sector moved first, establishing an Accreditation Council for Facilities for the Mentally Retarded within the JCAH (see p. 76). Al-though the Council was the first to develop standards for use in a formal accreditation program for residential facilities for the mentally retarded, the development of standards in this area has a much longer history.

In 1959, the American Association on Mental Deficiency's (AAMD) Project on Technical Planning in Mental Retardation began a major standards development project, producing the 1964 publication of *Standards for State Residential Institutions for the Mentally Retarded*.[31] The AAMD standards were presented as minimal service requirements, usually attainable within a 5- to 10-year period, to be used as a basis for self-evaluation. Along with this publication, AAMD established a committee to continue review and revision of the standards and to encourage their implementation by providing an objective evaluative service. AAMD thus began planning for the eventual establishment of a formal accreditation program. Federal grants were used over the next several years to develop instruments and provide for the evaluation of 134 state residential facilities for the mentally retarded.

Although AAMD initially attempted a global effort in the evaluation of residential services, the omission of standards relating to specific and important segments of programs and services was quickly recognized. Nursing was the first professional group to undertake measures to correct the omission. An ad hoc committee of nurses developed a statement, *Guidelines for Nursing Standards in Residential Centers for the Mentally Retarded*,[11] which was incorporated as a supplement to the AAMD evaluation instrument. Other disciplines, such as physical therapy and recreation, quickly followed suit, and further program service standards were added to the original document.

By 1966, AAMD had formed a National Planning Committee on Accreditation of Residential Centers for the Retarded, inviting representatives from five other professional and service associations to join in the effort to improve the quality of residential services. The broadening of support beyond

AAMD was of significance because it included representatives of the consumers of residential services. Later when JCAH offered a consolidated approach through the establishment of accreditation councils, the National Planning Committee moved to establish the Accreditation Council for Facilities for the Mentally Retarded (AC/FMR).* This was the first council to be established under the expansion of JCAH's accreditation programs.

In 1971, the AC/FMR published *Standards for Residential Facilities for the Mentally Retarded* and established the voluntary accreditation program.[30] There are more than 2,000 separate items in these residential standards, divided into specific categories related to the components of structure and process in quality assurance.

In 1973, AC/FMR published *Standards for Community Agencies,* which was used to accredit community facilities that provide services to persons with mental retardation and other developmental disabilities.[27] These standards also focus on the necessity for an individual program plan and are applicable to all specialized services, generic agencies, and planning and coordinating agencies. In January of 1977, AC/MR-DD began circulating the seventh draft of *Standards for Services for Developmentally Disabled Persons,* a document that represents a merger of *Standards for Community Agencies* and *Standards for Residential Facilities.* After extensive review from potential users, the Council and JCAH adopted and ratified this comprehensive standards document. The Council's goal is to provide for the accreditation of a coordinated, comprehensive, individualized system, placing emphasis on program effectiveness and follow-through of services. AC/MR-DD standards have focused on process and outcome of programs rather than on their structure, thus requiring agencies to have

effective methods of program delivery and evaluation, comparing outcomes with goals and providing for the review and modification of agency operations as needed.

The federal *Standards for Intermediate Care Facilities,* modeled after the accreditation standards, includes a section on facilities that serve the mentally retarded.[33] Many persons who are severely disabled because of their mental retardation and in need of specialized residential programs are eligible for federal support under Title XIX (Medicaid) of the Social Security legislation. Residential facilities capable of providing appropriate services may elect to participate in Title XIX programs as an intermediate care facility. To do so, they must meet both state and federal standards for active habilitative programming. States participating in Title XIX programs are required to establish licensing standards for the intermediate care facilities (ICF). Since compliance with these federal standards brings substantial financial rewards to states participating in the Medicaid program, there has been a significant effort across the country to meet ICF standards.

In the evolution of measures to provide quality assurance in residential programs, outcome criteria will be developed and utilized as the best evaluation tool. Peer review activities also must be employed with the intermediate care standards, providing a review of the appropriateness of the placement of each resident. In addition, there must be an independent professional review of the adequacy of the services being provided. Nurses are increasingly engaged in all of these activities. Some of them are working to meet the standards within the residential facility. Others are employed as surveyors and program review specialists in state agencies or professional standards review organizations responsible for the monitoring process.

DEVELOPMENT OF NURSING STANDARDS IN QUALITY ASSURANCE PROGRAMS

The tasks that must be accomplished in developing sound quality assurance pro-

---

*In 1976, the Council's name was changed to the Accreditation Council for Services for Mentally Retarded and Other Developmentally Disabled Persons (AC/MR-DD).

grams in services to mentally retarded persons represent a challenge to all professionals involved. Nursing may be in the forefront in developing the knowledge and skills necessary to participate and achieve results in this area. Much work has already been done in developing standards and devising measures to evaluate process and outcome. Existing standards of professional nursing practice and standards for nursing service structure and function will need to be examined and applied appropriately. Additional standards must be developed to reflect quality practice requirements in specific service settings. Wherever the nurse is engaged in professional practice to serve the mentally retarded population, the need exists for the development and application of specific standards for that setting. These standards must define and establish criteria to evaluate structure, process, and outcome, and outline the protocol for peer review methods. All are essential elements in assurance of quality nursing services for the consumer.[12] Nursing services provided to mentally retarded individuals must meet standards of quality equivalent to those available in every other area of nursing practice.

Nursing service departments should provide written statements of philosophy, objectives, job descriptions for each nursing position, statements of qualifications for those positions, and functional nursing procedures and policies. Organizational outlines delineating nursing responsibility and communication channels are also an essential element in the development of standards relating to nursing services structure and process.

Process standards may be developed in relation to the specific activities of nursing or the needs of the clients being served. Phaneuf has developed a process model that provides standards to be used in retrospective audit and can be used in a variety of settings.[22] These standards are based on the seven functions of nursing practice.[13] This method of audit can be useful in assessing the quality of care that has been documented

and increasing staff acceptance of the need for documentation. However, in view of the vital need for outcome evaluation, process audit should not be the first order of priority for program evaluation.

Although the needs for standards, methods of program evaluation, and peer review are clearly recognized as essential to any organized plan for accountability, these elements can never replace the personal and professional standards of the individual nurse who is responsible for providing quality service to each client. The professional ethics and value system of every nurse engaged in providing services to mentally retarded persons are of vital importance in determining the nature and quality of that service. The experiences gained in the educational system that prepares professional nurses contribute to development of values.

Participation with peers in organizations such as the American Nurses' Association or the Nursing Division of the American Association on Mental Deficiency is also important. For example, the code of professional ethics of the American Nurses' Association must be internalized by the nurse in order to have impact on the nature of professional activity.[3] The same is true of the *Standards of Nursing Practice* and those specific standards of practice that have been developed by the various divisions of the American Nurses' Association.[28] In every delineation of standards, there is a direct or indirect reference to the nurse's accountability to the client. The American Nurses' Association Division on Psychiatric-Mental Health Nursing Practice offers a significant additional standard relating to the nurse's responsibility for continued educational and professional development as well as a contribution to the professional growth of others.[29] This standard, if internalized and acted on by the nurse, will have an impact on the nature of the internal values system and the strength of beliefs concerning problematic areas of professional practice. Exposure to these basic issues in nursing practice can be secured through educational programs.

If practicing nurses are to keep pace with the demands of the times that require professionals capable of collaborating with other disciplines in identifying client needs, determining outcomes, and designing goal-oriented interventions, further formal or continuing education must be pursued. Cooper describes the need for increasing attention to interdisciplinary continuing education based on mutual respect and sharing.[4] Further attention must also be directed toward evaluation and self-appraisal wherein the learner carefully considers personal and professional goals, learning needs, assessment of potential resources, and evaluation of achievement. The ultimate responsibility for continued learning rests with the professional person who makes a lifelong commitment to personal development.

THE PROCESS OF ASSESSMENT AND THE NURSING ROLE

Stevens describes nursing assessment as usually combining the use of physical examination techniques, observation, and interview.[32] The use of structured assessment tools represents a way of assuring a standard of quality in categorizing the most important aspects of the individual, his or her strengths, and needs. Nurses use assessment tools in order to assure that the process of assessment is both systematic and complete. A number of other disciplines also employ assessment tools in order to develop a knowledge base on which to make programmatic decisions. In mental retardation programs, one area of interrelated concern is the assessment of adaptive behavior. For example, the nurse is concerned with the ability of the individual to perform self-care activities necessary for daily living and for maintaining health. This area of interest is also common to some occupational therapists, physical therapists, psychologists, and pediatricians. The ability of the individual to communicate in a meaningful way is of concern to every team member as well as to the speech pathologist. The manner in which the family copes with problems presented by the handicapped member concerns all the professionals but is also of particular interest to the social worker. A mutually developed assessment process will promote the growth of each team member's ability to identify strengths, needs, and problems. It will expand their knowledge of normative behavior and enhance the team's ability to identify deviations from expected programmatic outcomes. When one proceeds from an expanded knowledge base, the quality of the process in establishing realistic goals for the individual and the family can be greatly improved.

Lack of a precise approach or failure to utilize a standardized format for data collection can be a serious problem to the nurse who is participating as both a practitioner and an equal member of the interdisciplinary team. Many models, which may be helpful in developing a role in a specific service setting, are available to aid the nurse in assessment and data collection.[1, 9, 15, 25, 32] For example, the nursing assessment tool developed by Fuller and Rosenaur was designed for use in a primary care clinic serving ambulatory populations, encompassing all age ranges and the health-illness continuum.[9] Barnard and Erickson offer another model for nurses working with young mentally retarded children and their families. A parent interview, a developmental assessment, and observations of behavior and play are their methods for gathering data used to establish a development plan with the child's family.[1] The nurse is also advised to seek data such as previous evaluations, medical records, educational reports, and other sources that may provide additional assistance in understanding the problem.

As nurses use the data in intervening to remediate health concerns and problems caused by developmental deviation, they must also be aware of the need to prevent additional handicaps. Judicious and timely intervention, particularly in the early years of development, is of critical importance. The child's extremely rapid intellectual and physical development in the first 5 years of life dictates that early identification and intervention must be provided for children at risk. Careful monitoring of function and an effective nursing plan that includes the provision of anticipatory guidance should be provided to clients of all ages.

DESIGNING THE PLAN FOR INTERVENTION

Nurses in a Massachusetts program serving newborns at risk have defined areas for interventions. This program is described in Chapter 19. There are a number of other intervention models that have been described in both acute care and long-term care situations. In many instances, the purpose of intervention is to increase the capability of the primary care provider (parent or surrogate) to more effectively provide for the needs of the child.[7, 10, 14, 24] Eddington and Lee developed guidelines for interventions using suggestions sequenced according to development in order to elicit certain behaviors.[6]

This approach to delivery of service is not unique to nursing. Finnie, an occupational therapist, has described methods for parents to use in handling cerebral palsied children to enhance their motor functions.[8] Norton, another therapist, has data suggesting that mothers can function effectively as cotherapists in providing a home program of neurodevelopmental, sensory integration therapy.[19] Other resources that offer guidelines to assist parents or surrogates in methods that will foster development include the *Washington Guide for Promoting Development in the Young Child,*[1] the curriculum guide of the Portage Project,[23] and the Central Wisconsin Center *Growth and Development Deck.**

Planning and implementing a coordinated, interdisciplinary program of intervention involve far more skill, creativity, and imagination than is apparent from the available guidelines. In the process of interdisciplinary planning, it is necessary to look at where the client is and forecast the future in both short- and long-range terms. The team must develop priority factors before determining the structure of the program. It is essential to consider the perceptions of the client's and family's priorities. The success or failure of any program often depends on its response to the primary problems as the client perceives them.

Major areas of concern in programming for individuals with mental retardation are: life support and positive health, gross and fine motor functioning and the development of daily living activities, communication, development of a positive concept of self, socialization and the ability to participate in community life, participation as a citizen, and the exercise of human and civil rights. Unless there is concern for all of these parameters in the development of the habilitation plan for the client, the program may be lacking in the essential elements for the normalization of the individual. The desired outcomes of the interdisciplinary plan should relate to helping the person achieve greater control of the environment, increasing the complexity of behavior, and maximizing the human qualities of that person.

The nursing contribution to the interdisciplinary plan should include observations, assessments, and interpretations of: basic health care and health maintenance needs, including prevention; growth and development factors; strength and limitations in coping abilities; and social and environmental factors. Through utilization of professional knowledge, the nurse's activities in the design and implementation of the plan may include continuous or selective observation and assessment, teaching of the client, the parent or surrogate, or performing direct services related to the care and management of the client needs.

Whatever the nurse's actions on behalf of the client and family, evaluation will be needed to assess the effectiveness of the activity in achieving the desired goal and to assess the quality of the process in relation to standards of practice. If the nurse releases some traditional functions to other professionals, or if the nurse assumes roles usually

---

*Copies are available from Central Wisconsin Center for the Developmentally Disabled, 317 Knutson Dr., Madison, Wis. 53704.

performed by other disciplines, the evaluation and accountability of all professionals involved in the plan must be carefully exercised to assure that standards of quality and legal requirements are maintained.

The purpose of any plan is to bring about behavior that will lead to desired outcomes. Because of the many disciplines and agencies that might be involved at any given time, the plan must be dynamic, able to take in additional information, and be easily modified to reflect changing needs and conditions. The interdisciplinary plan serves as an organizer of care, training, education, and counseling. It establishes priorities through the process of reviewing the facts and perceptions of client needs. Objectivity is an important quality of any intervention program, and the team plan forces this issue through the interactive process. The unique qualities of each individual must be considered in developing the plan. Greater consistency of service is also accomplished through a comprehensive team plan. With stated goals and defined interventions, there is less opportunity for chance events to occur. The individual plan also provides essential directions that could not be offered by the client or the professionals on a regular and consistent basis. Serving as a reminder to all staff involved in the program, the plan provides continuous support for the conservation and efficient use of time. New members of the team can use the written plan to familiarize themselves with the priorities of need and the methods to be used to assist the client.

In the process of developing the intervention plan, the team must work through professional differences to develop a sense of trust and a spirit of cooperation, or the plan cannot be implemented. Finally, and perhaps most important, the plan's behavioral goals provide a means of evaluating the progress of the client and the effectiveness of the plan in influencing the direction and rate of development. Assessment of goal achievement is also a means of evaluating movement toward desired outcomes.

Criteria for assessing the quality of the interdisciplinary plan should include these considerations:

1. Is it specific in terms of the goals to be accomplished and the methods or approaches to be used? Is it related to the needs identified through the assessment process?

2. Is it realistic? Does it respond to the expressed needs of the client and the family? Based on present knowledge, can it be expected to resolve needs and promote function? Does it reflect the utilization of current knowledge and skills?

3. Is it attainable? Can it be accomplished with currently available resources? Is there consideration for the client's/family's ability to tolerate physical and emotional stress and to develop improved coping abilities?

4. Is it understandable to the client, the family, and all others who may be involved? Are unusual terms or techniques employed that should be defined or described in more common words?

5. Does it reflect current assessments of needs and problems?

The most difficult part of the development of the interdisciplinary plan appears to be the articulation of goal statements in measurable or observable terms. Even educators, many of whom have been provided with academic preparation in the development and use of individually prescribed learning goals for each student, experience difficulty in working with the team to develop interdisciplinary goal statements. The problem is greater in planning for the more severely retarded and physically handicapped client where objective assessment data are more difficult to obtain and broad expressions of goal statements are not pertinent. The goals must be measurable and attainable. Implied in these criteria is consideration for the time frame in which the goals should be accomplished. Mager defined questions to be answered in the goal statement as[17]:

1. Where is the client going? (performance)

2. When will the client arrive? (condition)
3. How will it be known? (acceptable performance criterion)

If the goal is not sequentially appropriate, there is a greater chance for large gaps in required intervention to achieve the desired behavior. This can cause failure in program effectiveness and result in increasing the problems and frustrations among those being served. If goals are not realistic and attainable, similar problems may result. Determining goals consistent with the assessment data may seem to be an obvious condition; however, this can be an area of neglect if the professionals involved have not pooled their assessment data and carefully analyzed the problem and the directions to be pursued in remediation.

The development of approaches designed for goal achievement provides the team members with an opportunity to consider theoretical frameworks and the related patterns and styles of interventions. Methods and techniques of providing service and the individual abilities of team members must be shared as appropriate approaches to goal achievement are developed. The team's determination of how to accomplish the goal should reflect both creativity and practicality by the best use of available resources. The plan should provide specific and detailed information concerning methods to be used in a form that is readily understandable to those who will deliver the services. Information concerning data collection is an important but often forgotten element of the plan. Descriptions of methods and approaches should supply direction for data collection. From this data, the team will be able to determine if the plan is working. When problems arise, questions must be raised as to the appropriateness of the goal, correctness of the assessment data, or the effectiveness of the intervention.

THE NURSING CONTRIBUTION IN RESIDENTIAL SETTINGS

Nurses have long been associated with the medical model in the delivery of residential services to individuals. Nurses and physicians are now being regarded with some suspicion in the development of service delivery models in which educational and developmental programs have been emphasized. Historically, nursing has had a long association with the severely or profoundly retarded population. Presently, thousands of nurses are employed in residential institutions across the United States where more than 70% of the total population receiving services are either severely or profoundly mentally retarded persons.[26]

Although today's nurses may point out that their professional education is focused on health, health maintenance, and the prevention of illness or disability, the traditional view of nursing with an emphasis on the care of the sick is difficult to dispel. Barnard has stated that nursing is increasingly concerned with engineering the environment and developing a plan that will allow the individual to have the most effective rate of developmental progress. Nursing intervention is designed to present environmental stimulation in ways that maximize its perception by the individual.[18] Blake also refers to the nursing responsibility for modifying the environment in the particular ways required by the individual or the family for satisfaction of needs and for adaptation to frustrations in a constructive manner.[2]

The need for nursing intervention and the application of new knowledge in practice have been described by Patterson and Rowland as essential to salvaging the human potential currently unrecognized among the mentally retarded population. Their view perceives the nurse as an educator, designing services congruent with the model of human development and habilitation. They condemn the use of clinical labeling to obscure the deviancy and human qualities of the mentally retarded individual.[20] Change is considered essential in order to avoid the negative results of such labeling, since it has been demonstrated that professional workers' expectancies directly influence the clients' behaviors. Role expectations for profoundly retarded individuals need to be examined in order to remove the dehumanizing or nonfunctional roles that have previously been assigned to them. According to

Wolfensberger, realistically high and occasionally normal expectancies must be developed in relation to specific areas of functioning and must be based on individual considerations.[34] Nursing services for individuals with developmental disabilities need to be designed and delivered with the expectation that goal achievements in health, independence, and individuality are attainable when quality services prevail.

SUMMARY

The focus of this chapter has been to present a discussion of the use of standards in quality assurance programs in residential settings for the mentally retarded. The history of the development of these standards as well as the development of nursing standards for quality assurance were reviewed. Examples of the use of nursing standards were presented. The contributions of nurses in implementing services that meet internal and external standards were emphasized. Throughout the chapter, the need to be accountable for services provided to the mentally retarded was stressed.

REFERENCES

1. Barnard, K., and Erickson, M.: Teaching children with developmental problems, ed. 2, St. Louis, 1976, The C. V. Mosby Co.
2. Blake, F.: Support of the person(s) in "accidental crisis," Madison, Wis., 1968, School of Nursing of the University of Wisconsin at Madison.
3. Code for nurses with interpretive statements, Kansas City, Mo., 1974, American Nurses' Association.
4. Cooper, S.: This I believe about continuing education in nursing, Am. J. Nurs. **20:**579, 1972.
5. Donabedian, A.: Some issues in evaluating the quality of nursing care, Am. J. Public Health **59:**1833, 1969.
6. Eddington, C., and Lee, T.: Sensory-motor stimulation for slow-to-develop children; a home-centered program for parents, Am. J. Nurs. **75:**59, 1975.
7. Fink, D.: Effective patient care in the pediatric ambulatory setting; a study of the acute care clinic, Pediatrics **43:**927, 1969.
8. Finnie, N.: Handling the young cerebral-palsied child at home, New York, 1970, E. P. Dutton & Co., Inc.
9. Fuller, D., and Rosenaur, J.: A patient assessment guide, Nurs. Outlook **22:**460, 1974.
10. Godfrey, A.: Sensory-motor stimulation for slow-

to-develop children; a specialized program for public health nurses, Am. J. Nurs. **75:**56, 1975.
11. Guidelines for nursing standards in residential centers for the mentally retarded, an Ad Hoc Committee Project, Una Haynes, Project Director, Subcommittee on Nursing, 1968, American Association on Mental Deficiency.
12. Guidelines for review of nursing care at the local level, Kansas City, Mo., 1976, American Nurses' Association.
13. Lesnick, M. J., and Anderson, B. E.: Nursing practice and the law, ed. 2, Philadelphia, 1955, J. B. Lippincott Co.
14. Lewis, C. W., and others: Activities, events, and outcomes in ambulatory pediatric care, N. Engl. J. Med. **280:**645, 1969.
15. Little, D., and Carnevali, D.: Nursing care planning, Philadelphia, 1969, J. B. Lippincott Co.
16. Long-term care; working toward accountability, how do you audit long-term care? J.A.H.A. **50:**69, 1976.
17. Mager, R.: Preparing instructional objectives, ed. 2, Belmont, Calif., 1975, Fearson Publishers, Inc.
18. Murray, L., and Barnard, K.: The nursing specialist in mental retardation, Nurs. Clin. North Am. **1:**631, 1966.
19. Norton, Y.: Neurodevelopment and sensory integration, Am. J. Occup. Ther. **29:**93, 1975.
20. Patterson, E., and Rowland, G.: Toward a theory of mental retardation nursing, Am. J. Nurs. **70:**531, 1970.
21. PEP manual, ed. 2, Chicago, 1974, Joint Commission on Accreditation of Hospitals.
22. Phaneuf, M.: The nursing audit; profile for excellence, New York, 1972, Appleton-Century-Crofts.
23. Portage Guide to Early Education; the Portage Project, Portage, Wis., 1972, Cooperative Educational Service Agency No. 12.
24. Pothier, P.: Therapeutic handling of the severely handicapped child, Am. J. Nurs. **72:**321, 1971.
25. Ryan, B.: Nursing care plans; a systems approach to developing criteria for planning and evaluation, J. Nurs. Admin. **3:**50, 1973.
26. Scheerenberger, R.: Current trends and status of public residential services for the mentally retarded, Madison, Wis., 1974, National Association of Superintendents of Public Residential Facilities.
27. Standards for community agencies, Chicago, 1973, Accreditation Council for Facilities for the Mentally Retarded, Joint Commission on Accreditation of Hospitals.
28. Standards of nursing practice, Kansas City, Mo., 1973, American Nurses' Association.
29. Standards of psychiatric and mental health nursing practice, Kansas City, Mo., 1973, American Nurses' Association.
30. Standards for residential facilities for the mentally retarded, Chicago, 1971, Accreditation Council for Facilities for the Mentally Retarded, Joint Commission on Accreditation of Hospitals.

31. Standards for state residential institutions for the mentally retarded, Project on Technical Planning in Mental Retardation, monograph supplement, Am. J. Ment. Defic., Jan. 1964.
32. Stevens, J.: The nurse as executive, Wakefield, Mass., 1975, Contemporary Publishing, Inc.
33. U.S. Department of Health, Education, and Welfare, Social and Rehabilitation Service, Medical Assistance Program, part 249 Standards for intermediate care facilities, Federal Register, 39, No. 12, Jan. 17, 1964, pp. 2221-2234.
34. Wolfensberger, W.: Normalization; the principle of normalization in human services, Toronto, 1972, National Institute on Mental Retardation.

Nursing approaches to care

CHAPTER 8

Genetic counseling

LUCILLE F. WHALEY

Will it happen again? This is a universal concern of families in which there is a member who is mentally retarded. Persons who seek professional advice regarding the probability that a condition might recur in their family come from all ethnic groups and socioeconomic levels. The question is often asked by young couples contemplating marriage or childbearing who are concerned about mental retardation in one of their families, no matter how remote the relationship. They may need guidance regarding cousin marriage. Both may be members of a population at risk for a disease known to produce retardation and may wish to determine whether they are carriers of the harmful gene. Couples planning to adopt will seek advice concerning the genetic background of a prospective child. More often, persons who inquire about the possibility of recurrence are parents of a mentally retarded child who are concerned that they might produce another similarly affected child. In this situation, advice may be sought before the couple decides to have another child, when the mother is already pregnant, or after another child has been born. Occasionally the question becomes an ethical, legal, or moral one that involves sterilization, artificial insemination, termination of a pregnancy, incest, or disputed paternity.

There is seldom a simple answer to the question. It would be convenient if mental retardation could always be attributed to a specific, identifiable cause. However, the causes are manifold. It has been demonstrated that both heredity and environment contribute to the development of intelligence and that both genetic and nongenetic factors, acting separately or in combination, can interfere with this development. A genetic origin is being recognized for an increasing number of disorders known to be associated with significant mental impairment, and a variety of environmental agents have been implicated in mental retardation, particularly when they exert their effect during critical periods in development. However, these known, discrete causes are found in only a small percentage of persons having mental retardation. In most instances the etiology of mental retardation is so obscure or multifaceted that the probability of recurrence can be predicted only on an empiric basis.

MENTAL RETARDATION

Intelligence, like stature, is a quantitative trait that is expressed in the population (as defined by IQ determination*) from very low to very high according to the normal, bell-shaped distribution curve. This variation in

---

*The relative merits of IQ determination and the arbitrary cutoff score as criteria for defining retardation are not of concern here.

intellectual capacity is produced by *polygenic* inheritance. Polygenic refers to a number of genes at different positions (loci) on the chromosomes that individually do not produce a large effect. They are minor genes, each of whose small effect combines with the others to produce a given trait, in this case intelligence. Studies consistently indicate that *with a relatively uniform environment* this variation in general intelligence observed in individuals is largely due to the additive effects of many small genes. The remainder is contributed by environmental factors, such as past intellectual stimulation and formal education.

People do not mate randomly with respect to general intelligence. Since most individuals tend to mate with persons of similar intellectual level, the same types of genes are transmitted through generation after generation, and the greater the overlap of genes, the greater the similarity in intelligence between relatives. The closer the relationship, the more genes these persons will have in common (Table 8-1). An increased incidence of low IQ among relatives is characteristic of the mildly retarded (IQ 52 to 68). Although estimates vary from study to study, the overall findings indicate that 13% to 30% of retarded individuals have at least one retarded sibling, 25% to 60% have at least one retarded parent, and 16% to 42% have at least one retarded child. Risk esti-

Table 8-1. Proportion of genes in common in various relationships

Relationships	Proportion of genes in common (as percentage)
First-degree relatives	
Parent, child, sibling	50%
Second-degree relatives	
Grandparent, grandchild, uncle, aunt, nephew, niece, half sibling	25%
Third-degree relatives	
First cousins	12.5%
Second cousins	6.25%

mates of retardation in these families are based on empiric figures derived from such studies. When both parents are retarded, it can be expected that approximately 55% to 60% of all offspring will be retarded, 35% to 40% will be normal but below average, and about 4% will approach average or better intelligence.[10]

It should also be pointed out that children of parents with less intellectual endowment do not always live in an environment that stimulates development of whatever intellectual potential they may have. Most familial retardation occurs in the lowest economic and social levels with the accompanying inadequate income and generally unfavorable social conditions that are reflected in poor housing, nutrition, and medical care. Interpersonal stimulation is deficient or distorted.

It would be expected, based on the characteristics of the normal curve, that the distribution of IQs in the population would be balanced, with the bulk centered around the average and a smaller percentage at each of the extremes. The variation of IQs *does* follow a normal distribution in the IQ ranges above about 70. However, in the IQ ranges below 50 to 70, there is an excess of individuals over the number that would be expected by chance. Observations also indicate that normal siblings of profoundly retarded individuals are more intelligent than siblings of the mildly or moderately retarded, and superior mental abilities occur with twice the frequency in relatives of the profoundly retarded than among relatives of less retarded persons. The types of persons who contribute to the excess of mental retardation in the lower IQ ranges indicate that other factors have in some way interfered with normal development.[13, 14]

Etiology of mental retardation

In regard to etiology, it is possible to divide mental retardation into two large categories. First, there are those individuals who represent a position on the lower end of the normal intelligence distribution curve. In this group, there is no recognized pathology aside from the decreased intellectual functioning. Most cases involve a mild degree of mental retardation and are probably responsible for the largest proportion of familial retardation. There is an excessive amount of slowness in siblings of mildly retarded persons. This group constitutes approximately 75% to 90% of all retarded individuals, and it is not often that advice is sought regarding risks to relatives of these persons.[5, 12] Occasionally, bright parents may be concerned that their child is developing slowly, or the question arises when an infant with an older retarded sibling is being considered for adoption. Recurrence risk estimates for persons in this group are based on observed frequencies in families in which there is a member with mental retardation of unknown etiology (Tables 8-2 and 8-3).

The second large category includes those individuals whose mental retardation is the result of gross interference with the normal process of development. Although these cases constitute a smaller percentage of the total number of retarded individuals, they account for the greatest number of those who are severely retarded. Since the cause of the condition is due to known etiological agents (either genetic or environmental), in most instances the risk of recurrence can be estimated with a high degree of accuracy. It is this group (primarily the hereditary disorders) that involves genetic counseling services.

Environmental factors that produce mental retardation include:

1. Intrauterine causes, such as radiation or maternal infections
2. Fetal or postnatal anoxia and birth injuries
3. Childhood trauma
4. Postnatal or childhood infections
5. Kernicterus due to severe or prolonged neonatal jaundice

Genetic disorders with harmful effects on intellectual development are:

Table 8-2. Empiric risk figures for normal or retarded persons who have had at least one retarded child*

Type of union	Number retarded after first retarded child	Percentage
1. Retarded × retarded	32 out of 76	42.1%
2. Retarded × normal or unknown	63 out of 317	19.9%
3. Normal × normal		
a. One normal parent with one or more retarded siblings	18 out of 139	12.9%
b. One normal parent with all siblings known to be normal	6 out of 104	5.7%

*Data from Reed, E. W., and Reed, S. C.: Mental retardation; a family study, Philadelphia, 1965, W. B. Saunders Co.

Table 8-3. Empiric risk figures for normal persons who have not had any children*

Type of union	Chance that the first child will be retarded (as percentage)
1. a. Normal (with retarded sibling) × retarded	23.8%
b. Normal (with retarded sibling) × normal	
(1) First parent had only one retarded sibling	1.8%
(2) First parent had two or more retarded siblings	3.6%
2. Normal (with all siblings normal) × normal	0.53%

combined average = 2.5%

*From Reed, E. W., and Reed, S. C.: Mental retardation; a family study, Philadelphia, 1965, W. B. Saunders Co.

1. Disorders due to a single gene substitute in either single or double dose
2. Chromosome abnormalities
3. Congenital malformations of the central nervous system due to multiple genetic factors unrelated to those which contribute to the normal intellectual variation

Many of these conditions cannot be categorized as strictly genetic or entirely environmental. In such situations the genetic component, relatively unaltered during a lifetime, produces an adverse effect only when influenced by environmental factors. For example, although an enzyme deficiency is present in PKU, the deleterious effects do not take place until the affected infant ingests sufficient amounts of the protein phenylalanine. Thus, the course and outcome of the disease often can be altered significantly by diet modification. Likewise, kernicterus is not a genetic disorder, but the incompatible blood antigens, which are inherited by the mother and fetus, can precipitate a reaction that produces damage to the central nervous system. Even the natural intellectual capabilities can be varied by environmental factors. For example, it is well documented that the child with normal intelligence who receives little environmental stimulation during early development can be greatly impaired in certain aspects of intellectual functioning, and it is possible to increase the intellectual abilities of some retarded persons by providing them with early and appropriate stimulation. Also, inadequate nutrition during critical periods of development is now known to produce irreversible damage to the brain.

Regardless of where they practice, the extent of their preparation, the roles in which they are engaged, or the degree of independence they are permitted, nurses who are involved with families in which there is a mentally retarded member need some understanding of the genetic and environmental agents known to contribute to mental retardation, the mechanisms by which these agents produce a deleterious effect, and the basic principles of genetic counseling.

GENETIC DISORDERS ASSOCIATED WITH MENTAL RETARDATION

The genetics of mental retardation are complex, and many mechanisms operate to produce the varied clinical manifestations. Although the genetically influenced causes of mental retardation constitute a small percentage of all retarded persons, they are primarily responsible for the severely and profoundly retarded. During the past few years the etiological factors in retardation have been greatly clarified, particularly those related to the inborn errors of metabolism and chromosomal aberrations. Through advances in biochemistry and cytogenetics, a specific cause has been identified for an increasing number of disorders with mental retardation as part of the symptom complex.

To facilitate a discussion of the genetic contribution to mental retardation, several terms used to describe inherited conditions need to be clarified.

Congenital: A condition present at birth; may be due to genetic causes, nongenetic (environmental) causes, or a combination of these.
Genetic: A condition due to an alteration in the genetic material, either a single deleterious gene or a chromosome abnormality.
Inherited (heritable, hereditary): Synonymous with genetic, although often used in the past to describe a disorder that appeared in parent and offspring over several generations.
Familial: A disorder that "runs in families" or is present in more members of a family than would be expected by chance.
Homozygous (homozygote): Possessing similar genes for a given trait.
Heterozygous (heterozygote): Possessing dissimilar genes for a given trait.

Single gene disorders

Disorders due to a single gene on either autosomes or X chromosomes are individually rare, although approximately 135 have been identified that have some degree of mental retardation as part of the clinical manifestations. Collectively they account for only about 2% of institutionalized retarded persons. Those that can be directly

		Heterozygous parent Aa	
	Gametes	A	a
Homozygous normal parent aa	a	Aa Affected	aa Normal
	a	Aa Affected	aa Normal

Fig. 8-1. Offspring ratio of an individual with a dominant trait mated to a normal individual. Capital letters represent the dominant gene.

		Heterozygous parent Aa	
	Gametes	A	a
Heterozygous parent Aa	A	AA Affected	Aa Affected
	a	Aa Affected	aa Normal

Fig. 8-2. Offspring ratio from a mating between two parents heterozygous for the same dominant trait.

attributed to a single mutant gene are distributed in families according to the basic Mendelian inheritance patterns—dominant, recessive, and X-linked. Each individual possesses two genes that determine any given trait, but not all genes operate with equal vigor. When a pair of genes are dissimilar, a competition will exist between them for expression in the individual. As a result of this competition, one may mask or conceal the other. The trait that is manifest in the individual (and the gene that produces the effect) is referred to as *dominant;* that which is hidden and not manifest is *recessive*. The dominant trait is always displayed in the individual, and it is usually impossible to tell whether the person is heterozygous or homozygous for the trait. To be expressed, a recessive trait must always be homozygous (unless the gene is located on an X chromosome).

Some generalizations have been observed regarding diseases and malformations due to a single gene. Disorders due to structural defects seem to be primarily the result of dominant genes, whereas a recessive inheritance pattern is seen in most metabolic disorders. Severe mental retardation is associated with many of the disorders with a recessive inheritance pattern and are collectively referred to as the *inborn errors of metabolism*. In these diseases, defective gene action results in deficiency of an enzyme required for an essential metabolic process. This produces physical effects of greater or lesser consequences, including mental retardation.

Autosomal dominant inheritance. Although there are factors that complicate a prediction in many disorders due to a dominant gene on an autosome, for most conditions a prediction is clearcut. The first case in a family usually appears as a fresh mutation and, depending on the degree of disability the condition imposes on the individual, will either die out or continue to be passed through several generations. A person who carries a dominant gene is always clinically affected, and there is a 50% chance that any offspring will have a similar defect (Fig. 8-1). In the highly unlikely event that both parents are affected by the same dominant defect, the ratio of affected offspring is 3:1 (Fig. 8-2).

Characteristics of a condition due to a dominant gene on an autosome are[15]:

1. Males and females are affected with equal frequency.
2. Affected individuals will have an affected parent (unless due to a fresh mutation).
3. Half the children of a heterozygous affected parent will be affected.

4. Normal children of affected parents will have normal children.
5. Traits can be traced vertically through previous generations—a positive family history.

Examples are tuberous sclerosis, Huntington's chorea, Apert's syndrome, and Lowry syndrome.

Some difficulties arise in relation to dominant disorders. Although a parent may appear to be free of a condition, on careful examination he may prove to carry the gene but exhibit a very minor manifestation of the disorder. Some disorders do not appear in all persons who carry the gene, which accounts for the apparent ''skipping'' of generations of dominant conditions. In others, such as Huntington's chorea, the clinical manifestations do not appear until the individual has reached an age characteristic of the particular disease. In the case of Huntington's chorea, an individual will have passed the gene to offspring before displaying any evidence of the disease.

Autosomal recessive inheritance. Since a normal gene will dominate and therefore mask a gene for a recessive trait, most persons who are heterozygous for the trait remain undetected in the population. An individual who is affected with an autosomal-recessive disorder will always have two defective genes (are homozygous) for the trait. Recurrence risk estimates for autosomal-recessive disorders, such as PKU or galactosemia, are most important in regard to subsequent siblings of an affected child. In recessive inheritance, the affected child has received two defective genes (one from each parent). Therefore, the recurrence risk is 1 in 4 of an affected child for each pregnancy (Fig. 8-3). There is relatively little risk to other relatives, although there is a two-thirds chance that unaffected siblings of the heterozygous couple will also be heterozygous for the defective gene.

Characteristics of a condition due to a recessive gene on an autosome are[15]:

1. Males and females are affected with equal frequency.
2. Affected individuals will have unaf-

Fig. 8-3. Offspring ratio from a mating of parents heterozygous for a recessive trait.

fected parents who are heterozygous for the trait.
3. One fourth of the children of two unaffected heterozygous parents will be affected.
4. Two affected parents will have affected children exclusively.
5. Affected individuals married to unaffected individuals will have normal children, all of whom will be carriers.
6. There is usually no evidence of the trait in antecedent generations—a negative family history.

Examples are PKU, galactosemia, maple syrup urine disease, Tay-Sachs disease, Wilson's disease, Hurler's syndrome, and Sanfilippo syndrome.

The risk of an autosomal-recessive disorder in a child is increased in matings between persons who are related. The closer the relationship, the more genes the parents have in common, and therefore the higher the risk (see Table 8-1). This is particularly applicable in regard to disorders that appear more frequently in the population as a whole.

X-linked inheritance. Genes on the X chromosome are transmitted according to the principles of heredity just as they are on the autosomes. However, since sex chromosomes differ from autosomes in both morphology and gene content, the inheritance patterns of X-linked disorders will vary ac-

A — Carrier mother / Normal father

Gametes	X	X̲
X	XX Normal daughter	X̲X Carrier daughter
Y	XY Normal son	X̲Y Affected son

B — Normal mother / Affected father

Gametes	X	X
X̲	X̲X Carrier daughter	X̲X Carrier daughter
Y	XY Normal son	XY Normal son

Fig. 8-4. Sex differences in offspring ratios in X-linked recessive inheritance. **A,** Mother is a carrier. **B,** Father is affected. 0 = recessive gene on an X chromosome. (From Whaley, L. F.: Understanding inherited disorders, St. Louis, 1974, The C. V. Mosby Co.)

cording to the sex of the individual who carries the gene. The outstanding characteristic of X-linked inheritance is that genes on the X chromosome have no counterpart on the Y chromosome. Therefore, a characteristic determined by a gene on the X chromosome is *always* manifest in the male who carries it. A female who inherits a defective gene on one X chromosome will usually receive a normal gene on the chromosome from the other parent. One of the most significant aspects of X-linked inheritance is the absence of father-to-son transmission. The father gives his one X chromosome to his daughters.

In X-linked dominant disorders, the pedigree pattern superficially resembles the autosomal dominant disorders with a significant difference; an affected male transmits the trait to all his daughters but to none of his sons.

Characteristics of X-linked dominant inheritance are[15]:

1. Affected individuals will have an affected parent.
2. All the daughters but none of the sons of an affected male will be affected.
3. Half the sons and half the daughters of an affected female will be affected.
4. Normal children of an affected parent will have normal offspring.
5. The inheritance pattern shows a positive family history.

A well-known example is vitamin D–resistant rickets.

In X-linked recessive disorders, the significant risk is related to male offspring of a female carrier. A male who receives the defective gene will always display the disorder, whereas the female with a normal dominant gene to oppose the abnormal gene will be clinically normal. However, she can transmit the defective gene to half her offspring, including the sons, all of whom will be affected (Fig. 8-4, *A*). An affected male with an X-linked disorder that does not lead to early death or incapacitation will transmit the defective gene to all his daughters who will be carriers. His sons will be both clinically and genetically normal for the disorder (Fig. 8-4, *B*).

Characteristics of an X-linked recessive disorder are[15]:

1. Affected individuals are principally males.
2. Affected individuals will have unaffected parents.
3. Half of the female siblings of an affected male will be carriers of the trait.
4. Unaffected male siblings of an affected male cannot transmit the disorder.
5. Sons of an affected male are unaffected.
6. Daughters of an affected male are carriers.

7. The unaffected male children of a carrier female do not transmit the disorder.

Examples are Lesch-Nyhan syndrome, Lowe's syndrome, Norris disease, Hunter syndrome, and X-linked hydrocephalus.

Chromosomal aberrations

An aberration is defined as a deviation from that which is normal or typical. In relation to the chromosomes, it can be a deviation in either structure or number, and the consequences can be observed in the individual. A structural aberration involves loss of genes, addition of genes, rearrangement of the genes within a chromosome, or exchange of genes between chromosomes. A deviation in chromosome number involves the gain or loss of an entire chromosome. Since the development of improved techniques for the study of chromosomes, a number of disorders that have mental retardation as a major manifestation have been associated with chromosome abnormalities. The majority of the abnormalities accounted for in the literature is related to variation in chromosome number, although there is evidence that with technical advances the structural abnormalities may assume greater significance in human disease. The largest number of chromosome abnormalities that have been identified are those in which there is a duplication of a chromosome.

The complex nature of cell division makes it highly susceptible to mechanical error, particularly during the critical processes of gamete formation and in the early divisions of the zygote following fertilization. Normally during cell division, the chromosomes duplicate and separate, and each of the two newly formed chromosomes become part of two identical daughter cells. This separation is called *disjunction*; failure of this process is *nondisjunction*. In the latter, the duplicated chromosomes fail to separate and remain attached during cell division. Consequently, there is an unequal distribution of chromosomes between the daughter cells. Of the two resulting cells, one will be a *monosomy*, containing only one member of a chromosome pair; the other will be a *trisomy* and contain an extra chromosome in the involved group. The most notable example of a disorder due to an extra chromosome is trisomy 21, or Down's syndrome.

Down's syndrome. The majority of cases of Down's syndrome (approximately 70%) are attributed to nondisjunction during gamete formation (meiosis). In most instances, it is a random event; however, there is a direct correlation between chromosome aberrations and advancing maternal age. For example, the incidence of Down's syndrome in young mothers is approximately 1 in 1,000 births. At age 35 years, the incidence increases to 1 in 300. From the age of 40, the incidence rises sharply to become 1 in 30 to 50 in those who are over 45 years of age.[6] Paternal age does not appear to be a factor.

Another source of trisomies is nondisjunction in somatic cells of the fertilized ovum or embryo (mitotic division). The nondisjunction can occur at the first or any subsequent mitotic division. When the division occurs at the first division, a trisomic cell and a monosomic cell will continue to divide and produce a trisomic individual. If the nondisjunction occurs at a later division, after more than one normal cell has already been produced, the result will be a *mosaic* — an individual composed of both normal and trisomic cells. The extent of the clinical manifestations is determined by the tissues that are involved and may show considerable variation. This is especially true in relation to the degree of mental retardation, which may be extremely severe or relatively mild.

Approximately 5% of persons with Down's syndrome are the result of translocation, a phenomenon in which a 21 chromosome becomes attached to another chromosome, usually of the D group or another G group chromosome. During cell division the translocated chromosome, which contains the genetic material of both the D and G chromosomes, will duplicate intact and travel to one daughter cell. When combined with a normal cell at fertilization, the resulting zygote will contain extra chromosome material, although the total chromosome count will be 46. In this situation, maternal age is no factor. Parents of an affected child are generally in the younger age group, have a history of spontaneous abortions of previous pregnancies, or have a family history of spontaneous abortions. Often one parent is found to be a carrier with a normal phenotype and a chromosome complement of 45. When a parent has a translocation involving a D and a G group chromosome, the chances for an affected offspring are theoretically 1 in 3 (Fig. 8-5). However, most authorities estimate the probability to be in the order of 1 in 5 when the mother is a carrier and less than 1 in 20 when the father carries the translocation.[9]

A very few cases of translocation Down's syndrome occur when the two members of the number 21 chromosome are fused together in a somatically normal individual. Because these cells contain the normal amount of genetic material, the individual is normal in every other respect. Such a person can produce nothing but affected offspring because the gametes that are formed will contain only the translocated chromosome 21 that creates the trisomy or else will have no 21 chromosome. Offspring with no 21 chromosome are nonviable.

Although the translocation forms of Down's syndrome are uncommon, the re-

currence risk is significantly higher than in the nondisjunction variety. Cytogenetic studies for identification of carriers are vital for purposes of counseling, particularly in young persons in whom the "maternal age effect" is unlikely to operate and who are more likely to want more children. It is also helpful in evaluating cases in which there is a history of repeated abortion.[7]

Most persons with Down's syndrome are sterile; however, there are recorded cases where females with the disorder have been fertile and produced offspring, both normal and affected. Theoretically, there is a 50% risk of an affected offspring with each pregnancy; actually, the incidence is considerably less. There are some, as yet unknown, selective forces that decrease the viability of trisomic embryos, as evidenced by a high percentage of trisomic abnormalities aborted early in pregnancy.[1]

Other autosomal aberrations. In addition to Down's syndrome, a fairly large group of disorders produces varying degrees of mental retardation that are associated with gross errors of chromosome constitution. These disorders are characterized by alterations in the genetic material that give rise to discrete features by which they are readily recognized, particularly in regard to the trisomies. Some are trisomy syndromes due to duplication of chromosomes. Others are deletion

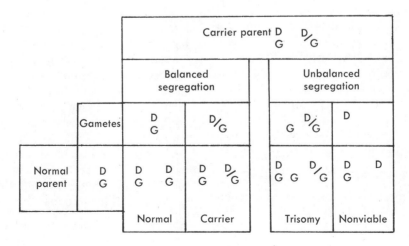

Fig. 8-5. Offspring ratio from a mating of a parent with a translocated G group chromosome (D/G) to a normal parent.

syndromes due to loss of significant amounts of genetic material. Some of the aberrations of autosomes include the cri du chat syndrome due to deletion of the short arm of chromosome 5; Edward's syndrome, a trisomy of the E group chromosome 18; and Patau's syndrome, a trisomy of a D group chromosome, probably 13.

Sex chromosome abnormalities. Anomalies of sex chromosomes are an important source of mental retardation. Less consistent in their effect on the central nervous system, trisomies of the sex chromosomes do not produce the profound effects that are associated with the autosomal trisomies, although some degree of mental retardation accompanies a large percentage of them. They can be the result of nondisjunction during either meiosis or mitosis, and the disorders that occur most frequently involve duplication of the X chromosome. Examples of sex chromosome trisomies are: the 47, XXY, or Kleinfelter's syndrome; the 47, XXX, triple-X, or "super female"; and the XYY syndrome.

Sex chromosome abnormalities have varied clinical and chromosomal characteristics. The multiple sex chromosome complement can vary from 1 to 6 X chromosomes, and mental abilities vary from normal to profoundly retarded. For instance, retardation occurs in approximately 51% of 47, XXY males, 100% in 48, XXXY or XXXXY males, and is a consistent finding in the 47, XXX female. In the only known viable monosomy, the 45, X female or Turner's syndrome, about 10% are mentally retarded. In general, there is a direct relationship between the number of X chromosomes and the severity of mental retardation. Except for the XXX female, who has somewhat diminished fertility, persons with sex chromosome abnormalities are infertile.

ESSENTIALS OF GENETIC COUNSELING

A comprehensive definition of genetic counseling has been prepared by a group of eminent medical geneticists and states that

genetic counseling is a communication process which deals with the human problems associated with the occurrence, or the risk of occurrence, of a genetic disorder in a family. This process involves an attempt by one or more appropriately trained persons to help the individual or family (1) comprehend the medical facts, including the diagnosis, the probable course of the disorder, and the available management; (2) appreciate the way heredity contributes to the disorder, and the risk of recurrence in specified relatives; (3) understand the options for dealing with the risk of recurrence; (4) choose the course of action which seems appropriate to them in view of their risk and their family goals and act in accordance with that decision; and (5) make the best possible adjustment to the disorder in an affected family member and/or to the risk of recurrence of that disorder.*

Rapid advances in the fields of biochemistry and cytology that have identified genetic etiologies for an increasing number of diseases and disorders have been accompanied by an increased need for genetic counseling services. Unfortunately, at the present time there are too few qualified persons and facilities accessible to a large number of persons needing such services, and another large number of persons needing services are either unaware that these services are available or do not know where to go for genetic counseling. When expert counseling is not available, families may become victims of well-meaning but uninformed quasiprofessionals or misguided relatives and acquaintances. Nurses should become familiar with facilities in their areas where genetic counseling is available and should learn the basic principles of heredity. In this way they will be able to direct these families to needed services and to be active participants in the counseling process. Genetic counseling services are primarily associated with applied human genetics units in health agencies and institutions. The majority are located in large hospitals, medical centers, major universities, and medical schools, most of which have facilities for the diagnosis and treatment of genetic diseases and

---

*From Fraser, F. C.: Genetic counseling, Am. J. Hum. Genet. **26:**636, 1974. Used with permission of the University of Chicago Press, publishers. Copyrighted by the American Society of Human Genetics.

birth defects. Genetic counseling is also part of the services of many government agencies, voluntary organizations, and institutes. There are several sources where an up-to-date list of genetic counseling services can be obtained. The National Genetics Foundation maintains a network of genetic counseling and treatment centers throughout the United States and Canada to provide patients and their families with counseling services. The National Foundation–March of Dimes (abbreviated The National Foundation) not only publishes a *Directory of Genetic Services* but also contributes significantly to professional education and research related to genetic defects and provides extensive programs directed toward teaching and disseminating genetic information. A directory of genetic counseling centers is issued by some state public health departments, and information is available through the Bureau of Maternal and Child Health of the Department of Health, Education and Welfare, the American Public Health Association, and the National Association for Retarded Citizens, Inc. Other sources include the numerous state and local organizations that are concerned with mental retardation.

Objectives of genetic counseling

Carter has outlined three objectives of genetic counseling: (1) to advise parents of risks of an abnormality in any future children, (2) to alert the medical profession to the possibility of a special risk in an unborn child, and (3) to ultimately reduce the number of children who are born with a serious handicap.[2, 3]

Advising parents. More than ever before, parents plan for and feel responsible for their children. They are entitled to accurate information regarding risks and to have this information presented to them in language they can understand and in the proper perspective. That is, they need to know the risks in their particular situation and how it relates to the random risk of severe abnormality in any child. It has been found that when parents understand the risks involved, they normally make sensible decisions regarding family planning.

Special risk situations. When health personnel are alerted to the possibility of an inherited disease in a family, this knowledge facilitates the early detection and subsequent treatment of the disease. This is increasingly important as more treatments are becoming available for genetically determined diseases and is especially true in situations where treatment is effective only when initiated early. History of a condition in an older sibling, such as PKU and galactosemia, provides a clue for specific and thorough testing for the condition in a newborn. In this way, an early dietary regimen can be instituted when indicated.

Reducing numbers of affected children. Since it is now possible to detect the carrier state in an increasing variety of single gene defects, this aspect of genetic counseling is assuming greater importance and offers hope in reducing the incidence of disabling disease. Persons with a family history of one of these hereditary disorders or those in an ethnic group at risk for a particular disease (for example, Tay-Sachs disease) are able to ascertain before initiating a pregnancy whether they are carriers of the gene for a severe defect. In these instances, the genetic counselor is able to advise the couple of the risk related to any pregnancy with a high degree of accuracy. New techniques for prenatal diagnosis of chromosomal aberrations and an increasing number of the inborn errors of metabolism have created a means for detecting the presence of an abnormal fetus early in pregnancy, which provides a couple who may have a defective child with the option to terminate the pregnancy.

Information essential to genetic counseling

Unlike a medical prognosis that predicts the outcome of a disease process, a genetic prognosis directly involves other persons: the affected child, other family members, relatives, and future offspring. Therefore, it is essential to perform a thorough evaluation of each situation. Effective genetic counseling is based on information from several sources from which the counselor derives risks of recurrence.

Accurate diagnosis. The initial and most important component in the counseling process is an accurate diagnosis. Mental retardation is a manifestation of such a variety of genetic and environmental causes that it is often difficult to distinguish one from the other. There are disorders with similar clinical manifestations that display different patterns of inheritance (genocopies). For example, gargoylism can be inherited as an autosomal recessive disorder (Hurler's syndrome) or as an X-linked recessive disorder (Hunter's syndrome). Nongenetic factors may produce an effect similar or identical to one due to a genetic disorder (phenocopies). For example, maternal infections (such as rubella and toxoplasmosis) are known to be damaging to the central nervous system in the unborn child. Not all retardation affecting more than a single member of a family is hereditary. Inadequate stimulation by a retarded parent may cause a child to appear retarded when he may, in fact, be in the normal range of intelligence. However, when a condition is found in definite proportions in families (for example, persons related by descent) and absent in unrelated individuals (spouses, in-laws) the likelihood of a genetic disorder must be considered.

Family history. A careful, detailed family history is necessary to the counseling process. Not only does it provide a picture of the *proband* (the affected person, or *index case*) in relation to other members of the kindred but may also serve to identify other persons in the kindred who are similarly affected. Analyzing the pattern of affected persons in a family may assist in confirming a tentative diagnosis. Observation of the frequency and relationships of the disorder among relatives helps to determine a level of risk in multifactorial inheritance (disorders due to combined genetic and environmental causes).

The person who takes the family history must allow a liberal amount of time. In the case of an affected child, it is best when the interview includes both parents in order to elicit information about relatives on both sides of the family. Medical records, family Bibles, and photograph albums are helpful sources, and interviewees should be instructed to bring such items if they are available. It may be necessary to consult other members of the family, although the reliability of information and informants may vary greatly, especially in regard to whether more distant relatives were or were not affected. The manner in which the information is elicited determines to a large degree the attitude and cooperation of the informant and, hence, the amount of information that is forthcoming. The amount of education and level of understanding vary widely among informants. There may even be reticence on the part of the informant, particularly if the disorder is considered to be a "skeleton in the closet." Sometimes true relationships may be concealed, such as illegitimacy. Information concerning first-degree relatives is most important, and the data on these should be complete. It is not uncommon to discover conditions in the family, other than the one under investigation, that may require therapy.

The family history is recorded in the form of a pedigree chart, or family tree, using standard symbols to indicate persons, relationships, and significant details related to them (Fig. 8-6). Situations that concern consanguineous marriages, multiple marriages, or any other complex relationships require extra care in order to outline the relationship accurately. There should be notations about the age, date and place of birth, and death and cause of death where possible. Sometimes the place of birth and racial background are significant. For example, the incidence of Tay-Sachs disease in Ashkenazic Jews from Eastern Europe is higher than in Jews from other geographic origins.

Construction of the pedigree chart begins with the proband, who is designated with an arrow, and the outcome of all the mother's pregnancies (Fig. 8-7). Marriages are represented by a bar, with males usually indicated on the left. Siblings, including

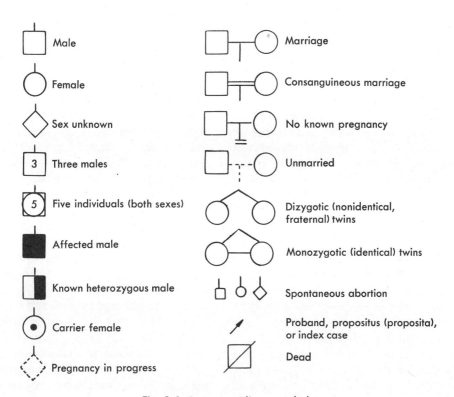

Fig. 8-6. Common pedigree symbols.

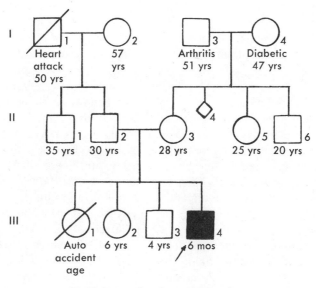

Fig. 8-7. Sample of a pedigree chart.

stillbirths and abortions, are designated by arabic numerals from left to right in order of birth. Generations are represented by roman numerals, the earliest at the top. Any abnormalities of the pregnancies are noted, such as high blood pressure, bleeding, anemia, convulsions, excessive weight gain, exposure to x-rays, or infectious diseases. The outcome of previous marriages may be important, and such facts as history of radiation exposure of the father should not be overlooked. Next the medical histories of the maternal relatives are explored, beginning with mother's siblings and including any other outcomes of her mother's pregnancies. Details concerning the general health or death of the maternal grandparents, nieces, nephews, uncles, aunts, and first cousins are included in a family history if the mother has information about them. The relatives on the father's side are explored in the same manner. It is important at this point to determine whether the couple might be related in any way.

When the family history is completed, the pedigree will reflect either a *positive family history,* in which other relatives are affected with the same disorder, or a *negative family history,* in which the proband is an isolated case. It is at this point that the counselor employs an understanding of the principles of genetics, a knowledge of the risks related to multifactorial inheritance, and up-to-date information on genetic diseases in order to counsel families regarding their specific problem.

Estimation of recurrence risks

The mode of inheritance determines the degree of risk in the major categories of genetic disorders. In general, the more definite and clearcut the genetics, the greater the risks; as the causative factors become more obscure, the outlook is more hopeful. Unfortunately, knowledge of the causes of mental retardation is so limited that a definite etiology can be assigned in only about 20% of cases and a possible etiology in another 20%. Fully 60% of cases remain unclassified, however. Broadly, the risks can be categorized as (1) random risks, (2) high risk of 1 in 10 or greater, and (3) moderate risk of better than 1 in 10 and usually less than 1 in 20.[11]

Random-risk situations. The random risk for a disorder of some type in any pregnancy is considered to be approximately 1 in 30, for a gross abnormality of the brain, 1%. Conditions that are due to environmental agents and, therefore, are unlikely to recur in another pregnancy are regarded as random risks. Examples include mental retardation due to maternal infections, fetal anoxia, or birth trauma. In these instances, the environmental agent affects the developing embryo or the fetus, not the germ cells.

When an individual is affected with a genetic disease as the result of a fresh mutation, subsequent siblings and other relatives will not be at risk for the disorder. However, the mutant gene can be transmitted to children of the affected person, and the risks to such children are estimated in relation to the mode of its inheritance. Dominant conditions are often due to a new mutation.

Most of the chromosome abnormalities, such as Down's syndrome, are considered random risks. However, after the birth of a child with a chromosome aberration, the risk of recurrence is estimated to be about double the random risk for another mother of the same age. Also, the risk of Down's syndrome rises remarkably with increased maternal age.

High-risk situations. The majority of genetic disorders that carry a high risk of recurrence are due to mutant genes. In the dominant conditions the risk is 1 in 2, or 50% if one parent is affected; for a recessive disorder the risk is 1 in 4, or 25%; and in X-linked disorders the risk is more complex and depends on the sex of the parent who carries the gene and the sex of the offspring (see X-linked inheritance, pp. 94-95).

A minority of disorders with a high risk of recurrence involve the chromosome anomalies in which a parent is the carrier of a balanced translocation (see Down's syndrome, pp. 96-97). Special problems are associated with the syndromes involving a structural anomaly, such as the cri du chat syndrome. It is felt that many of these cases arise as a result of a balanced translocation in a parent, but more cases must be investigated before a definite risk can be predicted.

Moderate-risk situations. Moderate-risk conditions are those multifactorial polygenic disorders that appear to run in families but for which no definite inheritance pattern can be identified. The risk is less than 1 in 10 but is substantially greater than the random risk in the population as a whole. Estimates in these disorders are *empiric*. That is, estimates are not based on genetic theory but on prior experience and observation much the same as a meteorologist bases a weather prediction. To arrive at an empiric risk estimate, the counselor applies a knowledge of frequencies that have been observed in families with a similar condition (in this case mental retardation) to the incidence of the disorder in the family under consideration. Since these risks are only estimates based on incidence in other families, the figures are undoubtedly exaggerated in some families and underestimated in others. The bulk of mental retardation falls into this category, and the recurrence risks are related to the familial incidence as discussed earlier.

Multifactorial disorders that affect the development of the central nervous system (for example, anencephaly, microcephaly, encephalocele, or hydrocephaly secondary to spina bifida) are variable in incidence. The risk of recurrence is increased with each such child that is born in a family, but it varies widely according to the investigator and the area in which the investigation is conducted. In general, recurrence risks for a central nervous system defect after one affected child (with any of these defects) are 1 in 25 to 40; after two such children, the risk is 1 in 10 to 15; following three such children, the risks become high at 1 in 3 to 5.[8]

Interpretation of risks

When explaining risk estimates, the counselor does not attempt to make recommendations or decisions for the clients, who are usually parents who have experienced the birth of a retarded child. The counselor provides appropriate and accurate information about the nature of the disorder, the extent of the risk involved, and the probable consequences but leaves the final decision to the persons concerned. It is sometimes difficult not to allow personal bias to interfere or to have a preconceived idea about the course of action a given client should take. All alternatives should be discussed, including sterilization, artificial insemination, birth control methods, and adoption. In some instances, genetic information will increase the family's distress. In others, their anxiety will be reduced. Their response will depend on their makeup and the meaning that the specific condition has for that particular family. On the basis of counseling information and their own goals, most parents tend to make sensible decisions.

It is helpful to explain risks in different ways and to use examples from games of chance to make clients understand the meaning of probabilities. Most persons do not have an adequate knowledge of genetics and human biology, which inhibits their comprehension of these concepts. However, few people have not had experience with flipping coins, baseball pools, lotteries, horse racing, and so on. Flipping a coin can be used effectively to illustrate the probabilities in single-gene disorders, and a weather report is a well-known example of an empiric risk estimate.

It is important to impress on the family that *each pregnancy is an independent event*. It is not uncommon for parents, told that a recessive disorder carries a 1 in 4 risk of recurrence, to feel secure with one affected child. They incorrectly reason that, since they already have one affected child, the next three will be unaffected. "Chance has no memory." The risk is 1 in 4 for each and every pregnancy.

A proposed marriage between blood relatives frequently involves the genetic counselor. There is considerable disagreement among authorities regarding whether there is a significant risk of mental retardation in the offspring of such a mating. The question is especially difficult regarding first-cousin marriage. A high incidence of postnatal mortality and an increase in mental retardation reflect the common genetic factors; however, the actual risk is relatively small, and many couples accept it. Certainly, the more genes two people have in common, the greater the probability that there will be an increase in identical polygene complexes in their children.

The nurse and genetic counseling

Nurses skilled in counseling techniques are in an ideal position to help meet the counseling needs of families in which there is a genetic disease or disorder. Public health nurses work with families in a close, sustained relationship and have earned the family's confidence and trust. The genetics nurse specialists, with advanced preparation in genetic theory, are assuming a prominent position on counseling teams. Practitioners in a variety of specialty areas are constantly involved with genetic defects, including mental retardation. Nurses are frequently the persons who recognize clues that indicate a genetic-related problem, who assist the family in obtaining the needed services for diagnosis and treatment, and who provide follow-up care.

Counseling services. The most efficient counseling service consists of a group of specialists that may include physicians, geneticists, psychologists, biochemists, a cytologist, nurses, social workers, and auxiliary personnel. The services are most often under the leadership of a physician, trained in medical genetics, who assumes responsibility for the medical aspects of the group.[4] The counseling service may serve only as a referral group, or it may conduct a regular clinic service. Most often, it is associated with a large medical center. Numerous specialty clinics deal with specific genetic disorders and provide their own genetic counseling services. Unfortunately, most units are concentrated in and around large metropolitan areas. As a result, counseling is not always accessible to a large number of persons who would benefit from the services.

A nurse is frequently the family's initial contact with a counseling service. An intake interview is conducted before the primary counseling session or diagnosis in order to assess the needs of the family and attempt to reduce their anxiety. In the process of the interview, the nurse takes a family history for pertinent information and explains the clinic procedures carefully. Many families are concerned about such things as whether they will be required to undress, whether blood is to be drawn, or whether they can accompany the child during the visit. Families who have a relaxed and nonstressful initial discussion are able to gain more from a counseling session.

Follow-up care. The success of counseling is measured by the way the family uses the information presented to them. Maintaining contact with the family or referral to an agency, usually the public health agency in their locality, that can provide a sustained relationship is one of the most important aspects of the counseling process. Some families do not choose to have follow-up visits, but in most instances it makes the family feel that they have not been abandoned, and it facilitates the process of adjustment to the problem.

Follow-up visits to the counseling service or in the home provide the family with the opportunity to ask questions that they did not ask on the previous visits. Often the family has not really "heard" the information presented to them or has misinterpreted what they have heard so that it may be necessary to repeat and reinforce counseling. In some disorders, a diagnosis of one family member places relatives at risk and is an indication for further screening. In a disorder such as PKU that requires conscientious diet management, it is important to make certain that the family understands and follows the advice regarding therapy. Subsequent children must be carefully observed to detect early symptoms.

Nurses should be prepared to help families arrive at tentative decisions regarding the future, including family planning and plans for an affected person (such as placement or education). Families can be directed to agencies and clinics specializing in a specific disorder that can provide services in the form of equipment, medication, and correction of physical problems that often accompany some forms of retardation (for example, heart defects associated with Down's syndrome). The location of infant stimulation programs, educational facilities, and parent groups are all a part of the nurse's resources. The nurse's role in follow-up care encompasses all those aspects of mental retardation that constitute the major focus of this book.

Psychological aspects of genetic counseling

It requires time and understanding to deal with the emotional tension and anxiety generated in families who are faced with the prospect of mental retardation, particularly when it is an inherited disability. Knowledge of, and the ability to cope with, the range of psychological responses and all their ramifications are essential components of the nursing role in genetic counseling. Many of these factors determine the degree to which a counselor's message is understood and influence the family's attitudes and the use they make of counseling information. It is the awareness and understanding of these feelings and attitudes that makes the difference between a genetic informant and a genetic counselor.

Timing of counseling is very important. Some families may not be ready to listen right after a diagnosis is made; many do not listen effectively the first time information is presented to them. There may be numerous blocks to getting information across to the clients. They may be so angry or frightened that they do not hear what is being said to them; they may feel guilty or embarrassed, or somehow inferior or inadequate. It may be necessary to wait a week or more to allow the family sufficient time to absorb the initial impact of the situation before they are ready to assimilate any new information or begin problem solving.

It is important early in the counseling to get a clear understanding of the family's initial concerns, their state of knowledge about the disorder, and their attitudes and beliefs

concerning the condition and mental retardation. Clients vary in the amount of education they have had and their level of understanding. It is important to determine the kind and amount of information they need or want. Some are not even sure they should be at a counseling service. Whether the clients are parents who have given birth to an affected child, relatives of an affected individual, or persons who have been identified as carriers of a deleterious gene, they have feelings, attitudes, and fears.

Guilt and self-blame are very natural and universal reactions. Nurses must deal with feelings of guilt about carrying "bad genes" or having "made my child retarded." Often the counselor is in a position to absolve the parents of guilt by explaining the random nature of segregation during both gamete formation and fertilization. Sometimes there is comfort in knowing that everyone carries some defective genes and that it is mere chance that a particular couple happens to carry the same abnormal gene. Reactions may be different in situations where one member can pinpoint the "blame," whereas there is some measure of reassurance for the couple to know that it is not just one of them who is responsible for the defect. The impact of a hereditary "taint" often creates intrafamily strife, hostility, and marital disharmony, sometimes to the point of family disintegration. Relatives frequently cease reproduction after the diagnosis of mental retardation in a partner's family, no matter how remote the relationship or the etiology of the defect. Although people may understand the situation on an intellectual level, it may not help them on an emotional level. A large and important part of the nurse's role in genetic counseling is that of a sympathetic and supportive listener.

The way a family responds to the probability of mental retardation will depend a great deal on the burden, actual or perceived, that the condition places on them. A burden is considered to be the total amount of distress created by the birth of an affected child—the anticipated burden as well as the threat of disability.[9] A risk that is reassuring to one may be threatening or intolerable to another. Also, two individuals will respond differently to a hazard that both perceive as threatening. There are those who are fatalistically willing to accept the "will of God." Others who have experienced the problem of a mentally retarded person are unwilling, under any circumstances, to face the prospect of another affected child. One couple may choose to have children in the face of a high risk, whereas another couple may consider even a moderate risk too much to hazard. The prospect of inevitable death from any disorder is distressing, but to prepare to lose an anencephalic child at birth is quite different than to anticipate loss of a child with Tay-Sachs disease at age 3, or the lifelong disability created by nonfatal mental retardation. All of these factors confront a family when they must make a decision about whether to risk a pregnancy that might result in a defective child. The longer the duration of the disability, the greater the financial and emotional burden.

A frequent barrier to an objective use of information is religious attitude toward conception and the opposition to sterilization and abortion in situations where there is a high risk of recurrence or where prenatal diagnosis has indicated a defective fetus. Another is the rights of the individual—the right of the fetus to come to full term and the rights of parents to conceive. A person with a high risk of producing a disabling condition in an offspring may feel that he is entitled to the same rights as anyone else, including the right to procreate children.

Sometimes nurses themselves may create barriers with their own biases. Some diseases have a special impact on a nurse, and in such cases it is difficult to be nonjudgmental. Families may become defensive if they feel the nurse is bringing undue pressure to bear on their decision. Others may pressure the counselor to make the decision for them. "What would you do if you were in this situation?" is a common question. There are instances where some nurses (intentionally or unintentionally) influence families. In genetic counseling, the families should be given all the facts and possible consequences and assisted in their problem solving, but the decision concerning a course of action should be their own.

SUMMARY

A significant number of disorders can be positively attributed to a genetic etiology. Although prevention of retardation has been disappointingly limited in most instances, there are many conditions for which a prediction can be made regarding recurrence risks with a high degree of accuracy. The nurse who has some understanding of the role heredity plays in mental retardation is in a better position to recognize situations in which genetics is a factor, interpret genetic information for the clients, and intervene appropriately to provide assistance for clients and their families.

REFERENCES

1. Carr, D. H.: Chromosomes and abortion. In Harris, H., and Hirschhorn, K., editors: Advances in human genetics ed. 2, New York, 1971, Plenum Publishing Corp.
2. Carter, C. O.: Genetic counseling. In Allen, R. M., Cortasso, A. D., and Toister, R. P., editors: The role of genetics in mental retardation, Coral Gables, Fla., 1971, University of Miami Press.
3. Carter, C. O.: Genetic counseling. In Berg, J. M., ed.: Genetics counseling in relation to mental retardation, Elmsford, N.Y., 1971, Pergamon Press, Inc.
4. Epstein, C. J.: Who should do genetic counseling, and under what circumstances? In Bergsma, D., and Neel, J. V., editors: Birth defects; original article series, vol. IX, No. 4, April 1974.
5. Gottesman, I. I.: An introduction to behavioral genetics of mental retardation. In Allen, R. M., Cortasso, A. D., and Toister, R. P., editors: The role of genetics in mental retardation, Coral Gables, Fla., 1971, University of Miami Press.
6. Hirschhorn, K.: Chromosome abnormalities I; autosomal defects. In McKusick, V. A., and Claiborne, R., editors: Medical genetics, New York, 1973, H. P. Publishing Co., Inc.
7. Holtzman, N. A.: Prevention of retardation of genetic origin, Pediatr. Clin. North Am. **20:**151, 1973.
8. Kirman, B. H.: Genetic counseling of parents of mentally retarded children, In Berg, J. M., editor: Genetic counseling in relation to mental retardation, Elmsford, N.Y., 1971, Pergamon Press, Inc.
9. Leonard, D. O., Chase, G. A. and Childs, B.: Genetic counseling; a consumer's view, N. Engl. J. Med. **287:**433, 1972.

10. Reisman, L. E., and Matheny, A. P., Jr.: Genetics and counseling in medical practice, St. Louis, 1969, The C. V. Mosby Co., Chapter 13.
11. Roberts, J. A. F.: An introduction to medical genetics, ed. 5, New York, 1970, Oxford University Press, Inc., Chapter 12.
12. Scott, C. I., and Thomas, G. H.: Genetic disorders associated with mental retardation, Pediatr. Clin. North Am. **20:**121, 1973.
13. Smith, G. F.: Clinical aspects of genetics in mental retardation. In Allen, R. M., Cortasso, A. D., and Toister, R. P., editors: The role of genetics in mental retardation, Coral Gables, Fla., 1971, University of Miami Press.
14. Stevenson, A. C., and Davison, B. C. C.: Genetic counseling, Philadelphia, 1970, J. B. Lippincott Co., Chapter 11.
15. Whaley, L. F.: Understanding inherited disorders, St. Louis, 1974, The C. V. Mosby Co., Chapter 2.

CHAPTER 9

Prenatal care

CAROL DOWLER

The current goal of obstetrical care is the reduction of perinatal mortality and morbidity. This would affect both pregnant women and the children who result. Statistics for the United States from 1973 demonstrate that there are 25 perinatal deaths for every 1,000 births.[2] Readings project even higher perinatal morbidity figures, but the exact number is unknown because of the vast range of factors considered under morbidity, such as documented mental retardation, seizure disorders, cerebral palsy, or the more subtle compromises, such as moderate decreases in IQ, minimal brain dysfunction, or learning disabilities.

Although the causes of mental retardation and other developmental disabilities are varied and numerous, a large number of high-risk problems can occur during the prenatal period and have the potential of resulting in a damaged child. Etiological factors resulting in developmental disabilities, such as genetic disorders, poor thermoregulation of the newborn, poor oxygenation, and care of high-risk infants, are explored in other chapters of this book.

The environment of the developing fetus is composed of the mother's reproductive organs and birth canal as well as the placenta and, ultimately, the mother's supporting body systems. The developing fetus is highly susceptible to damage resulting from any alteration of its normal environment.

During the first trimester of pregnancy, the fetus is particularly vulnerable to damage of its developing organ systems. It is known that the damage that occurs during sequential fetal development cannot later be remedied during development to result in a normal child. Therefore, it is imperative to prevent any alterations of the fetal environment that could result in an abnormality.

Over the past 10 years, new methods for detecting fetal anomalies early in pregnancy and fetal distress before or during labor have been developed to improve perinatal care and mortality and morbidity statistics. As methods such as amniocentesis, fetal challenge tests, and biochemical assessments of fetal by-products continue to become more and more a part of maternity care, nurses will find their roles in preventive antenatal care increasing. Tests such as these make it possible to predict many conditions that cause developmental disabilities and, in many cases, to prevent them by appropriate intervention.

The purpose of this chapter is to highlight the nurse's role in preventing fetal mortality and morbidity. It explores the nurse's role in antenatal clinical assessment, early identification of prenatal high-risk factors, and antenatal diagnostic testing. Prenatal factors that may result in developmental disabilities, such as maternal infections and medical problems, are presented.

ANTENATAL CLINICAL ASSESSMENT

Since nurses are often the family's initial contact with the health care system, it is of utmost importance that they completely assess each pregnant woman. In some settings, clinical nurse specialists or nurse midwives may perform these assessments. In other settings the physician will do so. It is the nurse's responsibility, however, to assure that a thorough examination is completed on each pregnant woman and that all findings are documented and used in planning appropriate care. A complete assessment of the mother should begin as soon as pregnancy is suspected or confirmed. Initial assessments should include a complete health interview with attention to:

- Past medical-obstetrical history
- Current health status
- Family history of genetic disorders, anomalies, or developmental disabilities
- Observation of psychoemotional response to pregnancy
- Educational needs
- Social-financial needs
- Nutritional status, including an assessment of the basic four food group intake

On the patient's initial visit, the nurse should also be certain that:

- A complete physical examination of all body systems is performed.
- Basic laboratory data are completed (such as complete blood cell count, hemoglobin/hematocrit value, blood type and Rh factor, rubella titer, and serological evaluation).
- A tuberculin test is performed.
- A vaginal examination is performed and that gonorrhea cultures and a Pap test are done.
- Special laboratory tests are completed as necessary (such as TORCH— toxoplasmosis, other, rubella, cytomegalovirus, and herpes) in positive histories, including an amniocentesis for genetic studies before the fourteenth week of pregnancy in mothers over 30 years of age and on all mothers with a family history of genetic disorders.

Assessments performed during each follow-up visit should include:

- A blood pressure reading taken while the patient is lying on her left side. Attention should be directed to ominous signs of hypertension. This could be determined by a resting blood pressure above 140/90. A more dependable indicator is a 30 mm Hg or greater rise in the systolic reading and a 15 mm Hg or more rise in the diastolic reading.[7]
- Weight, with attention given to decreases as well as increases. For a patient of ideal weight for height at time of conception, weight gain should be 2 to 4 pounds during the first 13 weeks of pregnancy and an average of .9 pounds each week during the second and third trimesters. Total weight gain should be 22 to 27 pounds.[5]
- Urine checks for protein, glucose, and ketones to rule out ominous signs of diabetes, kidney disease, negative nitrogen balance, or preeclampsia.
- A hematocrit value every 4 to 6 weeks, or at least at 26 to 28 weeks and 36 weeks of gestation. Repeat values help to differentiate true anemias from the condition referred to as pseudoanemia of early pregnancy, such as a hematocrit value below 30% with a hemoglobin level of 10.5 gm or less per 100 ml.[7]
- Fetal assessments, including determination of (a) fetal activity; (b) fetal growth via fundal assessments from the eighth to tenth week through the thirty-sixth week of gestation; and (c) fetal heart tones. Fetal heart tones should be determined by using a 1 full–minute count beginning at 10 to 12 weeks of gestation if an electronic doppler is used. If a stethoscope is used, they can be taken at 17 to 18 weeks of gestation. Notations should be made of the rate, pattern, and location of the fetal heart tones.

Finally, at 36 weeks of gestation, the nurse should see that all mothers have a repeat gonorrhea culture, a beta-streptococcal culture, vaginal examinations to assess the status of the cervix, and reporting of any abnormalities. Appropriate intervention should be initiated as soon as abnormalities are detected; however, the nurse should be alert to detecting abnormalities early.

EARLY IDENTIFICATION OF HIGH-RISK FACTORS

The second role of the nurse in preventive antenatal care is the early recognition of mothers and fetuses at risk. Risk factors are present in pregnancies in which the fetus has a significantly increased chance of death, either before or after delivery, or a potential for some chronic physiological or developmental disability.

Maternal high-risk factors that are known to contribute to fetal mortality and morbidity may be grouped into four broad categories: (1) past obstetrical high-risk factors, (2) present pregnancy-related factors, (3) maternal medical health factors, and (4) psychosocial factors.[8]

Past obstetrical, high-risk factors

Past obstetrical factors considered significant in antepartum assessment interviews include:
- A history of two or more spontaneous first or midtrimester abortions
- A history of premature delivery
- A history of intrapartum complications, such as fetal distress, abruptio placentae, and abnormal fetal position
- A history of pregnancy-related toxemia
- A history of congenital anomalies, developmental disabilities, or genetic defects
- A history of perinatal death due to fetal demise, stillbirth, or neonatal or infant death in the first year

Present pregnancy-related factors

Present pregnancy-related factors associated with the outcome of newborn disability or death include:
- Maternal age under 16 years or over 30 years
- Primiparas over 30 years of age
- Excessive multiparity greater than four
- Bleeding after 20 weeks' gestation

- Premature labor or premature rupture of membranes
- Multiple gestations
- Postmaturity
- Rh incompatibility or other antibody sensitization in maternal blood
- Toxemia
- Intrauterine growth delay (SGA babies)
- Abnormal fetal position, including breech
- Incompetent cervix
- Hydramnios (excess amniotic fluid) or polyhydramnios (amniotic fluid in excess of 2,000 ml)

Maternal medical health factors

Acute or chronic medical health disorders are the third group of high-risk factors that may contribute to poor fetal outcomes. Maternal medical factors include: (1) maternal conditions that result in fetal hypoxia, (2) maternal infections, (3) maternal-fetal nutrition or nutrient transport disorders, and (4) maternal conditions that result in fetal trauma.

Maternal conditions that may cause hypoxia in the fetus during pregnancy or delivery are diabetes, cyanotic heart or lung disease, excessive smoking, chronic hypertensive disease, poorly controlled seizure disorders, and anemia. Hypoxic morbidity occurs when conditions exist that prevent the adequate perfusion of blood through maternal or fetal vessels. For example, sclerotic vessels are often seen in women who have had diabetes for a long time. Hypoxic morbidity also occurs when there is a decrease in the oxygen saturation levels of maternal-fetal blood.

Another situation resulting in hypoxic morbidity is an abnormal, intermittent transport of oxygen across the maternal-fetal placental barrier. Insufficient oxygen transport can occur during labor when intermittent decreases in uterine blood flow that are secondary to uterine contractions and preexisting borderline placental function may compromise the fetus's already decreased oxygen supply.[2]

Systemic, vaginal, or intrauterine infections are the second group of maternal medical health disorders that may result in fetal mortality or morbidity. Fetal involvement occurs when organisms invade via placental transfer or ascend into the uterus via the cervical os. The severity of illness in mothers is not the factor most closely correlated to embryonic or fetal damage. For example, infants with rubella syndrome may result from mothers who were not aware of exposure to the illness and who did not notice symptoms of illness during the pregnancy.

Infections documented as precursors of fetal mortality and morbidity include[1]:

- Pyelonephritis
- Pneumonias
- Rubella, especially in the first trimester of pregnancy
- Vaginal infections
- Toxoplasmosis
- Syphilis
- Varicella
- Tuberculosis
- Rubeola
- Coxsackie viruses
- Cytomegalovirus
- Infectious hepatitis
- Asian flu
- Mumps
- Listeriosis
- Herpesvirus hominis

The third group of maternal medical health disorders related to poor fetal outcome are the maternal nutritional-fetal nutrient transport disorders. Conditions where the fetus may receive improper or inadequate nutrients in utero include:

- Maternal obesity, defined as a weight gain of 20% or more above ideal weight for height at the time of conception
- Excessive weight gain above 22 to 27 pounds (10 to 12 kg) for a woman of ideal weight at time of conception, with or without other signs of preeclampsia
- Inadequate weight gain, below recommended American College of Obstetrics and Gynecology weight patterns[5]
- Diabetes where excess carbohydrates increase fetal weight

- Inadequate intake of any or all of the basic four food groups

Maternal malnutrition is thought to result in intrauterine death, malformations, or growth retardation. However, an excess of certain vitamins during pregnancy may also result in developmental abnormalities.

The last group of maternal medical health factors to be considered are those disorders or agents that may alter fetal development or cause excess trauma to the fetus during labor or delivery. They include:

- Exposure to high doses of radiation during fetal development
- Ingestion of certain chemicals or drugs during fetal development (such as thalidomide, steroids, or folic acid antagonists)
- Precipitous, uncontrolled delivery
- Prolonged labor, as in cephalopelvic disproportion, transverse arrest, or cervical stenosis
- Pregnancies/deliveries not managed by competent staff in equipped centers

Embryonic or fetal development may be altered by exposure to certain chemicals, drugs, or radiation of the mother during pregnancy. In the case of radiation exposure, large doses are required to result in malformation, growth retardation, intrauterine death, or postnatal functional deficit, whereas relatively small doses may result in gene mutation or chromosomal aberrations. Chemicals and drugs make up the largest category of agents that can adversely alter fetal or embryonic development. There is a wide variation in the ways that different chemicals or drugs act on the developing body systems. Although there is a known correlation between certain abnormalities and drugs (as in the case of thalidomide), other drugs (such as anticonvulsants, anorexogenics, or oral hypoglycemics) are only suspected of having adverse effects on the embryo or fetus.[9] Further studies are needed in this large category of maternal risk factors to continue to isolate agents responsible for defects and prevent abnormalities by patient education and counseling.

Inadequate prenatal care and delivery

have been included here in response to the increasing social desire to avoid proper antenatal care and hospital deliveries. Inadequate prenatal care and poorly managed labor and delivery in settings where emergency measures cannot be instituted have been recognized as major causes of poor fetal outcome for many years. These situations can result in intracranial hemorrhage with permanent destruction of brain tissue.

Psychosocial high-risk factors

The fourth category of maternal high-risk conditions is linked to the psychosocial realm. They include:

- Income level of the family
- Quality and quantity of antenatal care received
- Social intactness of family
- Family structure
- Family psychological well-being
- History of institutionalization
- Parenting capacities of the mother
- Status of pregnancy (unwanted or wanted)
- History of abuse or neglect

The psychosocial realm reflects how well a mother and her fetus can cope with the world, its demands, and each other. It also takes into account the environment of the mother and her baby-to-be and what potential the environment provides for the baby's growth and development after birth. Finally, it identifies the resources that the mother has had at her disposal to provide care and how she views herself, her pregnancy, her baby, the baby's father, and their future as a family.

ANTENATAL DIAGNOSTIC TESTING

The third role of the nurse in preventing fetal mortality and morbidity is participation in antenatal diagnostic testing, the interpretation of findings, appropriate interventions, and providing patient education and support. Antenatal testing performed to assess maternal-fetal placental intactness, sufficiency and fetal reserve, and maturity includes the nonstress test, the oxytocin

challenge test, ultrasound or echogram, urinary estriol determinations, and amniocentesis.

Nonstress heart rate testing is used to assess the fetal reserve of mothers when oxytocin challenge tests are contraindicated. This test consists of monitoring the fetal heart rate and spontaneously occurring contractions. A fetus with good heart rate variability, accelerations of heart rate with fetal movements, and no late decelerations with spontaneous contractions is considered a reactive fetus whose prognosis is excellent.[3]

A nonreactive stress test demonstrates poor heart variability, no accelerations with or without fetal movements, and late decelerations of heart rate with spontaneous contractions. Fetal prognosis is poor and delivery should be immediate if fetal survival is to be assured.

The oxytocin challenge test is a test of placental sufficiency and fetal reserve.[3, 4] The test is used to evaluate placental function from the thirty-fourth week of gestation to term in mothers with the problems of diabetes, hypertension (chronic or pregnancy-induced), toxemia, chronic renal disease, postdatism, intrauterine growth delay, previous stillbirths, chronic heart disease, or sickle cell anemia.[3]

The oxytocin challenge test is performed in the labor and delivery area of the hospital. The mother is placed in a semi-Fowler's, or left lateral, position with external fetal monitoring equipment in place. A baseline strip is then obtained for 15 minutes, with attention to clarity of the fetal heart rate pattern, variability, and contractions. Three or four spontaneous contractions within 10 minutes produce a readable strip and complete the test.

If no contractions are noted, a 500-ml 5% dextrose in water infusion is started with a scalp vein needle, and a second infusion of 5% dextrose in water with 5 units of oxytocin (Pitocin) is piggy-backed into the first intravenous infusion by an infusion pump. The dosage of Pitocin is slowly increased 1 to 2 drops every 15 to 20 minutes until three to four moderate contractions in 10 minutes are observed. Once contractions are noted, the intravenous infusion is discontinued, and monitoring persists until contractions cease.

Interpretation of data obtained from the oxytocin challenge test is either positive, negative, suspicious, or unsatisfactory.[4] The oxytocin challenge test is considered positive when persistent late decelerations occur with normal uterine contractions. Fetal maturity studies and delivery should be performed immediately, if feasible.

The oxytocin challenge test is considered negative when no decelerations occur with adequate contractions. The test indicates good fetal reserve and should be repeated in 1 week in high-risk mothers. The test is considered suspicious when occasional late decelerations occur. No immediate action is taken, but the test should be repeated in 2 or 3 days.

An oxytocin challenge test is considered unsatisfactory when the test is not interpretable because of a poor-quality tracing or inadequate uterine contractions. Patients with unsatisfactory tracings should have the test repeated in 24 hours. Although nurses may have received additional training to conduct this test, they need to bear in mind the supportive aspects of their role. This is especially true for patients having a positive, suspicious, or unsatisfactory test result.

Ultrasound or echogram is an antenatal diagnostic procedure that uses high-frequency sound waves to make a picture of the fetus. Sound waves are directed into the body, and echoes are received intermittently by a dual-purpose doppler. As sound waves bounce off fetal and adjacent structures, a white-gray-black picture is produced that gives five valuable pieces of information: (1) the gestational age of the fetus by measurements of the biparietal diameter, (2) estimates of fetal growth when echoes are done serially during the first and second or third trimester, (3) placental localization, (4) diagnosis of multiple fetuses, and (5) presence of certain neurological defects,

such as hydrocephalus, spina bifida, or anencephaly.[6]

Biochemical assessments

The biochemical assessment of fetal well-being is accomplished by urinary estriol determinations and amniotic studies.[6] Urinary estriol determinations are endocrinological tests of fetal-placental function. Estriol is a hormonal substance produced by the fetus and placenta in increasing quantities as pregnancy advances. It is the best indicator of the fetus's survival potential. Marked changes, less than 8 mg/24 hours in falling serial values, or constantly low readings are ominous signs of fetal distress. Estriol values in urine seem to be affected by the urinary output (amount) and the nutritional status of the mother. They do not always indicate poor growth of the fetus, and single determinations are useless.

The second biochemical test of the fetus and its environment is amniocentesis. Amniocentesis is a relatively low-risk method of obtaining samples of amniotic fluid for study. Many laboratory studies can be performed on amniotic fluid that reflect fetal biochemical function, certain chromosomal abnormalities, and maturity. Laboratory studies of fetal amniotic fluid include[1]:

- Creatinine levels
- Sodium levels
- Protein levels
- Lecithin-sphingomyelin (L/S) ratio
- 17-ketosteroid values
- Pregnanediol levels
- Sex chromatin studies
- Chromosomal studies

SUMMARY

Three of the major roles of the nurse in preventing fetal mortality and morbidity have been discussed. Early and ongoing assessment, recognition of maternal high-risk factors, antenatal testing and interpretation, followed by appropriate interventions and patient education, are the keys to reducing the occurrence of poor fetal outcome and improving prenatal care.

REFERENCES

1. Babson, G., and Benson, R.: Management of high-risk pregnancy and intensive care of the neonate, St. Louis, 1971, The C. V. Mosby Co.
2. Butler, J. M., and Parer, J. T.: Is intensive intrapartum monitoring necessary? J. Obstet. Gynecol. Nurs. **5:**4s, 1976.
3. Chapman, N. L.: Antepartum assessment; the oxytocin challenge test and nonstressed heart rate testing, J. Obstet. Gynecol. Nurs. **5:**74s, 1976.
4. Chez, R. A.: The oxytocin challenge test, Contemp. Obstet. Gynecol. **6:**29, 1975.
5. Holey, E. S.: Promoting adequate weight gain in pregnant women, Am. J. Maternal-child Nurs. **2:** 86, 1977.
6. Jones, M. B.: Antepartum assessment in high-risk pregnancy, J. Obstet. Gynecol. Nurs. **4:**23, 1975.
7. Lerch, C.: Maternity nursing, ed. 2, St. Louis, 1974, The C. V. Mosby Co.
8. Ohio State University High-risk Perinatal Project; high-risk factors, Columbus, Ohio, 1976, Ohio State University.
9. Wilson, J. G.: Environment and birth defects, New York, 1973, Academic Press, Inc.

ADDITIONAL READINGS

American College of Obstetrics and Gynecology: Fetal heart rate monitoring; guidelines for monitoring, terminology, and instrumentation, A.C.O.G. Technology Bulletin No. 32, Sept./Oct., 1976, The College.
Galloway, K. G.: Placental evaluation studies; the procedures, their purposes, and the nursing care involved, part 2, Am. J. Maternal-child Nurs. **1:**300, 1976.
Martin, C. B., and Gengerich, B.: Uteroplacental physiology, J. Obstet. Gynecol. Nurs. **5:**16s-25s, 1976.
Sahin, S. T.: The multifaceted role of the nurse as a genetic counselor, Am. J. Maternal-child Nurs. **1:**211, 1976.

CHAPTER 10

Care of the newborn

LUELLA STEIL

Although the basic principles of modern newborn care were first established in the 1890s by a French obstetrician, Pierre Budin, it has not been until the last 15 years that the field of neonatology has developed into an entity of its own.[10] Historically, there was an attitude of resigned acceptance of high neonatal mortality. This attitude has now changed to one of concern not only for survival but for the quality of survival. Fortunately, there is growing evidence that as survival rates have been improved by techniques, the quality of survival has also been improved. Before the advent of neonatal intensive care units, about 85% of babies in the birth-weight range of 500 to 2,000 gm who managed to survive had some neurological or intellectual impairments, such as mental retardation. Follow-up data on survivors of modern neonatal intensive care show that 85% test normal.[16]

The nurse has an important role in the improvement of neonatal mortality and morbidity. The nurse is the one member of the health care team who is with the patient for an extended period of time and is responsible for making the majority of observations and carrying out prescribed therapy. Because of this unique position as a major contributor to the care of the newborn, the nurse must have adequate knowledge and understanding of the principles of newborn care so that accurate judgments can be made with confidence. Thus, the neonatal nurse has the responsibility of helping to reduce the incidence of mental retardation by contributing to its prevention in the perinatal period.

Although the etiology of mental retardation is not always identifiable, there are certain factors during the perinatal period that are already known to result in this condition. For example, fetal hypoxia, inappropriate resuscitation, or improper thermoregulation may result in brain damage. This chapter focuses on delineating the proper techniques that should be utilized to prevent mental retardation or other handicapping conditions. The newborn is not really new but just newly born. The status of the infant admitted to the newborn nursery from the delivery room is dependent on the complex interplay of genetic, intrauterine, intrapartal, and other maternal factors, as well as the kind of obstetric, pediatric, and nursing care that has been given.[6] The care of the newborn actually begins before conception and includes prenatal, intrapartal, and postnatal phases of the childbearing cycle. The previous chapter discusses the importance of prenatal care in the prevention of perinatal mortality and morbidity. Therefore, this chapter begins with labor and delivery room care and includes care of the newborn in the hospital nursery. It does not cover all aspects of fetal and newborn care or go into detail concerning specific diseases. It does, however, deal with those principles of care that have a major effect on neonatal mortality and morbidity, particularly mental retardation. Although methods of application may differ with individual situations, the principles are the same for both the normal and high-risk patient.

CARE OF THE NEWBORN IN LABOR AND DELIVERY

The goal of labor and delivery room nursing is the delivery of a healthy baby to a healthy mother in a safe and satisfying manner. A high-risk pregnancy is one that has the potential for producing death or disability of mother or fetus.[10] Knowing those factors that make a pregnancy high risk and knowing what might occur when these factors present themselves enable the nurse to anticipate what problems might occur during the birth process and thus be prepared to deal with them as soon as possible. In obstetrics, early intervention assures a more successful outcome of pregnancy and reduces the incidence of mentally and physically handicapping conditions in the newborn. Table 10-1 is a list of maternal high-risk factors.

Care of the fetus during labor

The progress that has been made in obstetrics toward the reduction of maternal mortality and morbidity has not been matched by similar results in perinatal mortality and morbidity. This lack of improvement in perinatal mortality and morbidity is an indication of the limited value of the classical criteria for evaluating the status of labor to determine fetal stress.[15] These traditional observations have been concerned

Table 10-1. High-risk pregnancy factors*

Patient	Medical history	Previous pregnancy history	Pregnancy-related medical conditions (past or present)
Teenage (<16 at conception)	Hypertension	Grand multiparity	Toxemia
Elderly (>40 at conception)	Renal disease	Previous surgical delivery	Bleeding after 12 weeks' gestation
Underweight or overweight (2 SD† from mean when compared to standard chart appropriate for race and/or ethnic group)	Diabetes	Previous prolonged labor (>24 hours)	Multiple pregnancy (present)
	Cancer	Previous fetal loss	Abnormal presentation or position of fetus (present)
	Thyroid disease	Previous live premature infant	Hydramnios
	Cardiovascular disease	Previous infant death in first week of life	General anesthesia during pregnancy
Low socioeconomic status	Rh sensitization	Previous "damaged" infant (birth trauma, cerebral palsy, mental retardation, etc.)	Administration of certain drugs to mother (propylthiouracil)
	Tuberculosis		Anemia (Hb <8 gm/100 ml)
	Lupus erythematosus		Indifference to health needs (multiple missed appointments, failure to follow recommendations)
	Mental retardation		
	Alcoholic or narcotic addict		
	Major psychoses		
	Neurologic disease		
	Severe anemia (sickle-cell, thalassemia)		

*From Klaus, M. H., and Fanaroff, A. A.: Care of the high-risk neonate, Philadelphia, 1973, W. B. Saunders Co.
†SD = Standard Deviation.

with the duration of labor: frequency, duration, and quality of labor contractions as determined by the examiner's hand; intermittent auscultation of fetal heart tones; presence or absence of meconium in the amniotic fluid; maternal blood pressure; and presence or absence of vaginal bleeding. The only observations that could still be considered of any value are the latter two. Both maternal hypotension and vaginal bleeding lead to fetal hypoxia and possible subsequent brain damage.

From the standpoint of the fetus, the defined normal duration of labor for the primigravida and multiparous patient is unacceptable. For example, if the fetus is already compromised by a maternal complication, such as diabetes mellitus or Rh isoimmunization, it may not be able to tolerate even a few minutes of labor. Therefore, normal labor should be defined as that degree of labor that is not hazardous to fetal well-being.[2]

Recently, divergent opinions have been expressed concerning the passage of meconium in utero. Traditionally, it has been thought to be due to a hyperperistaltic response of the bowel and anal sphincter relaxation in response to hypoxia. Hon has suggested, however, that it could be due to vagal hypertonus rather than hypoxia. The increased incidence of perinatal morbidity with the presence of meconium may be due more to intrapartum aspiration.[15] However, the presence of meconium in the amniotic fluid should continue to be considered a sign of possible fetal distress and suggests closer monitoring of the fetus.

If auscultation of the fetal heart is carried out every 15 minutes, counted for 30 seconds, and then averaged to express the beats per minute, only 3% of available information is obtained.[15] Fig. 10-1 points out this fact very explicitly. In addition, it is difficult, if not impossible, to evaluate fetal response to the stress of a contraction. Also, in an evaluation of more than 24,000 labors, it was found that intermittent auscultation of fetal heart tones was of no value in determining early fetal distress.[15] The advent of continuous electronic monitoring has made it possible to record the fetal heart rate in relation to the intensity and duration of uterine contractions. This gives the physician and nurse a more accurate evaluation of fetal status and labor process.

External (indirect) monitoring consists of the application of sensing devices to the maternal abdomen. These devices, known as transducers, detect uterine contractions and fetal heart tones and translate them into electrical impulses that are recorded on graph paper. The external method of monitoring is used when the membranes have not ruptured and the cervix is not dilated.[2]

Internal (direct) monitoring is a more efficient means of obtaining fetal heart rate and uterine contraction data. This is accomplished by the application of an electrode to the fetal scalp and the introduction of a polyethylene catheter, filled with sterile water, into the uterus by the transcervical route. As with external monitoring, the fetal heart rate and uterine contractions are recorded on graph paper. Internal monitoring is used when the membranes have been ruptured, and the cervix is at least 1 cm dilated.[2]

The graph produced by the fetal monitor permits the assessment of fetal heart rate in

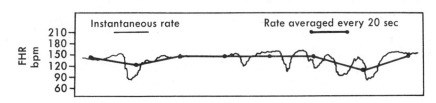

Fig. 10-1. Auscultation of fetal heart versus beat-to-beat recording. (From Hon, E. H.: An atlas of fetal heart rate patterns, 1968, New Haven, Conn., Harty Press.)

relation to the intensity and duration of uterine contractions. Changes in fetal heart rate patterns are divided into two categories: changes related to contractions and changes not related to contractions. The fetal heart rate may stay the same, accelerate, or decelerate with uterine contractions. Acceleration and deceleration patterns may occur unrelated to the uterine contractions. Although fetal heart rate accelerations have not been studied extensively, there is indication that they may give some evidence of fetal status. Accelerations associated with each uterine contraction seem to be the earliest sign of fetal distress. They often precede the development of a later deceleration pattern that is associated with fetal hypoxia. Variable accelerations or those occurring without any relationship to uterine contractions are probably associated with fetal movement.[2]

The most important patterns for consideration in management of labor and delivery are the deceleration type. There are three basic patterns, illustrated in Fig. 10-2. The early deceleration pattern is recognized by the fact that the onset begins at the same time as the uterine contractions, and the fetal heart rate returns to its previous baseline at the end of the contraction. This pattern is thought to be due to head compression and has not been associated with depressed or acidotic fetuses. When the pattern of deceleration begins late in the contracting phase of the uterus and returns to baseline after the contraction is over, it is called a late deceleration pattern. It is thought to be associated with uteroplacental insufficiency and has been associated with fetal acidosis and death. Variable decelerations occur with no regular relationship to the uterine contractions, are considered to be due to cord compression, and can be associated with fetal asphyxia and death.[2]

Continuous changes in the baseline heart rate provide less information about fetal status but should be viewed with suspicion if tachycardia (greater than 160 beats per minute) or bradycardia (less than 120 beats per minute) occurs. Fluctuations in the baseline

pattern are referred to as the beat-to-beat variability. A loss of beat-to-beat variability may also indicate a problem. The frequent underlying causes of these problems are: excessive uterine activity, maternal fever, hypotension and drugs, fetal asphyxia, and immaturity of the fetal nervous system.[2]

When the technique of electronic fetal monitoring was first introduced, it was used primarily for those obstetrical cases identified as high risk. However, there is growing evidence that possibly all patients in labor should receive the benefits of fetal monitoring. In studies conducted by C. J. Hobel and associates, it was shown that 30% of a low-risk obstetric group had to be reclassified as high-risk in labor, and the babies of this group did poorer on developmental testing at 1 year of age than did the babies of high-risk mothers who had low-risk labors. Other studies have shown that 25% of fetuses who have difficulty in labor cannot be predicted on the basis of prenatal high-risk identification.[15] Data such as these are leading to a strong opinion among professionals that all fetuses are at risk during the stress of labor and that they should receive the same modern surveillance that adults receive in life-threatening situations.

Electronic fetal monitoring has not been in use long enough to determine its effects on long-term morbidity. There are not yet any follow-up programs on newborns and infants who were monitored as fetuses.[2] However, studies have indicated a lowering of fetal mortality with use of fetal monitoring. Also, the same fetal heart patterns that indicate fetal hypoxia in human fetuses have been demonstrated in animal studies. In these studies, when the fetal hypoxia was permitted to persist, the fetal animal developed brain damage similar to that found in humans.[2] From this data, it can be assumed that fetal monitoring allows for early detection of fetal hypoxia, permitting appropriate intervention to alleviate it, and thus preventing brain damage and mental retardation.

The utilization of fetal monitoring in the labor room often depends on the nurse's will-

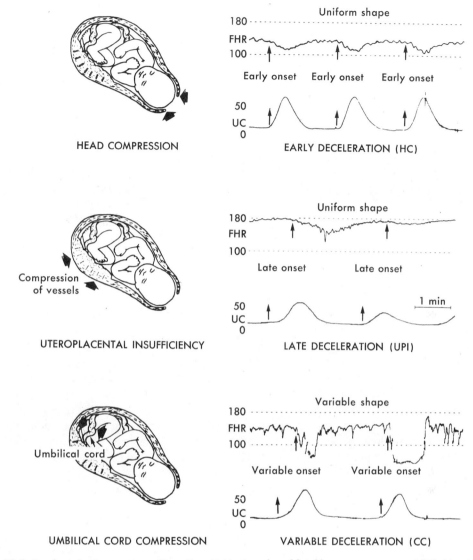

HEAD COMPRESSION — EARLY DECELERATION (HC)

Uniform shape
180
FHR
100
Early onset   Early onset   Early onset
50
UC
0

UTEROPLACENTAL INSUFFICIENCY — LATE DECELERATION (UPI)

Uniform shape
180
FHR
100
Late onset   Late onset
50
UC
0
1 min

Compression of vessels

UMBILICAL CORD COMPRESSION — VARIABLE DECELERATION (CC)

Variable shape
180
FHR
100
Variable onset   Variable onset
50
UC
0

Umbilical cord

Fig. 10-2. Fetal monitoring patterns. (From Hon, E. H.: An atlas of fetal heart rate patterns, 1968, New Haven, Conn., Harty Press.)

ingness to accept and use it. There are hospitals equipped to do fetal monitoring whose monitor is not used. Lack of knowledge interferes most with the acceptance of monitoring. Thus, it is important that both the medical and nursing staff receive education in its use. In-service education programs are available at most institutions that use the monitoring device. Classroom teaching is followed by supervised clinical experience. The collection of sample tracings in a notebook kept in the obstetric department is useful in providing practice for staff in reading fetal monitor tracings.[5] Once the staff becomes comfortable with the procedure, utilization increases.

Equipped with knowledge of fetal monitoring, nurses have the responsibility of knowing what to do with it. Nurses trained to recognize an abnormal fetal heart rate have the opportunity to avert tragedy or to be prepared before it occurs. When an ominous pattern occurs, the nurse notifies the physician and takes the following corrective measures:

1. Changes the patient's position to either relieve the pressure on the umbilical cord or to correct supine hypertension. (Left lateral position is preferable.)
2. Elevates the patient's legs to correct maternal hypotension due to causes other than the vena cava syndrome (supine hypotension).
3. Administers oxygen by way of a face mask.
4. If oxytocin is being used to induce or stimulate labor, discontinues the infusion.
5. Is prepared for an operative delivery.

Often, conservative treatment corrects the situation, and operative delivery is avoided.[2]

When the fetal monitor is used, it is important to nurse the patient and not the machine. The monitor does not replace the personal care a nurse gives to the patient but frees the nurse to give more direct care to the mother. Since women in labor are often anxious and frightened, explanations of procedures should be given. Any family member or support person who is present should also be included when explanations are given. The purpose of fetal monitoring and how it is done should be thoroughly explained. Luckner demonstrated in an unpublished study that the majority of patients and their families responded favorably to fetal monitoring when adequate nursing support was given.[12]

Currently, monitoring of all fetuses in labor is not possible, but it is a goal toward which to work. Improvement in machinery and techniques is continually being researched and developed. As the equipment used to monitor labor becomes more compact, easier to use, and more comfortable for the patient, its use will increase. The commitment of the obstetrician, the obstetrical nurse, and the hospital administrator to improved quality of care for the fetus will also increase use of the electronic fetal monitor. This kind of commitment can be seen in community hospitals where nurses with

proper training have assumed the major responsibilities for carrying out both direct and indirect fetal heart monitoring.[5]

The sampling of fetal scalp blood is another technique for diagnosing fetal distress. Biochemical evaluation of the blood for the pH is of value in the detection of fetal hypoxia. The use of this technique is more involved than fetal heart rate monitoring. It is intermittent, requires skill to perform, and requires the continuous availability of a biochemical technician. Currently, the use of fetal scalp blood sampling in concurrence with fetal monitoring is available only in high-risk perinatal centers. Fortunately, there is a strong correlation between the fetal scalp blood pH and fetal heart rate patterns. As fetal heart rate patterns become more ominous, fetal acidosis increases.

There is some additional basic knowledge required to aid the nurse in the anticipation, recognition, treatment, and prevention of problems during labor. This includes having an adequate understanding of the principles of human reproduction, the mechanisms of labor, the concepts of prepared childbirth, and the nursing process.[6] By understanding the normal, the nurse can more easily recognize the abnormal. Knowledge of the prepared methods of childbirth permits the nurse to more adequately support prepared patients and promote use of the methods by unprepared patients through on-the-spot teaching. This has the effect of reducing the amount of analgesia and anesthesia needed that could adversely affect the fetus. The use of the nursing process permits the nurse to assess each patient as an individual and plan appropriate care rather than force the patient to adhere to rigid routines.

Delivery room care of the newborn

Even though many problems can be anticipated through high-risk identification in labor, not all delivery room emergencies can be predicted. Any hospital that assumes the responsibility for obstetrical care must provide a properly equipped delivery room service and an adequately trained professional staff who can deal efficiently and effectively with any crisis when it occurs. In the provision of adequate staff, it must be remembered that maternal and newborn complications can occur simultaneously, and appropriate resuscitation measures require two or more people.[10]

Aspects of care of the newborn in the delivery room that influence its long-term outcome are: establishment and maintenance of respirations, prevention of hypothermia, and assessment and continued monitoring of the cardiovascular system. The process of being born and going from an intrauterine environment to an extrauterine environment is a major change for the newborn. It is a complex process that involves changes in organ systems and metabolic processes. Too often this fact is overlooked, particularly in the case of the "normal newborn." The strong cry of the infant immediately after birth brings sighs of relief from delivery room personnel, and this, coupled with a good Apgar score, leads to the assumption that it is a healthy infant. Little else is done to assess the status of the newborn, causing the danger that important information may be overlooked.[4] The attitude that all newborns are well until proved ill should be changed to state that all newborns are ill until proved well. This would lead to more thorough observation and assessment of newborns during the critical time of adjustment after delivery.

Because pediatricians are rarely available in the delivery room, the responsibility for initial observation, assessment, and immediate care frequently becomes the responsibility of the delivery room nurse.[18] Therefore, the delivery room nurse must have an adequate understanding of the process by which respirations are established, knowledge of thermal regulation, and the ability to recognize normal and abnormal conditions in order to assist the newborn through this most critical time of life. Some hospitals are beginning to employ a highly skilled neonatal nurse specialist to provide more comprehensive care to newborns in the delivery room and newborn nursery. This person is a registered nurse who has re-

Table 10-2. Apgar score*

Sign	Score		
	0	1	2
Heart rate	Absent	Below 100	Over 100
Respiratory effort	Absent	Weak, irregular	Good, crying
Muscle tone	Flaccid	Some flexion of extremities	Well flexed
Reflex irritability (catheter in nose)	No response	Grimace	Cough or sneeze
Color	Blue, pale	Body pink, extremities blue	Completely pink

*From Klaus, M. H., and Fanaroff, A. A.: Care of the high-risk neonate, Philadelphia, 1973, W. B. Saunders Co.

ceived extra training in newborn care, is capable of managing the care of the normal newborn, and can make appropriate referrals to physicians.

Apgar scoring. The Apgar score is a systematic assessment of the condition of the newborn at 1 minute and at 5 minutes after birth. It consists of an evaluation of heart rate, respiratory effort, muscle tone, reflex irritability, and color. Table 10-2 illustrates the Apgar system. The 1-minute Apgar score is of value in determining the presence or absence of asphyxia as well as giving some clue to the degree of asphyxia. The 5-minute Apgar score has proved to be a reliable predictor of long-term outcome.

The person who is providing care to the newborn is the one who should assign the Apgar score. The assessment requires physical contact with the infant. It is therefore impossible for an obstetrician to assign the score while repairing an episiotomy. The use of an automatic timer is helpful in reminding the person giving care to do the assessment at 1 minute and at 5 minutes. Posting of Apgar charts over the newborn cribs is another tool used in assuring accuracy of the evaluation.

Additional research is needed to clearly understand how respiration is initiated in the newborn. A combination of factors is thought to be involved. The slightly acidotic state of the newborn at the time of delivery has a stimulating effect on the respiratory centers in the medulla. The transition from a warm, watery environment to a cold, air environment is probably stimulating to the functions of respiration. The thoracic cage of the fetus is compressed while passing through the birth canal. It is believed that the recoil of the chest wall that occurs after delivery produces a small passive inspiration of air and subsequently leads to the first active breaths. In any event, if respiration does not begin soon after birth, active intervention is needed to avert brain damage.

Resuscitation. To provide adequate resuscitation measures, it is important to understand the pathophysiology of asphyxia. During asphyxia, the newborn is in a state of hypoxia and metabolic and respiratory acidosis. Fig. 10-3 shows the physiological changes that occurred during asphyxiation and resuscitation of rhesus monkey fetuses. It demonstrates that two kinds of apnea occur during asphyxia. Rapid gasps occur shortly after the onset of asphyxia and are followed by a period of primary apnea. During this phase respirations can be induced by sensory stimulation, and the heart rate drops. Primary apnea is followed by a series of deep gasps that gradually weaken and terminate with the last gasp, and secondary apnea occurs. During secondary apnea, respiration cannot be induced by sensory stimulation. Active resuscitation measures are required to prevent death. How long it takes to resuscitate depends on how soon resuscitation measures are begun after the last gasp. For every 1 minute between last gasp and onset of resuscitation, there are about 2 minutes to the first gasp and 4 minutes to the onset of rhythmic breathing.[10] This is an important concept to remember during resuscitation. Time seemingly passes slowly during an emergency, and there is

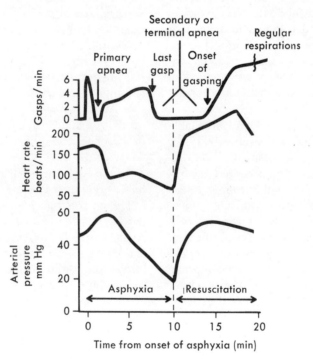

Fig. 10-3. Changes during asphyxiation of rhesus monkey. (From Klaus, M. H., and Faranoff, A. A.: Care of the high-risk neonate, Philadelphia, 1973, W. B. Saunders Co.)

often the tendency to stop resuscitation measures too soon.

Even though it is difficult to determine if an apneic newborn is in primary or secondary apnea, the Apgar score can be used as an estimate of degrees of asphyxia and to help determine what intervention is necessary. A newborn with an Apgar score of 7 or above rarely needs any resuscitation and should be kept warm and closely observed. An Apgar score between 3 and 6 usually indicates mild to moderate asphyxia and generally requires brief suctioning followed by bag and mask ventilation with oxygen for a short period of time before the infant's condition improves. If the Apgar score is below 3, aggressive resuscitation measures are needed.[10]

The steps taken to resuscitate an asphyxiated newborn are the same as for any asphyxiated person. The airway is cleared, and then ventilatory support is given, followed by circulatory support and correction of the metabolic acidosis. Important principles to remember in the provision of newborn resuscitation include gentle and brief suctioning of the airway. Valuable time can be wasted, and prolonged deep suctioning can produce a vagal response of bradycardia or cardiac arrhythmias.[7] If meconium-stained amniotic fluid is present, suctioning should be done under direct visualization with a laryngoscope. This assures clearing the airway of meconium to prevent it from being pushed into the lungs when positive pressure ventilation is applied.[2]

Ventilation can be done with either a pressure-controlled ventilator or ventilation bag. Both devices can be used with either a tight-fitting face mask or an endotracheal tube along with oxygen. In most cases, bag and mask ventilation is sufficient to bring about results. The rate of ventilation should be approximately fifty times per minute. When this method is used, an orogastric tube should be passed into the stomach to prevent overdistention with air.[2] If bag and mask ventilation does not improve the situation by evidence of an increasing heart rate, endotracheal intubation may be needed.[10]

However, an inexperienced person should not attempt to perform endotracheal intubation, because valuable time can be lost with unsuccessful attempts. The infant can be sustained with bag and mask ventilation until further assistance can be obtained. Endotracheal intubation is rarely resorted to at New York hospitals, for example, and infants rarely suffer any complications.[1]

Since there is no time to determine blood gas values, if a newborn has a 1-minute Apgar score of between 1 and 3 or has failed to respond to artificial ventilation, it is assumed that acidosis is present, and sodium bicarbonate should be infused by way of an umbilical vein catheter. An alternative method is to use a No. 25 scalp vein needle to provide infusion into the umbilical vein.[1] The usual dosage of sodium bicarbonate is 3 mEq/kg diluted with equal volumes of sterile water. If the heart rate continues to fall after these measures have been taken, then 1 to 2 ml of 1:10,000 epinephrine should be given into the umbilical vein. If the heart rate is absent or below 50 beats per minute, external cardiac massage should be started.[2]

Throughout the resuscitation procedure, the newborn should be kept warm. The newborn should be dried off immediately after delivery to prevent evaporative heat losses and placed under an overhead radiant warmer. The overhead warmer provides warmth while at the same time allowing easy access to the infant. Attempts should be made to identify the cause of asphyxia. The amount of narcotic the mother received during labor should be considered to determine if the infant needs to receive a narcotic antagonist, such as nalorphine (Nalline) hydrochloride or naloxone hydrochloride (Narcan). Stimulating drugs have no place in the treatment of neonatal asphyxia. All resuscitated newborns should be observed closely for any complications, such as pneumothorax, convulsions, and meconium aspiration. They should be monitored closely until blood gas values and vital signs are normal.[1]

The newborn infant is able to tolerate asphyxia better than an adult. This is probably due to the lower metabolic requirements of the immature brain. However, prolonged hypoxia will eventually overcome any compensatory mechanisms, and brain damage or death will occur.[10] Therefore, it is important to have a delivery room staffed with personnel trained to provide prompt and adequate resuscitation to prevent or minimize brain damage in the newborn. Nurses assigned to the delivery room should seek education and training that would enable them to deal with any situation that may occur. They also have the responsibility of assuring that the equipment and drugs needed for newborn resuscitation are kept readily available, are in good repair, and are in appropriate sizes and dosages for the newborn.

CARE OF THE NEWBORN IN THE NURSERY

All too frequently following admission to the newborn nursery, the infant has fallen into a period of limbo in which it is nobody's baby.[10] Several hours, or even a day, may elapse before the baby is seen by a pediatrician. If the infant appears normal, it may not be observed closely by the nursing staff.[4] The majority of neonatal deaths occur in special care nurseries; however, the majority of neonatal disease occurs in the normal, or limbo, nursery. It is estimated that 50% of all newborns have special problems and require close observation. Closer observation of all newborns leads to earlier detection and treatment of conditions that could have a damaging effect on the quality of survival.[18]

This realization of the need to more closely observe the newborn has led to the establishment of a transitional care nursery to which newborns are admitted directly from the delivery room. Here, under close surveillance by trained personnel, the infant is kept until a smooth transition has been accomplished, at which point transfer to a normal nursery or rooming-in setting is made. If during this time the newborn develops any complications, it is transferred to an appropriate intensive care setting.[10]

The growing shortage of physicians makes it impossible to have 24-hour in-house coverage in the transitional care nursery. Therefore, the nurse's role can be expanded in this setting to include activities that have traditionally been delegated to the physician. Nurses educated in the skills of physical examination and screening techniques help to fill the gap between delivery room care and the time when the newborn is first seen by a pediatrician.[4]

Not all aspects of routine nursery care are covered in this section. Only those aspects of newborn care that represent the greatest amount of change in theory, practice, and attitude over the last 15 years are discussed. These topics are gestational age assessment, thermal regulation, oxygen therapy, and newborn feeding. The changing trends in practice in these four areas have had positive effects on neonatal mortality and morbidity and probably contribute to prevention of mental retardation.

Gestational age assessment

One activity that is not routinely conducted on all newborn infants is gestational age assessment. Many "normal" newborns therefore slip through the newborn nursery with undetected clinical problems. Also, clinical problems that could be anticipated through the use of this assessment catch the nursery personnel off guard when they occur. It is important that all newborns be assessed for gestational age so that early detection can lead to early intervention in an effort to prevent long-term morbidity. With practice, the assessment is easy to do, and the nurse can be taught its technique.[4]

Prematurity in the past was based on birth weight alone. Infants weighing less than 2,500 gm were classified as premature. Those weighing over 2,500 gm were considered as term babies. When it was discovered that one-third of infants born with a birth weight of less than 2,500 gm were really undergrown term babies, the importance of relating birth weight to gestation and the need for a more appropriate classification of the newborn were recognized.[2] The clinical problems of the preterm infant are different from those of the intrauterine growth retarded infant, and the infant who is preterm but weighs the same as a term peer will also have different needs.[10]

It is now possible to categorize an infant according to weight and assessed gestational age using standard intrauterine growth charts and methods utilizing criteria based on the infant. The categories by weight are: appropriate for gestational age (AGA), small for gestational age (SGA), and large for gestational age (LGA). An infant is considered preterm, or premature, if born before 37

weeks' gestation, term if born between 37 and 42 weeks' gestation, and postterm if born after 42 weeks' gestation.[2] These parameters are determined by assessing the gestational age of the infant and plotting its weight on an intrauterine growth chart (Fig. 10-4). If the birth weight falls on or above the ninetieth percentile, the infant is considered LGA. If the birth weight falls below the tenth percentile, the infant is categorized as being SGA. If the birth weight is between the tenth and ninetieth percentiles, the infant is AGA. Fig. 10-5 gives an example of two in-

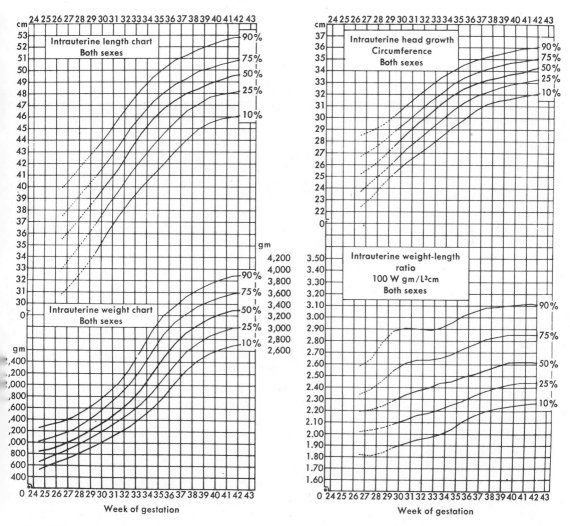

Fig. 10-4. Colorado intrauterine growth charts. (From Klaus, M. H., and Faranoff, A. A.: Care of the high-risk neonate, Philadelphia, 1973, W. B. Saunders Co.)

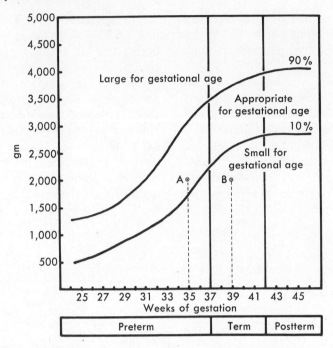

Fig. 10-5. Classification of newborn. (From Klaus, M. H., and Faranoff, A. A.: Care of the high-risk neonate, Philadelphia, 1973, W. B. Saunders Co.)

fants of the same weight who fall into different categories. Infant *A* is preterm and AGA. Infant *B* is term and SGA.

In order to determine gestational age, it is necessary to use one of several tools that have been developed over the past 15 years. Obstetrical measurements, such as date of the last menstrual period, fundal height, and quickening, may not always be accurate. Thus, it is necessary to use a method based on the infant. Studies by a group of French physicians under the direction of Minkowski have resulted in the use of a neurological evaluation to determine gestational age.[2] The method has been described by Dr. Amiel-Tison, and judgment of gestational age is made on the basis of posture, passive range of motion, active tone, righting reactions, and a variety of reflexes. Unfortunately, this method requires the infant to be alert and vigorous; thus, it is not always possible to do on the first day of life (when it is

needed most) due to depression, asphyxia, or neurological damage.[10]

Mitchell, Farr, and Dubowitz in England and Usher in Canada have used various external physical characteristics to determine gestational age.[2] Certain physical characteristics appear with progressing gestational age and are unaffected by intrauterine disease, such as growth retardation. The external physical characteristics can also be evaluated regardless of the condition of the infant at birth.

A scoring system that combines the neurological evaluation and the physical characteristics has been developed by Dubowitz and associates. Ballard has developed an abbreviated version of the Dubowitz system (Fig. 10-6). She has included in her scoring system only those neurological parameters that do not require an alert, vigorous infant. In addition, it is simple and practical to use.[10] With practice,

NEUROMUSCULAR MATURITY

	0	1	2	3	4	5
Posture						
Square window (wrist)	90°	60°	45°	30°	0°	
Arm recoil	180°		100°-180°	90°-100°	<90°	
Popliteal angle	180°	160°	130°	110°	90°	<90°
Scarf sign						
Heel to ear						

Apgars _____ 1 min _____ 5 min

Age at Exam _____ hrs

Race _____ Sex _____

B.D. _____

LMP _____

EDC _____

Gest. age by Dates _____ wks

Gest. age by Exam _____ wks

B.W. _____ gm _____ %ile

Length _____ cm _____ %ile

Head Circum. _____ cm _____ %ile

Clin. Dist. None_____ Mild _____

Mod. _____ Severe _____

PHYSICAL MATURITY

Skin	gelatinous red, transparent	smooth pink, visible veins	superficial peeling &/or rash few veins	cracking pale area rare veins	parchment deep cracking no vessels	leathery cracked wrinkled
Lanugo	none	abundant	thinning	bald areas	mostly bald	
Plantar Creases	no crease	faint red marks	anterior transverse crease only	creases ant. 2/3	creases cover entire sole	
Breast	barely percept.	flat areola no bud	stippled areola 1–2 mm bud	raised areola 3–4 mm bud	full areola 5–10 mm bud	
Ear	pinna flat, stays folded	sl. curved pinna; soft with slow recoil	well-curv. pinna; soft but ready recoil	formed & firm with instant recoil	thick cartilage ear stiff	
Genitals ♂	scrotum empty no rugae		testes descending, few rugae	testes down good rugae	testes pendulous deep rugae	
Genitals ♀	prominent clitoris & labia minora		majora & minora equally prominent	majora large minora small	clitoris & minora completely covered	

MATURITY RATING

Score	Wks
5	26
10	28
15	30
20	32
25	34
30	36
35	38
40	40
45	42
50	44

Fig. 10-6. Assessment of gestational age. (From Klaus, M. H., and Faranoff, A. A.: Care of the high-risk neonate, Philadelphia, 1973, W. B. Saunders Co.)

the nurse can learn to incorporate this assessment into the rest of the procedures performed on the newborn upon admission to the nursery. The nurse evaluates the newborn according to each one of the categories in the left-hand column and circles the result. The numbers at the top of each column are the value for the column. On completion of the evaluation, the nurse totals the scores for each circle and determines gestational age according to the maturity rating in the lower right-hand corner. Table 10-3 describes the neurological evaluation. The physical characteristics are self-explanatory.

Although this neurological assessment and other methods of gestational age assessment have an accuracy of only plus or minus 2 weeks, they are valuable tools in helping to anticipate, recognize, and treat

clinical problems in the newborn.[15] For example, hypoglycemia, pulmonary aspiration, and congenital anomalies are more common in SGA infants. Hyaline membrane disease and hyperbilirubinemia are more common in preterm, SGA infants. LGA infants in all categories are often infants of diabetic mothers and are prone to early onset of hypoglycemia. It is therefore important that all newborns are evaluated physically and neurologically as soon as possible after birth.[10] In order to meet this criteria, the nurse should be prepared to conduct gestational age assessment. In doing so, the nurse can identify infants who are at risk due to prematurity or discrepancy in weight for gestational age and alert the physician to facilitate early treatment in order to prevent handicapping conditions, such as mental retardation.[14]

Table 10-3. Techniques of neurological assessment*

Posture

With the infants supine and quiet, score as follows:
0 = arms and legs extended
1 = slight or moderate flexion of hips and knees
2 = moderate to strong flexion of hips and knees
3 = legs flexed and abducted, arms slightly flexed
4 = full flexion of arms and legs

Square window

Flex the hand at the wrist. Exert pressure sufficient to get as much flexion as possible. The angle between the hypothenar emenence and the anterior aspect of the forearm is measured and scored according to Fig. 10-6. Do not rotate the wrist.

Arm recoil

With the infant supine, fully flex the forearm for 5 seconds, then fully extend by pulling the hands and release. Score the reaction according to:
0 = remain extended or random movements
1 = incomplete or partial flexion
2 = brisk return to full flexion

Popliteal angle

With the infant supine and the pelvis flat on the examining surface, the leg is flexed on the thigh and the thigh fully flexed with the use of one hand. With the other hand, the leg is then extended and the angle attained scored as in Fig. 10-6.

Heel to ear maneuver

With the infant supine, hold the infant's foot with one hand and move it as near to the head as possible without forcing it. Keep the pelvis flat on the examining surface. Score as in Fig. 10-6.

Scarf sign

With the infant supine, take the infant's hand and draw it across the neck and as far across the opposite shoulder as possible. Assistance to the elbow is permissible by lifting it across the body. Score according to the location of the elbow:
0 = elbow reaches the opposite anterior axillary line
1 = elbow between opposite anterior axillary line and midline of thorax
2 = elbow at midline of thorax
3 = elbow does not reach midline of thorax

*Adapted from Klaus, M. H., and Fanaroff, A. A.: Care of the high-risk neonate, Philadelphia, 1973, W. B. Saunders Co.

Thermal regulation

Maintenance of the newborn in a proper thermal environment increases survival rates. Budin recognized the importance of temperature control in 1907. He had observed a higher survival rate among infants whose body temperature was maintained within a normal range.[10] However, it was not until the past 2 decades that an understanding of the physiology of thermoregulation in the newborn was developed. The newborn is now recognized as a homeotherm, capable of maintaining body temperature at a constant level despite changes in the environmental temperature. Reptiles, such as turtles, are examples of poikilotherms. Unlike homeotherms, they adjust their body temperatures to that of the environment.[10]

Body temperature is the measurement of the balance between heat production and heat lost to the environment. In cool environments, heat production increases; in warm environments, heat loss increases. The range of environmental temperature over which a newborn can maintain body temperature is severely restricted when compared with the adult. The newborn has decreased protection against heat loss due to a thinner layer of subcutaneous fat and, when compared with weight, a larger skin surface area. The adult can effectively increase heat production by increasing voluntary muscle activity or by shivering, an involuntary muscle activity. Heat loss can be increased by sweating. The adult also has the options of altering the environment or leaving it. The newborn cannot effectively shiver or sweat, nor does the newborn have the ability to control its own environment.[2, 13]

Probably the most important mechanism by which the newborn increases heat production is nonshivering thermogenesis. This is the increase in oxygen consumption and heat production in response to a cold environment. It is thought that the main energy source for this activity is the presence of brown fat. It is more abundant in the newborn, found at the base of the neck, between the scapulae, in the mediastinum, and surrounding the kidneys and adrenal glands. Brown fat cells contain many fat vacuoles rather than a single fat vacuole, as found in white fat. It also has numerous mitochondria, the cell organelles that contain enzymes for metabolism. These facts, plus a rich sympathetic nerve and blood supply, contribute to the high metabolic rate of brown fat.[10] The amount of brown fat is probably inadequate to provide all the heat-producing needs of the cold-stressed newborn.[2]

The nurse has an important role in the provision of a safe environmental temperature for the newborn. It is the nurse who is in constant attendance and who is available to continually monitor the environment and the infant's responses. Even slight variations in environmental temperature can have an effect on the baby. In order to protect the newborn from undue stress, the nurse needs a thorough knowledge of the mechanisms of heat loss and how to maintain appropriate thermal environments to meet the individual needs of each newborn.

Heat transfer from the body surface to the environment involves four major routes: (1) radiation (2) convection, (3) conduction, and (4) evaporation. Radiation is the transfer of heat from the body to a cooler surface that is not in contact with the body, independent of air temperature. For example, the air temperature of an old house in the winter may be 80° F, but a person will still feel chilled because of radiation of body heat to the cooler outside walls. Convection is heat loss due to air currents flowing over the body. Conduction is heat transfer that occurs when a warm body is placed in direct contact with a cold surface. When a wet skin surface is exposed to dry air, evaporation occurs and heat is lost.

The range of environmental temperature in which a newborn with normal body temperature has minimal oxygen consumption, and thus a minimal metabolic rate, is called the neutral thermal environment or range of thermal neutrality.[2] Fig. 10-7 shows this range along with the effect of environmental temperature on oxygen consumption. It is

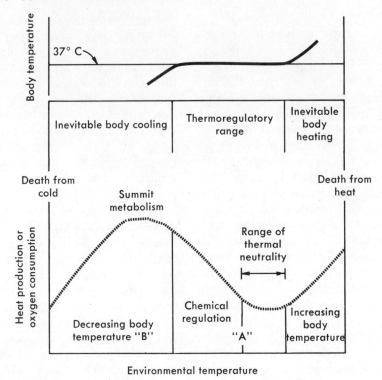

Fig. 10-7. Neonatal thermal environment. (From Klaus, M. H., and Faranoff, A. A.: Care of the high-risk neonate, Philadelphia, 1973, W. B. Saunders Co.)

important to note from this graph that the newborn is able to maintain a normal body temperature to a certain point in a cold environment. Thus, a normal body temperature is not an indication that the newborn is in a neutral thermal environment. No single temperature measurement can be used to determine adequate thermal protection. The temperatures of room air, the incubator, and the walls of the incubator must be considered. Also, no single range of environmental temperature is appropriate for all newborns. The neutral thermal range is individual, depending on size, age, and condition of the infant.[2] Table 10-4 is a general guide that can be used to estimate the neutral thermal environment when caring for an infant in an incubator. When this table is used, it should be noted that 1° C must be added to each temperature for every 7° by which the incubator air temperature exceeds the room temperature.[10]

It is of particular importance that hypothermia is avoided in the newborn. A negative thermal balance increases the incidence of hypoglycemia, metabolic acidosis, and reduced pulmonary perfusion in the infant.[2] In addition, it is difficult to rewarm a cold infant without producing apnea.[13] Hypoxia, secondary to apnea, may be a cause of central nervous system damage and mental retardation, particularly in the preterm infant.[9] Therefore, the nurse needs to be aware of situations that could cause hypothermia and to provide protection for the newborn. It is important to remember that the newborn does attempt to maintain a normal body temperature, but it does so at the expense of oxygen and calories that could be better used for physical and brain growth. Therefore, a newborn nursed outside the range of thermal neutrality has the potential of developing intellectual impairment.

Table 10-4. Neutral thermal environmental temperatures*

Age and weight	Starting temperature (°C)	Range of temperature (°C)	Age and weight	Starting temperature (°C)	Range of temperature (°C)
0-6 hours			72-96 hours		
Under 1,200 gm	35.0	34.0-35.4	Under 1,200 gm	34.0	34.0-35.0
1,200-1,500 gm	34.1	33.9-34.4	1,200-1,500 gm	33.5	33.0-34.0
1,501-2,500 gm	33.4	32.8-33.8	1,501-2,500 gm	32.2	31.1-33.2
Over 2,500			Over 2,500		
(and >36 weeks)	32.9	32.0-33.8	(and >36 weeks)	31.3	29.8-32.8
6-12 hours			4-12 days		
Under 1,200 gm	35.0	34.0-35.4	Under 1,500 gm	33.5	33.0-34.0
1,200-1,500 gm	34.0	33.5-34.4	1,501-2,500 gm	32.1	31.1-33.2
1,501-2,500 gm	33.1	32.2-33.8	Over 2,500		
Over 2,500			(and >36 weeks)		
(and >36 weeks)	32.8	31.4-33.8	4-5 days	31.0	29.5-32.6
12-24 hours			5-6 days	30.9	29.4-32.3
Under 1,200 gm	34.0	34.0-35.4	6-8 days	30.6	29.0-32.2
1,200-1,500 gm	33.8	33.3-34.3	8-10 days	30.3	29.0-31.8
1,501-2,500 gm	32.8	31.8-33.8	10-12 days	30.1	29.0-31.4
Over 2,500			12-14 days		
(and >36 weeks)	32.4	31.0-33.7	Under 1,500 gm	33.5	32.6-34.0
24-36 hours			1,501-2,500 gm	32.1	31.0-33.2
Under 1,200 gm	34.0	34.0-35.0	Over 2,500		
1,200-1,500 gm	33.6	33.1-34.2	(and >36 weeks)	29.8	29.0-30.8
1,501-2,500 gm	32.6	31.6-33.6	2-3 weeks		
Over 2,500			Under 1,500 gm	33.1	32.2-34.0
(and >36 weeks)	32.1	30.7-33.5	1,501-2,500 gm	31.7	30.5-33.0
36-48 hours			3-4 weeks		
Under 1,200 gm	34.0	34.0-35.0	Under 1,500 gm	32.6	31.6-33.6
1,200-1,500 gm	33.5	33.0-34.1	1,501-2,500 gm	31.4	30.0-32.7
1,501-2,500 gm	32.5	31.4-33.5	4-5 weeks		
Over 2,500			Under 1,500 gm	32.0	31.2-33.0
(and >36 weeks)	31.9	30.5-33.3	1,501-2,500 gm	30.9	29.5-32.2
48-72 hours			5-6 weeks		
Under 1,200 gm	34.0	34.0-35.0	Under 1,500 gm	31.4	30.6-32.3
1,200-1,500 gm	33.5	33.0-34.0	1,501-2,500	30.4	29.0-31.8
1,501-2,500 gm	32.3	31.2-33.4			
Over 2,500					
(and >36 weeks)	31.7	30.1-33.2			

*From Klaus, M. H., and Fanaroff, A. A.: Care of the high-risk neonate, Philadelphia, 1973, W. B. Saunders Co.

The greatest risk situation for exposing the newborn to the cold stress is a delivery room that is too often air conditioned for the comfort of the personnel. The newborn arrives in this environment (from one that is very warm) wet, naked, and exposed to all four mechanisms of heat loss. Even with a delivery room temperature of 25° C (77° F), a healthy, vigorous newborn with maximal increase in metabolic rate cannot keep up with the rate of heat loss of about 200 kcal/kg/minute.[2] Drying the infant immediately, providing radiant warmth, and preventing convective losses by swaddling with warm blankets or a plastic bag through which the infant can be seen help to minimize heat loss in the delivery room. Another very important heat source is the mother herself. An obvious solution to the problem is to warm up the delivery room. If a pediatric surgeon can perform delicate surgery on a newborn that may take hours at an 85° F temperature, then certainly delivery room personnel could learn to tolerate this temperature for the brief time they spend attending a delivery.

Oxygen therapy

Oxygen therapy is an area of newborn care that has seen a great deal of change in the past 2 decades. In the early 1940s, an improvement in incubator design permitted a maintenance of higher oxygen concentration than was possible in the 1930s. It was noted that the incidence of periodic breathing in the premature was decreased in high oxygen concentrations. This became a recommendation for clinical practice until the early 1950s when the use of high oxygen concentrations was associated with the occurrence of retrolental fibroplasia. A collaborative study carried out in 1954 showed a minimal incidence of retrolental fibroplasia in environmental oxygen concentrations below 40%. Thus, the rule that no newborn receive oxygen at a level of higher than 40% was established. In the 1960s, an increased incidence in hyaline membrane disease was observed in the years after the curtailment of the use of high oxygen concentrations.[11]

Retrolental fibroplasia is the result of prolonged vasoconstriction of the retinal vessels in response to high arterial blood oxygen concentration. This response is not observed when only the cornea of the eye is exposed to oxygen. Also, this response is not observed in the fully vascularized retina after 36 weeks' gestation.[10] Therefore, the more immature the infant, the greater the susceptibility to development of retrolental fibroplasia. The amount of oxygen in inspired air required to produce vasoconstriction is dependent on the individual infant's pulmonary and circulatory functions. In the case of lung disease or poor pulmonary perfusion, high concentrations of inspired oxygen will be required to maintain arterial oxygen at a level that prevents hypoxia. Some evidence suggests that immature infants with intact pulmonary and circulatory systems are at risk for retinopathy in oxygen concentrations between 25% and 40%. There is also suspicion that some infants are at risk in room air.[10] Therefore, the 40% rule is no longer appropriate when providing oxygen therapy to the newborn.[11]

The goal of oxygen therapy is to provide the newborn with adequate amounts of oxygen without giving too much or too little. Too much arterial oxygen causes retrolental fibroplasia. High concentrations (70%) of inspired oxygen given for a period of more than 4 to 6 days put the infant at risk for the development of bronchopulmonary dysplasia.[10] Too little oxygen leads to central nervous system damage, which may manifest itself as mental retardation or cerebral palsy. The exact, safe level at which the partial pressure of oxygen in the arterial system (Pa_{O_2}) should be maintained is as yet undetermined. One authority suggests that the Pa_{O_2} between 50 and 80 mm Hg is satisfactory.[2] Another authority suggests maintaining the Pa_{O_2} between 40 and 90 mm Hg but admits that the safe upper limit for the immature is unknown and that a Pa_{O_2} under 65 mm Hg may be more appropriate.[3] Follow-up studies on infants who received lower oxygen concentrations are needed when they reach school age to determine Pa_{O_2} levels appropriate for maintaining an infant's intellectual potential.[17]

Indications for oxygen therapy are resuscitation, apnea, and cyanosis in infants with pulmonary disease. The only appropriate way to provide added oxygen for prolonged periods of time is in a facility that has trained personnel and the capability of monitoring blood gas values to determine the minimal amount of oxygen needed to prevent hypoxia. Clinical observations are not always accurate, because some noncyanotic infants may be hypoxic.[3] At this time, determination of blood gas values is the only safe way to regulate oxygen therapy. Since most community hospitals do not have the capabilities of providing the needed support, newborns requiring oxygen greater than 40% for more than 4 hours should be transported to a facility that can provide these services.

The following are some basic principles of oxygen administration:

1. The provision of added oxygen requires separate line sources of compressed air and oxygen with a mixer valve.
2. It is impossible to maintain oxygen concentrations above 30% in an incubator due to opening of portholes and hood leaks. Therefore, a head hood should be used. A flow rate from 5 to 8 liters/minute is needed to prevent accumulation of carbon dioxide within the hood.
3. The oxygen should be humidified and warmed to the temperature of the incubator and should be checked hourly. Cold oxygen on the infant's face can cause hypothermia.
4. The environmental oxygen should be monitored hourly. The oxygen concentration should be analyzed and equipment calibrated daily.
5. Capillary blood obtained from a puncture of a warmed heel is inadequate for accurate determination of the Pa_{O_2}. Arterial blood obtained from a catheter in the umbilical, radial, or temporal artery is needed. The Pa_{O_2} should be measured at least every 4 hours on infants receiving greater than 40% oxygen.
6. As the infant's condition improves, the amount of inspired oxygen should be reduced slowly, no faster than 10% every hour, to avoid the "flip-flop" phenomenon. This is a greater than expected drop in the Pa_{O_2} when ambient oxygen is lowered, and a higher concentration of ambient oxygen may be needed than was originally given in order to return the Pa_{O_2} to the original level.
7. The ordering and measurement of oxygen according to flow rate is not appropriate since various flow rates produce various concentrations of oxygen depending on the equipment used, such as incubators, head hoods, funnels, or face masks.
8. Oxygen should be treated like any other drug. Before administration, the amount, side effects, and method of administration should be known.

The nurse has a major role in the administration of oxygen. In order to provide appropriate care, the nurse must have an understanding of principles of oxygen therapy and the methods of administration. This includes knowledge of the proper use and maintenance of equipment used to administer oxygen. As stated previously, the nurse is in constant attendance with the newborn and is therefore better able to detect subtle changes in the infant's responses to oxygen therapy than the physician who may see the infant once or twice a day. The appropriate management of the newborn requiring added oxygen is dependent on a close and collaborative working relationship between physician and nurse.[17]

Newborn feeding

Feeding and nutrition is a controversial topic in newborn care today. What to feed, when to feed, and how to feed are debated among those persons involved in perinatal care. Emotions, fads, and commercialism are all involved in determining newborn feeding practices.[10] Too often the needs of infants are overlooked, and they are forced to adhere to routine feeding practices that may be inappropriate to meet individual needs. It is not the purpose of this chapter to discuss controversial issues or to go into detail regarding the nutritional requirements of newborns. However, early feeding of the newborn is discussed. This is an area of general agreement among experts and an area that is clearly important in the prevention of mental retardation.

Hypoglycemia is a condition that occurs frequently in the newborn period. Infants born to diabetic mothers, preterm, or SGA infants are at highest risk for the development of hypoglycemia. The normal term infant can also develop hypoglycemia, particularly if allowed to become hypothermic. Newborn infants who have suffered asphyxia are also prone to hypoglycemia.[2] Too often the glycogen stored in the liver and the dietary sources of glucose offered the newborn are inadequate to meet physiological requirements. Hypoglycemia is a cause of motor and intellectual impairment. Because of these factors, it is no longer considered appropriate to delay the feeding of newborns for 12, 24, or 72 hours.[19] In addition to reducing the incidence of hypoglycemia, early feeding also reduces the degree of hyperbilirubinemia and dehydration. Infants weighing less than 1,500 gm showed a steep reduction in mortality when they were provided fluids and calories per intravenous feedings in the first 6 hours of life when compared with infants who were starved or given nasogastric feedings. A delay in the provision of fluids and calories to the newborn may also reduce the chance for normal development.[10]

The method by which the first feeding is given is dependent on the newborn's birth weight, gestational age, and general condition. In infants under 34 weeks' gestation, the gag reflex is not present, and the ability to coordinate sucking and swallowing is not present. These infants, as well as infants with pulmonary disease, should not be fed orally but instead should be started on parenteral fluids. The normal, healthy, term baby can be started on oral feedings if adaptation to extrauterine life is normal. The infant should be warm, breathing normally, and have good color, muscle tone, and cry. Term infants will often exhibit a readiness to feed by crying, rooting, and sucking of fists. Nurses who are experienced in caring for newborns have the ability to recognize when an infant is ready for oral feedings and can be given the responsibility for making this decision. Many infants will exhibit this readiness to feed within the first hour after birth. Term infants should probably receive their first feeding by 4 to 6 hours of age.[10]

The choice of the first feeding for the normal newborn is dependent on whether the infant is breast- or bottle-fed. The bottle-fed newborn has traditionally been given 5% glucose in water for the first feeding. This has been used as a precautionary measure in the event of an esophageal anomaly.[8] However, glucose in water instilled in the lungs of rabbits caused the same type of irritation as milk. Based on this fact, sterile water is now preferred for the first feeding. If the newborn tolerates this first feeding well, direct progression to a formula is made.[10]

Colostrum is considered to be an appropriate first feed for the breast-fed newborn. It is a physiological substance that does not produce irritating effects and is high in protein, vitamins A and E, and antibodies. In addition to these factors, colostrum has a laxative effect that promotes early evacuation of meconium, decreasing the reabsorption of bilirubin present in meconium. Also, there is a strong correlation between successful breast-feeding and the occurrence of the first feed within the first hour of life. Therefore, breast feeding should be instituted as soon as the conditions of mother and baby permit in order to promote breast-feeding success and to give the newborn the benefits of colostrum.[8]

SUMMARY

The field of neonatology, or care of the newborn, is new and rapidly changing. This chapter has dealt with only a small segment, and the reader is referred to current textbooks for more in-depth information. The topics discussed here are those that have experienced the greatest changes in practice in the past 15 years. They are also the areas that have had the greatest impact on the reduction of newborn mortality and morbidity, particularly mental retardation and other developmental disabilities. The important points made in this chapter are:

1. Monitor the fetus closely.
2. Resuscitate the newborn promptly.
3. Assess the newborn for gestational age.
4. Keep the newborn warm.

5. Provide the newborn with adequate oxygen.
6. Feed the newborn early.

The neonatal nurse has a major role in the provision of care to the newborn. Newborn nursing is a combination of theoretical knowledge and information gained from direct experience. The nurse needs to cultivate an ability to closely examine and observe the newborn for signs of impending difficulties. These signs may be very subtle, and the nurse in constant attendance with the newborn may be the first to recognize them. Because changes in newborn care are occurring rapidly, the neonatal nurse has the responsibility to keep up with current research in order to maintain proficiency.[6]

REFERENCES

1. Auld, P.: Resuscitation of the newborn infant, Am. J. Nurs. **74:**68, 1974.
2. Avery, G. B., editor: Neonatology, Philadelphia, 1975, J. B. Lippincott Co.
3. Babson, G. S., and Benson, R. C.: Management of high-risk pregnancy and intensive care of the neonate, St. Louis, 1971, The C. V. Mosby Co.
4. Cahill, B.: The neonatal nurse specialist; new techniques for the symptomatic newborn, J. Obstet. Gynecol. Neonat. Nurs. **3:**34, 1974.
5. Chagnon, L. J., and Heldenbrand, C. L.: Nurses undertake direct and indirect fetal monitoring at a community hospital, J. Obstet. Gynecol. Neonat. Nurs. **3:**41, 1974.
6. Clausen, J. P., and others: Maternity nursing today, New York, 1973, McGraw-Hill, Inc.
7. Cordero, L., Jr., and Hon, E. H.: Neonatal bradycardia following nasopharyngeal stimulation, J. Pediatr. **78:**441, 1971.
8. Countryman, B. A.: Hospital care of the breast-fed newborn, Am. J. Nurs. **71:**2365, 1971.
9. Daily, W. J. R., Klaus, M., and Meyer, H. B.: Apnea in premature infants; monitoring incidence, heart rate changes, and an effect of environmental temperature, Pediatrics **43:**510, 1969.
10. Klaus, M. H., and Fanaroff, A. A.: Care of the high-risk neonate, Philadelphia, 1973, W. B. Saunders Co.
11. Klaus, M. H., and Meyer, B. P.: Oxygen therapy for the newborn, Pediatr. Clin. North Am. **13:**731, 1966.
12. Luckner, K.: Patients' response to fetal monitoring, Toledo, Ohio, 1973, an unpublished study.
13. Lutz, L., and Perlstein, P.: Temperature control in newborn babies, Nurs. Clin. North Am. **6:**15, 1971.
14. McClean, F. H.: Significance of birthweight for gestational age in identifying infants at risk, J. Obstet. Gynecol. Neonat. Nurs. **3:**6, 1974.
15. McCrann, D. J., and Schifrin, B. S.: Fetal monitoring in high-risk pregnancy, Clin. Perinatol. **1:**229, 1974.
16. Schneider, J. M.: Regionalization of perinatal care, Sixty-sixth Ross Conference on Pediatric Research, Columbus, Ohio, 1974, Ross Laboratories.
17. Segal, S.: Oxygen; too much, too little, Nurs. Clin. North Am. **6:**39, 1971.
18. Sutherland, J.: The hospital between, Nurs. Clin. North Am. **6:**103, 1971.
19. White, M., and Keenan, W. J.: Recognition and management of hypoglycemia in the newborn infant, Nurs. Clin. North Am. **6:**67, 1971.

CHAPTER 11

High-risk infants and families

SUSAN BLACKBURN

Although the term "high risk" has traditionally been used to refer to premature infants, it now incorporates a wide variety of infants and families. The high-risk infant is one, regardless of birth weight or gestational age, whose extrauterine existence and potential for later development are compromised by prenatal, natal, or postnatal factors, and who is in need of special nursing and medical care.[11]

A variety of factors before and during pregnancy and after birth influence infants and place them at risk, including[11, 18]:

1. Preconceptual factors
   a. Family history
   b. Poor nutrition
   c. Chronic disease
   d. Socioeconomic problems
2. Prenatal factors
   a. Pregnancy complications, such as toxemia or infection
   b. Multiple birth
   c. Fetal growth aberrations
   d. Maternal medications during pregnancy
   e. Stressful events
   f. Lack of prenatal care
   g. Maternal age
3. Natal factors
   a. Complications of labor and delivery
   b. Anesthesia
   c. Fetal distress
   d. Premature labor
   e. Abnormal presentations
4. Postnatal factors
   a. Low Apgar score
   b. Birth injuries or trauma
   c. Congenital anomalies
   d. Neonatal medical and surgical problems

Approximately 10% of pregnancies carry a significant risk to the infant, and 3% to 5% of all births result in infants who need special or intensive care. These infants, although small in proportion to the total number of births, are a significant minority since they account for a large proportion of neonatal deaths and perinatally determined disabilities.[18] Although intensive care of the high-risk infant is costly, in the long run it is more expensive to do nothing. In comparison with the costs involved in providing care and rehabilitation for the brain-damaged individual, neonatal intensive care aimed at prevention of handicaps becomes relatively inexpensive.[13, 17]

Low birth weight infants comprise 60% to 70% of the newborns who require special care. As mentioned in Chapter 10, low birth weight infants are generally classified as either premature (that is, born at 37 or fewer weeks' gestation) or SGA (that is, infants whose birth weights are below the tenth percentile for their gestational age). Although an SGA infant may also be classified as premature, approximately 30% to 40% of all low birth weight infants are born at or near term.[11, 12]

These two groups of low birth weight infants are quite different, each requiring special nursing care and each at risk for developing unique problems. The premature infant has difficulty adapting to the extrauterine environment due to immaturity of major body systems. This immaturity is reflected in problems such as temperature instability, hyperbilirubinemia, respiratory distress, apneic episodes, and feeding difficulties. The SGA infant more commonly has problems with fetal distress, asphyxia, heat loss, meconium aspiration, and hypoglycemia.[7, 12]

Infants who are LGA (that is, birth weight above the ninetieth percentile for gestational age) and infants who are born after 42 weeks' gestation are also high risk. Other newborns requiring special care are those with metabolic problems, such as hypoglycemia, hypocalcemia, hyperbilirubinemia, sepsis, congenital malformations, birth injuries, cardiopulmonary problems, asphyxia, infants with surgical problems, and infants of drug-addicted mothers.[7, 11, 12]

NEWBORN SPECIAL CARE UNITS

Care of the high-risk infant and family requires a multidisciplinary team approach. The primary members of this team are the obstetrician, pediatrician, nurse, and social worker. Other health care professionals are involved depending on the individual needs of an infant or family.

Because of the high costs of staffing and operating newborn special care units, regional centers are being developed to provide consistent high-quality care and to meet community needs economically. One problem with the development of newborn special care units has been the uneven distribution and unnecessary duplication of units as hospital "status symbols."[8, 13, 14, 18]

Although organization of perinatal care in any state or region depends on the individual needs and characteristics of that area, regionalization usually results in the development of primary, secondary, and tertiary centers. Primary centers are responsible for the care and supervision of normal pregnancies and newborns as well as the more common obstetric and neonatal problems. Secondary centers provide services for many infants who require care that is specialized but not as intensive as that provided by the regional or tertiary center. Tertiary centers are responsible for normal pregnancies in their area as well as many high-risk pregnancies and newborns requiring intensive care.[8, 18]

One half to two thirds of the infants cared for in a regional center are referred by hospitals in a wide geographic area. Infants are transported in a heated mobile incubator via ambulance, helicopter, or airplane and are accompanied by a nurse-nurse or nurse-physician team. Since transporting a newly born high-risk infant is not an ideal situation for either the mother or her infant, some areas have begun to develop combined maternal-fetal and infant intensive care units.[3, 4, 11] Mothers identified as high risk before or during their pregnancy are cared for and delivered at a hospital that has facilities for evaluation and monitoring of the mother and fetus during pregnancy, labor, and delivery. In addition, this hospital has adjacent newborn special care facilities to provide immediate intensive care of the infant.

Nurses and other health care professionals in the regional center are actively involved in teaching and consulting with the staff of the community hospitals in their area. Initial education is usually directed toward early identification of infants in need of transfer, standardization of the care infants receive before the transfer, and facilitation of early transfer so that infants are not kept in hospitals with inadequate facilities until their condition has deteriorated. Educational efforts are also directed toward improving the care of infants who do not require intensive care and in sharing new knowledge and techniques. Many centers offer 24-hour telephone consultation for the nursing and medical staff of hospitals in their region.[3]

Educational programs to better prepare nurses and physicians for care of high-risk infants and families have become increasingly available in the past few years. Since few schools of nursing offer formal instruction in newborn intensive care, in-service, short-term continuing education programs, and education at the master's level are being developed.[15] These programs prepare nurses for a variety of roles from staff nurse to clinical specialist. Varied levels of expertise and knowledge are essential since it is often impossible for one nurse to meet the complex physical, developmental, and psychosocial needs of high-risk infants and their families, particularly in an intensive care setting where life-supporting functions must take first priority.

OUTCOME OF HIGH-RISK INFANTS

Establishment of newborn intensive care units in an area has tended to reduce neonatal mortality by 40% to 60%.[4, 8, 12, 18] Today, the majority of low birth weight and other high-risk infants survive. Among infants cared for in intensive care units, 90% of those weighing more than 1,500 gm (3 pounds, 5 ounces) and 70% to 75% of those weighing between 1,000 and 1,500 grams will survive.[14, 17]

With increasing numbers of high-risk infants surviving, a major concern is the quality of that survival. Are more infants surviving the neonatal period only to develop severe handicaps later? Numerous studies have demonstrated the prevalence of mental and neurological disorders among surviving infants.[5, 6, 11] Low birth weight remains the factor associated with the highest incidence of later problems. In recent years, however, there has been a striking reduction in the incidence of moderate and severe neurological and mental handicaps among infants cared for in intensive care units.[5, 6, 9] Although most of the children in recent follow-up studies have not yet reached school age, 70% to 90% of infants with birth weights below 1,500 gm have no detectable handicaps and are considered normal at 2 to 7 years of age.[5, 6, 9, 17]

The later status of infants who are potentially normal at birth depends to a large extent on the quality of the natal and postnatal care they receive. The changing prognosis

for high-risk infants is attributed to the development of neonatal intensive care units, increased knowledge of the pathophysiology of neonates, improved facilities for monitoring biochemical and physiological processes, and education of nursing and medical personnel.[6, 12]

During the last 15 to 20 years, there have been extensive changes in the care of high-risk infants. In the late 1940s and early 1950s, incubators capable of maintaining high oxygen concentrations became available. Between 1955 and 1959, the administration of intravenous fluids with correction of pH and provision of calories was begun and was in common use by 1964. Accompanying this was a gradual shift from early starvation of infants to early feeding. The importance of maintaining body temperature was not appreciated until the late 1950s. The use of artificial ventilation and monitoring equipment was introduced in the middle 1960s and is still being refined and modified.[15] Phototherapy for preventing and treating hyperbilirubinemia was begun about the same time. By the late 1960s, parents were routinely allowed to handle their infants and participate in the infant's care in many units.[12] Intravenous alimentation and the use of constant positive airway pressure are recent promising methods of managing nutritional and respiratory problems.[12, 13]

Hagberg summarizes the perinatal preventive measures that contribute to the reduction of handicaps among high-risk infants:

1. Improved obstetric techniques
   a. Less hypoxia
   b. Less trauma
2. Improved neonatal regimens
   a. Less hypoxia
   b. Less acidosis
   c. Less hypoglycemia
   d. Less hyperbilirubinemia
   e. Less hypocaloremia
   f. Less hypothermia
   g. Less hypernatremia*

---

*From Hagberg, B.: Pre-, peri-, and postnatal prevention of major neuropediatric handicaps, Neuropaediatrie **6:**334, 1975.

ROLES OF THE NURSE

Nursing has a critically important role in the management of high-risk infants and prevention of later sequelae. The nurse in the special care unit is with the infant 24 hours a day and is the main provider of care to both infant and family. Special care of the newborn covers a wide spectrum of activities ranging from the close observation of apparently well infants who are at risk for developing serious illness to the intensive care of infants whose survival is in doubt.[12] The nurse is often the first to observe signs of impending problems and begin diagnostic and therapeutic procedures.

Clinical functions of the nursing staff in a newborn special care unit fall into several general areas.[12] The first, and one of the most important, of these functions is the direct observation of infants. Severe problems may be detected in the earliest stages by an alert nurse long before any of the sophisticated monitoring equipment notes these changes.

The second general function of nursing is the use of electronic monitors to detect cardiovascular and respiratory difficulties. These instruments monitor heart and respiratory rates, temperature, oxygen concentration, and blood pressure.[12] Electronic monitors, mechanical respirators, and other such items, although important, should remain a secondary consideration because caring for babies in newborn intensive care first requires that the personnel perform with intensity.[12] Without well-trained medical and nursing staff, complex equipment is useless.

Nursing responsibilities in a variety of diagnostic and therapeutic procedures are expanding. For example, in some units the nurses routinely perform blood gas analysis and intubation. Nursing care routinely includes isolette care, gavage feeding, bottle feeding, monitoring of fluid and caloric intake, monitoring of weight, suctioning, care for infants receiving phototherapy and infants on respirators, resuscitation, and monitoring of blood gases, serum bilirubin, and blood glucose values.

The last two areas of nursing function in newborn special care units are the consideration of planning for the developmental needs of the infant and the promotion of parent-infant contact. These areas are almost exclusively dependent on skillful and creative nursing interventions. They are areas of increasing attention and concern.

There has been long-standing concern about the impact of the early environment—the standard hospital incubator—on the growth and development of low birth weight infants.[1, 19] The extrauterine environment differs significantly from the intrauterine one, particularly in the lack of appropriate sensory input that is thought to play an important role in the maturation and organization of the central nervous system.[19] Life in the uterus is very rich in tactile, auditory, and kinesthetic stimulation, which the infant experiences on a constant and predictable schedule.

In contrast to the uterine environment, the incubator environment falls far short. The infant is thrust before being ready into a world of constant bright lights, sudden loud noises, temperature changes, and cold hands. It is an environment without the containment and movement of the uterus, and one in which people poke, prod, and strike things into and onto the infant on a variable and unpredictable schedule. Infants have been given additional stimulation by the use of swings, tape recordings of mothers, patterned handling and stroking, and waterbeds.[1, 19]

At the University of Washington, the Premature Infant Refocus Project is currently using a rocking bed–heartbeat program to promote neurological organization in premature infants. It is anticipated that infants on the rocking bed program will be more responsive and predictable, thus fostering positive parent-infant interaction.[19]

Nurses caring for high-risk infants should provide them with a variety of experiences as part of routine care. These activities include placing brightly colored mobiles, toys, and pictures in the isolette. Rocking, holding, establishing eye-to-eye contact, talking, cuddling, providing sucking experience for infants who are not being fed, and using music boxes and radios are other experiences important for these babies. Nurses may perform these activities, but often they encourage parent involvement.

Finally, the nurse plays an important role in assisting the parents and infant in getting to know and trust each other. Hospital practices, home environment, and parents' caregiving abilities may have as significant an effect on the infant's outcome as perinatal complications.[4, 11]

It is increasingly apparent that the quality of a neonate's life depends not just on his physiologic and neurologic integrity. The stability and strength of his attachment to his family and his family to him also determine, in large measure, the degree to which he will achieve his potential as a self-confident, fruitful member of society.[*]

The birth of a small or sick infant is most often an unanticipated, unplanned-for event for which the family is emotionally unprepared. The shock of this event, coupled with the apprehension and concern surrounding labor and delivery, can precipitate feelings of disorganization, isolation, and inadequacy.[20]

The focus of care in neonatal intensive care units has changed over the past decade from a primarily infant-centered approach to one of providing care for both the infant and family. Many units now encourage maximum parental participation in the care of their infants. The nursing staff attempts to provide guidance and acceptance of parental feelings and reactions and to facilitate parent-infant interaction. This is no small challenge, considering the circumstances. Families must face the economic and emotional stresses of prolonged hospitalization and separation from their newborn and of eventually incorporating this child who has been singled out as special into the family.

One consequence of having a high-risk infant is that the early interaction between parent and infant is altered. Separation from

the infant in the neonatal period may interfere with the development of parenting behaviors, such as cuddling, eye-to-eye contact, and development of caretaking skills.[11] Early separation of parent and infant has been suggested as a possible etiological factor in the high incidence of battering and failure to thrive among children who were born prematurely or separated from their parents in the neonatal period.[10, 16]

Parents of high-risk infants are often in conflict between the behavior they feel is appropriate as parents and the behavior they are allowed to emit. For the first weeks or months of their child's life, they play a supporting rather than leading role.

You don't really become parents until you have them at home . . . till you can make the decisions and are responsible.

Most newborn special care units now have open visiting policies so that parents can visit and interact with their infant as often as they choose. The nursing staff attempts to promote parental involvement in caretaking activities, such as stroking, talking, holding, rocking, and playing with the infant and in feeding, burping, diapering, and bathing.

If an infant is unable to take oral feedings, mothers who plan to breast-feed are encouraged to express milk for the infant, which is then given to the infant by gavage. When an infant is critically ill, many mothers feel it is important for them to provide milk for the infant.

Right now it's the only thing I can do for my baby.

The extent to which any parent is involved with an infant's care depends on the infant's condition and the parent's readiness. The staff encourages parents by fostering a permissive atmosphere rather than a pushy one and by permitting parents to do as much for their baby as they feel they can comfortably.[20]

Many units also allow friends, relatives, and siblings to view the baby. The nursing staff often assists parents in dealing with the reactions of other children to the new baby. By coming to visit, the siblings can see for themselves that there really is a new baby.

Even with open visiting policies, long distances frequently separate the family and infant. Often, after several weeks or months, essentially strange infants are returned to families that may not feel much closeness to them. To diminish the effects of parent-infant separation, the regional center attempts whenever possible to transfer infants back to the community hospital as soon as they are stabilized.

Families must not only travel considerable distances to maintain physical contact with their infants but they are also expected to develop a relationship with their babies in an environment that often lacks privacy. Neonatal intensive care units can be frightening and overwhelming places for parents to visit. Often it is impossible to see the baby because of all the equipment, tubes, and people.

I took one look and ran out . . . looked like a zoo . . . something out of science fiction.

Kaplan and Mason proposed four psychological tasks that mothers of premature infants must accomplish in order to successfully master the experience. These tasks can be generalized to parents of any sick infant. The first task is anticipating grief or preparation for the possible loss of the infant. The parents must then face or acknowledge their failure to produce a full-term or healthy infant. The third and fourth tasks are the resumption of a process of relating to the infant and preparing themselves for caring for the baby through an understanding of its special needs and growth patterns. Parents must also recognize that these needs are temporary and will yield in time to more usual patterns. These tasks are not entirely separate and often exist side by side or overlap.[10]

Recently, nurses at the University of Washington have been involved in the development of parent support groups and in facilitating individual parent-to-parent interaction. Both mothers and fathers are involved in these groups. Parents who are presently going through the experience of having a small or sick baby and parents who have gone through similar experiences provide peer support for one another. Parents whose children are at home act as resources for newer parents whose infants are still in the hospital or are recently discharged, demonstrating that not only do the babies survive, but the parents survive as well!

Parent groups are available weekly for parents while their infant is hospitalized and focus on experiences during pregnancy, labor, and delivery, feelings surrounding the birth of the infant, explanations of medical problems and care the infants are receiving, and plans for taking the baby home. Monthly meetings with a focus on growth and development are available for parents whose infants are at home.

The group situation provides a place for parents to share their experiences and feelings and to develop appropriate methods of coping with them.

By bringing together people who are sharing, or are about to share, a common adaptive experience . . . we help equip them to cope with it. A man required to adapt to a new life situation loses some of his bases for self-esteem. He begins to doubt his own abilities. If we bring him together with others who are moving through the same experience, people he can identify with and respect, we strengthen him. The members of the group come to share, even if briefly, some sense of identity. They see their problems more objectively. They trade useful ideas and insights. Most important, they suggest future alternatives for one another.*

Parents respond positively to these groups and find them helpful:

. . . don't have to feel alone . . . things don't seem as scary . . . trial and error is no way to handle such a traumatic experience . . . relieved a lot of stress . . . by sharing with others I don't feel like such a freak . . . need time to let out your feelings . . . helps you sort out what is going on.

*From Toffler, A.: Future shock, New York, 1971, Bantam Books, Inc. Used with permission of Random House, Inc.

Regardless of whether done in a group setting or on a one-to-one basis, the nurse caring for the high-risk infant helps the family deal with many concerns and feelings. The most frequently expressed concerns among parents during the group discussion have been related to guilt over causing the baby's early birth or problem, appearance of the baby, the intensive care environment, finances, fear of having another baby with similar problems, concerns about later development and the sudden infant death syndrome, stress between parents, reactions of siblings and relatives, relations with health care professionals, father's involvement, and concerns over taking the baby home.

SUMMARY

The care of high-risk infants, those infants who are at risk both in terms of immediate survival and for later developmental problems, has been a matter of health care concern for the past 50 years. Low birth weight infants account for a major proportion of at-risk infants. Over the past 10 to 15 years, increased knowledge of the pathophysiology of neonates, improved facilities for monitoring biochemical and physiological processes, education of medical and nursing personnel, and the development of neonatal intensive care units have contributed to increased survival of low birth weight infants and lowered incidence of later developmental problems.[7, 12] Yet the low birth weight infant continues to be significantly more vulnerable for the development of later handicaps ranging from minimal neurological defects and learning problems to severe mental retardation.

High-risk infants and their families present a continuing challenge to the nurse. Neonatal nursing "is part of one of the most exciting, rewarding and emotionally draining fields" of health care.[7] The nurse must understand complex disease processes; anticipate and evaluate a wide range of clinical problems, operate sophisticated and ever-changing supportive equipment, deal on a daily basis with families in crisis with dying infants, grieving families, and with complex ethical issues.[7] Neonatal nursing must continue to deal with the changing and increasingly complex areas of physiological care, with meeting the developmental needs of infants, and in facilitating positive parent-infant interaction. By attending to these problems, nursing will continue to make significant contributions to the prevention of postnatal sequelae in high-risk infants.

REFERENCES

1. Barnard, K. E.: The effect of stimulation on the sleep behavior of the premature infant, Communicating Nurs. Res. **6:**12, 1973.
2. Caplan, G.: Support systems. In Support systems and community mental health, New York, 1974, Behavioral Publications.
3. Callon, H. F.: Regionalizing perinatal care in Wisconsin, Nurs. Clin. North Am. **10:**263, 1975.
4. Cranley, M. A.: When a high-risk infant is born, Am. J. Nurs., **75:**1696, 1975.
5. Davies, P. A., and Tizard, J. P. M.: Very low birth weight and subsequent neurological defect, Dev. Med. Child. Neurol. **17:**3, 1975.
6. Drillien, C. M.: Aetiology and outcome in low birth weight infants, Dev. Med. Child Neurol. **14:**563, 1972.
7. Fogerty, S.: The nurse and the high-risk infant, Nurs. Clin. North Am. **8:**533, 1973.
8. Harrison, L. K.: Making a good thing better; the regionalization of neonatal intensive care units, J. Obstet. Gynecol. Neonat. Nurs. **4:**49, 1975.
9. James, L. S.: Long-term follow-up studies of prematurely born infants, Pediatrics **80:**513, 1972.
10. Kaplan, D. M. and Mason, E. A.: Maternal reactions to premature birth viewed as an acute emotional disorder, Am. J. Orthopsychiatry **30:**539, 1960.
11. Klaus, M. H. and Fanaroff, A. A.: Care of the high-risk neonate, Philadelphia, 1973, W. B. Saunders Co.
12. Korones, S. B.: High-risk newborn infants; the basis for intensive nursing care, St. Louis, 1972, The C. V. Mosby Co.
13. Lucey, J. F.: Why we should regionalize perinatal care, Pediatrics **52:**488, 1973.
14. Schlesinger, E.: Neonatal intensive care; planning for services and outcomes following care, J. Pediatr. **82:**916, 1973.
15. Schneider, J. M., and others: Education of the perinatal nurse clinician, Nurs. Clin. North Am. **10:**285, 1975.
16. Stern, L.: Prematurity as a factor in child abuse, Hosp. Practice **8:**117, 1973.
17. Stewart, A. L., and Reynolds, E. O. R.: Improved prognosis for infants of very low birthweight, Pediatrics **54:**724, 1974.

18. Swyer, P. R.: The organization of perinatal care with particular reference to the newborn. In Avery, G. B., editor: Neonatology, Philadelphia, 1975, J. B. Lippincott Co.
19. University of Washington Premature Infant Refocus Project, HSMA Grant No. MC-R-530348-01-0, Rockville, Md., 1974, Maternal-Child Health Services, Health Services and Mental Helath Administration.
20. Warrick, L. H.: Family-centered care in the premature nursery, Am. J. Nurs. **71:**2134, 1971.

CHAPTER 12

Neuromotor development: assessment and implications

EDE MARIE BUERGER

In the United States, 20% of the population experiences brain damage in infancy that results in learning problems.[6] Of all cerebral palsied children, 35% are born prematurely and 85% have a history of anoxia, hemorrhage, infection, or hyperbilirubinemia.[42] Infants born before 37 weeks' gestation, small-for-date, with metabolic disorders, or with significant dysmorphology are at risk for developmental problems. This risk increases with infants from low socioeconomic groups.[46]

Insults to the central nervous system (CNS) are not frequently manifested until months or years after the precipitating cause occurred. Unusual motor and sensory patterns emerge as a result of the maturation of an abnormal nervous system. This emergence is correlated with maturation of the CNS. Insults affecting CNS maturation may occur in utero, during the birth process, or during the neonatal period. This chapter identifies those problems that occur during the last trimester of pregnancy and during the neonatal period.

NEUROPHYSIOLOGICAL MATURATION

As the fetus enters the last trimester, the nervous system is in a dynamic state as mat-

Note: I wish to express my sincere gratitude for the assistance in the preparation of this manuscript to Dr. T. Joe Willey, Ms. Marilyn Thunquest, and Ms. Noreen Burlew.

uration proceeds. With increasing gestational age, myelination will progress through the brainstem.[7, 37] Paroxysmal, asynchronized cyclic firing of the inspiratory-expiratory centers will shift to a more synchronized, modulated rhythm.[33] Brain weight and size will increase as individual neurons develop mature dendritic and axonal spines.[4] This proliferation provides a wealth of synaptic corrections, resulting in higher order integration and complexity.[41, 42] Bioelectrically, the ratio of active to quiet sleep rhythms on the electroencephalogram (EEG) will change toward longer, quiet sleep[44]; evoked potentials will become less prolonged[7]; and refractory periods will shorten.[16] Biochemically, there will be an increase in vesicles and in quantum production.[27] Separate distribution of cholinesterase and catecholamines will occur as neuronal cells of different shape and size develop.[6]

Functional correlates can be observed. The absence of myelin and small fiber diameters implies motor reactions with long latencies that are uncontrolled and generalized. Completion of myelination through the brainstem during the last trimester and through the central nervous system during the first 2 years after birth parallels the behavioral progression from general to specific action, from gross motor to specific refined control, and from undifferentiated general to integrated patterned movements. The proliferation of synaptic connections also accompanies the emergence of those self-controlled, modulated behaviors, such as socialization, self-quieting, and learning.

Synchronized firing of inspiratory-expiratory centers parallels a gradual shift from arrhythmic breathing patterns to rhythmic ones. More synchronized, quiet sleep rhythms and more mature alpha-wave activity on the EEG are frequently accompanied by such activities as alerting, habituation, and orientation. Prolonged refractory periods, prolonged evoked potentials, and vesicle and quantum production affect recruitment and fatigability of cortical responses. Thus, the implication is that afferent pathways are limited in their capacity to supply information to the cortex per unit of time. Maturation results in more information for the fetus to appreciate.

Sensory awareness emerges in two forms: protopathic and epicritic.[26] Protopathic awareness is the more primitive form and emerges early in utero. It is characterized by undifferentiated, massive impacts of noxious stimuli. When this system predominates, hyperactivity is aggravated, affect and somatic discomforts are heightened, and perceptual-motor development is retarded.[1] Epicritic awareness is a more mature form of tactile awareness and emerges later in utero and infancy.[19] It is characterized by discrimination of tactile contacts that are purposive, seeking manipulations. It is thought that this discriminative system inhibits the action of the protopathic (protective) system.[34] Thus, tactile defensiveness is decreased with maturation.

ENVIRONMENTAL INFLUENCE

During the first trimester, genetic factors play a key role in the development of a normal nervous system. As the fetus matures, environmental factors play an increasingly important role. Biologically, maternal nutrition is of primary importance, since poor nutrition is the primary cause of low birth weight infants throughout the world.[2] The possibility that neuromotor development may be impaired due to poor nutrition emphasizes the urgency of proper food intake during pregnancy. Prepregnancy weight also plays a significant role. Low prepregnant weight with limited weight gain during pregnancy is associated with high neonatal mortality.[17]

Other factors that biologically affect fetal outcome during the first trimester include severe and prolonged emotional stress, neglected antenatal care, close spacing of pregnancies, maternal age and parity, history of miscarriage or abortion, maternal smoking, excessive use of unprescribed drugs, and heredity.

Throughout pregnancy, the fetus is subjected to a variety of repetitive environmental stimuli. Maternal blood flow through the aorta and peristalsis produce auditory rhythm that is magnified by amniotic fluid. Maternal movements, such as walking and breathing, provide a rhythmic, tactile motion against the fetal skin and external ear, thereby inducing vestibular, kinesthetic, and tactile stimulation. Maternal circadian rhythm affords the fetus a rhythmic, biochemical environment. In contrast, a consistent atmospheric pressure (somewhat similar to weightlessness) and temperature offer a more constant sensory environment.

All environmental stimuli are thought to alter the emerging nervous system development. Such repetitive, long-term stimulation results in neurophysiological changes. Salient effects are: an increase in white matter of cortex, an increase in myelination, action-directed dendritic and axonal spine growth, an increase in vesicles and in quantum production, development of a parallel level of sensorimotor coordination, and production of a more efficient neural conduction through symbiosis.[24, 26, 32, 36] Furthermore, Grimwade and others state that stimulation of fetal nervous pathways not only influences maturation of nerve cells and development of reflexes but also causes improvement in blood supply to the brain.[23]

PRONENESS AND ASSESSMENT

Proneness is identifying an implied increased probability of handicap in childhood. It is evident that proneness screening and assessment must take into account the dynamic state of the maturing nervous system. Maternal-child nurses can now move beyond identifying existing problems to predicting problems. Such a process involves two levels of perception. The first level is identifying the elements or conditions that interfere with or alter the health status of the newborn. Predictive nursing includes being sensitive to indicators that give reliable estimates of proneness for unfavorable developmental outcomes. The second level is assessment of developmental dysfunction.

In the development of a proneness profile, no one variable gives a complete answer. Interactions of characteristics and events should be examined closely. The University of Washington is presently studying methods for screening and assessing proneness to developmental problems in over 189 infants. Findings indicate that the following variables and interactions must be considered during screening[3]:

1. Perinatal health states of mother and infant, including complications of pregnancy, delivery, and the neonatal period.
2. Characteristics of the caregiver, including temperament, educational level, personality, perception of life situation, and perception of infant.
3. Characteristics of the infant, including alertness, type of activity pattern, and sensory threshold level.
4. Behaviors of caregiver and infant as they are observed interacting with one another.

Moreover, it is evident from the above that nurses are engaged not only in preventing later learning and behavior problems but also in treating acquaintance process (maternal-infant familiarizing) and adaptation (maternal-infant adjustment to each other) during the first 3 months of infancy.

Screening occurs primarily when the infant interacts with the health care system. Proneness screening should be initiated in the newborn nursery. Such a health care delivery service thereby requires improved agency linkage between acute care institutions and community resources.

As previously mentioned, the second level of perception is identifying cases of developmental dysfunction and abnormalities. In the assessment phase, the nurse should consider the following:

1. Home health status, including environmental health, safety, comfort, and stimulation.
2. Characteristics of the caregiver, including adaptation to a new infant, sensitivity to infant cues, methods of alleviating distress, and provisions for growth.
3. Characteristics of the infant, including adaptation and response to environment, ability to give interpretable cues, and developmental progress.

Case-finding skills of public health nurses are an important component of our present health care system. Programs of assessment could fit into already operational immunization programs for children. Some 85% of all children in the United States now receive their infant series of diphtheria-pertussis-tetanus (DPT) vaccine,[13] whereas 66% of those who are less than 5 years of age receive polio and measles vaccines[48]; hence, an assessment process that adapts to this health care mechanism is reasonable.

TOOLS AND IMPLICATIONS
Perinatal health states

Perinatal health states are most frequently discussed in the medical history, including all complications and high-risk illness factors. Screening data include Apgar scores and maternal or infant illness and should indicate proneness. Babson and Benson's *Management of High-Risk Pregnancy and Intensive Care of the Neonate* provides a survey of perinatal health states and their implications as an assessment tool.[2]

Characteristics of caregiver

Caregiver characteristics take into account the influence of the parents' view of infant behavior on developmental outcomes. Research has demonstrated that as high as 25% of variances in cognitive development in children may be associated with maternal education.[3, 47] Parental educational level also influences the methods used to teach tasks to the infant. Assessment of how mothers teach their infants a task appropriate to their age is useful. The nurse should observe the type and amount of opportunities the mother provides for problem solving by the infant, the type and amount of information given to the infant, and the quality of reinforcement or feedback given.

It is becoming more evident that parents' perceptions are major determinants in shaping the environmental response to the child. Broussard and Hartner have illustrated that a mother's perceptions of her newborn in-

Table 12-1. Neonatal perception inventory*

You probably have some ideas of what most little babies are like. We would like to know what those ideas are. Please check the blank you think best describes the *average* baby.

	A great deal	A good bit	Moderate amount	Very little	None
How much crying do you think the average baby does?	___	___	___	___	___
How much trouble do you think the average baby has in feeding?	___	___	___	___	___
How much spitting up or vomiting do you think the average baby does?	___	___	___	___	___
How much difficulty does the average baby have with bowel movements?	___	___	___	___	___
How much difficulty do you think the average baby has in sleeping?	___	___	___	___	___
How much trouble do you think the average baby has in settling down to a predictable pattern of eating and sleeping?	___	___	___	___	___

You have had a chance to visit and care for your baby while he has been ill. Please check the blank you think best describes your baby.

	A great deal	A good bit	Moderate amount	Very little	None
How much crying has your baby done?	___	___	___	___	___
How much trouble has your baby had feeding?	___	___	___	___	___
How much spitting up or vomiting has your baby done?	___	___	___	___	___
How much difficulty has your baby had in sleeping?	___	___	___	___	___
How much difficulty has your baby had with bowel movements?	___	___	___	___	___
How much difficulty has your baby had in settling down to a predictable pattern of eating and sleeping?	___	___	___	___	___
Values	5	4	3	2	1

*Adapted from Broussard, E., and Hartner, M. S.: Further considerations regarding maternal perception of the first born. In Hellmuth, J., editor: Exceptional infant, vol. 2, New York, Brunner/Mazel, Inc., pp. 442-443.

fant, and later the infant at 1 month of age, are predictors of the child's subsequent development (see pp. 169-170).[10, 11] Furthermore, it reflects the effect of maternal confidence on perception of the infant. That is, if the mother is pleased and rewarded with the interaction with her infant, she is most likely to feel a positive perception of the baby. This relationship fosters and main-

tains more positive mothering behaviors. A questionnaire that has been adapted from Broussard and Hartner's work may be used (Tables 12-1 and 12-2).[11]

Results are obtained by totaling the scores for the "average baby" and for "your baby." After the latter score is subtracted from the first, the difference indicates the mother's perceptions of her baby as related

Table 12-2. Neonatal perception inventory*

Now that you have had your baby at home for _____ weeks, we would like to know what your ideas are about babies. Please check the blank you think best describes the *average* baby.

	A great deal	A good bit	Moderate amount	Very little	None
How much crying do you think the average baby does?	___	___	___	___	___
How much trouble do you think the average baby has in feeding?	___	___	___	___	___
How much spitting up or vomiting do you think the average baby does?	___	___	___	___	___
How much difficulty does the average baby have with bowel movements?	___	___	___	___	___
How much difficulty do you think the average baby has in sleeping?	___	___	___	___	___
How much trouble do you think the average baby has in settling down to a predictable pattern of eating and sleeping?	___	___	___	___	___

You have had a chance to live with your baby for _____ weeks now. Please check the blank you think best describes your baby.

	A great deal	A good bit	Moderate amount	Very little	None
How much crying has your baby done?	___	___	___	___	___
How much trouble has your baby had feeding?	___	___	___	___	___
How much spitting up or vomiting has your baby done?	___	___	___	___	___
How much difficulty has your baby had in sleeping?	___	___	___	___	___
How much difficulty has your baby had with bowel movements?	___	___	___	___	___
How much difficulty has your baby had in settling down to a predictable pattern of eating and sleeping?	___	___	___	___	___
Values	5	4	3	2	1

*Adapted from Broussard, E., and Hartner, M. S.: Further considerations regarding maternal perception of the first born. In Hellmuth, J., editor: Exceptional infant, vol. 2, New York, 1971, Brunner/Mazel, Inc., pp. 444-445.

to any other infant. A negative score indicates that the mother believes her infant's behavior is less than average, or more negative than most infants. A positive score indicates that she thinks her infant is like most newborns.

Many researchers have demonstrated the importance of early attachment between mother and infant during the first month of life.[5, 30, 31] A description of maternal acquaintance and adaptation processes may be found in works by Rubin and Kennedy.[29] Based on identification of maternal-infant discord, nursing interventions may be devised to assist the mother in understanding her baby. Therefore, assessment and intervention phases begin immediately after birth and continue until the infant reaches 1 month of age.

Temperament and personality play key roles in parental emotional orientation and annoyance levels. They influence a parent's decision as to what constitutes an infant's problem. Broussard and Hartner have designed a test that may be administered with the 1-month-old perception inventory.[11] This test measures individual problems in infant behavior as perceived by the parent (Table 12-3).

The score is calculated by totaling the values with high face validity. In other words, higher scores indicate higher levels of the mother's annoyance by her child.

Characteristics of infant

Infant characteristics can best be evaluated by using the Brazelton Neonatal Behavioral Assessment Scale.[8] (For more information regarding Dr. Brazelton and his assessment scale, see pp. 167-168.) This scale assesses behavioral responses as the infant matures and adjusts to the environment. Variances in alertness, motor activity, and sensory threshold indicate proneness.

When the Brazelton scale is combined with motor tests appropriate for age, the examiner has adequate data to assess the infant's developmental progress, sensorimotor and cognitive levels, interactional adaptation, and acquaintance ability. Therapeutic intervention programs can then be developed. Infant disposition influences effective mothering and all therapeutic programs; the uniqueness of each infant should be emphasized to the mother.

Infants are capable of responding to the environment and of selective discrimination.[18] Thus, the infant controls which stimuli will be repeated. Important factors are: (1) how the infant obtains, integrates, and responds to information; (2) what assists the infant in reacting; and (3) what influences participation in acquaintance with the caretaker.[14] Infant responses to graded visual and auditory stimulations and infant activity levels and self-controlling behaviors are Brazelton scale items that are valuable in the assessment of these areas.

The infant's visual and auditory responses provide data regarding sensitivity and attentiveness to new stimuli, ability to habituate

Table 12-3. Degree of bother inventory*

Listed below are some of the things that have sometimes bothered other mothers in caring for their babies. We would like to know if you were bothered about any of these. Please place a check in the blank that best describes how much you were bothered by your baby's behavior in regard to these.

	A great deal	Somewhat	Very little	None
Crying	___	___	___	___
Spitting up	___	___	___	___
Sleeping	___	___	___	___
Feeding	___	___	___	___
Elimination	___	___	___	___
Lack of a predictable schedule	___	___	___	___
Other: (specify)				
a.	___	___	___	___
b.	___	___	___	___
c.	___	___	___	___

*Adapted from Broussard, E., and Hartner, M. S.: Further considerations regarding maternal perception of the first born. In Hellmuth, J., editor: Exceptional infant, vol. 2, New York, 1971, Brunner/Mazel, Inc., p. 448.

SUMMARY OF BRAZELTON SCALE SCORING*

Visual and auditory stimulation

1. Response decrement to light
2. Response decrement to rattle
3. Response decrement to bell
4. Response decrement to pinprick
5. Orientation response to inanimate visual
6. Orientation response to inanimate auditory
7. Orientation response to animate visual
8. Orientation response to animate auditory
9. Orientation response to animate visual and auditory

Activity (or maturational) levels

10. Alertness
11. General tonus
12. Motor maturity
13. Pull-to-sit
15. Defensive movements
20. Activity
21. Tremulousness
22. Amount of startle during exam
26. Hand-to-mouth facility
27. Smiles

Self-controlling (or variability) behaviors

14. Cuddliness
16. Consolability with intervention
18. Rapidity of build-up
19. Irritability
24. Lability of states
25. Self-quieting activity

*Adapted from Brazelton, T.: Neonatal behavioral assessment scale. In Clinics in developmental medicine, vol. 50, London, 1973, Spastics International Medical Publications (partial listing of Brazelton scale scoring).

STEP SCALE FOR RECIPROCAL CREEPING*

Infant can:

Step 1

   a. Raise head when placed on stomach

Step 2

   a. Lift head with weight supported on elbows

   b. Hold head while being pulled to a sitting position

Step 3

   a. Lift head and support weight on hands (arms straight)

   b. Lean forward while sitting

Step 4

   a. Roll over (back to stomach)

   b. Roll over (stomach to back)

Step 5

   a. Creep (stomach on ground)

   b. Raise up on all fours

   c. Creep (reciprocal)

*Used with permission of Athleen B. (Godfrey) Coyner, R.N., M.S., F.A.A.N., MCH Consultant, Utah State Division of Health, Salt Lake City, Utah. Incomplete table presented here.

information, primary exploratory behaviors, level of curiosity, and discriminative skills. The infant's activity levels and self-controlling behaviors provide data about sensory threshold capacities, patterns of nonverbal communication, anticipatory tolerance levels, behavioral response capacities, and socializing skills.

Examiner expectations of the infant's general tonus, motor maturity, and reflex responses should be appropriate to the infant's chronological age. The infant born prematurely is tested and measured according to gestational age plus chronological age at the time of the examination. For example, using a modified version of Brazie and Lubchenco's gestational age scoring inventory (Fig. 12-1), the examiner would evaluate the level of functioning in posture, tone, and various reflexes, including plantar grasp, galant, nystagmus, and ankle tonus.[9] Furthermore, the examiner must assess the premature infant's capacity for robustness, endurance and exhaustion, control of input in awake states, and self-organization.

The infant is further evaluated according

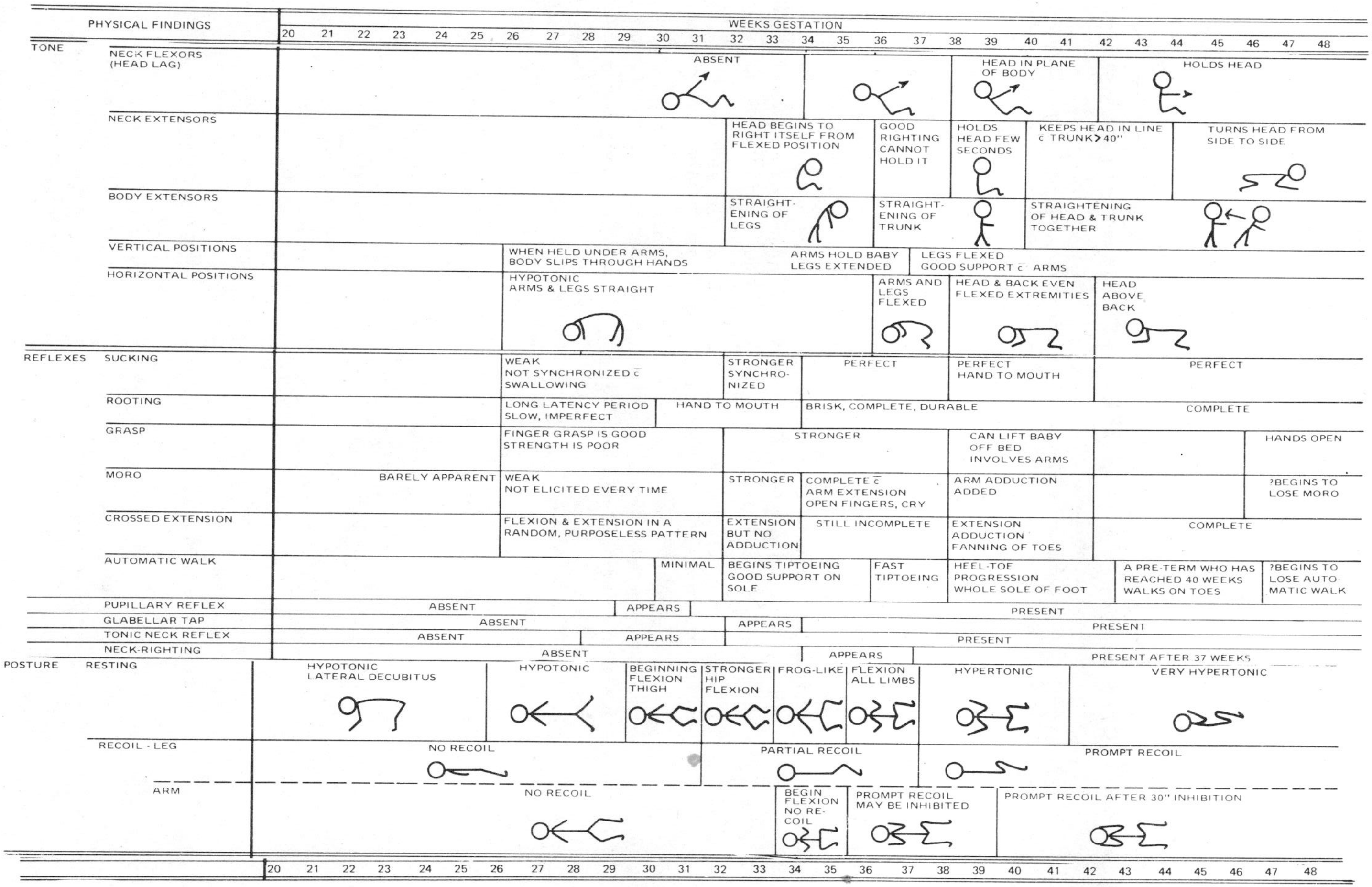
PHYSICAL FINDINGS
WEEKS GESTATION
20 21 22 23 24 25 26 27 28 29 30 31 32 33 34 35 36 37 38 39 40 41 42 43 44 45 46 47 48
TONE
NECK FLEXORS (HEAD LAG)
ABSENT
HEAD IN PLANE OF BODY
HOLDS HEAD
NECK EXTENSORS
HEAD BEGINS TO RIGHT ITSELF FROM FLEXED POSITION
GOOD RIGHTING CANNOT HOLD IT
HOLDS HEAD FEW SECONDS
KEEPS HEAD IN LINE c̄ TRUNK > 40"
TURNS HEAD FROM SIDE TO SIDE
BODY EXTENSORS
STRAIGHTENING OF LEGS
STRAIGHTENING OF TRUNK
STRAIGHTENING OF HEAD & TRUNK TOGETHER
VERTICAL POSITIONS
WHEN HELD UNDER ARMS, BODY SLIPS THROUGH HANDS
ARMS HOLD BABY LEGS EXTENDED
LEGS FLEXED GOOD SUPPORT c̄ ARMS
HORIZONTAL POSITIONS
HYPOTONIC ARMS & LEGS STRAIGHT
ARMS AND LEGS FLEXED
HEAD & BACK EVEN FLEXED EXTREMITIES
HEAD ABOVE BACK
REFLEXES
SUCKING
WEAK NOT SYNCHRONIZED c̄ SWALLOWING
STRONGER SYNCHRONIZED
PERFECT
PERFECT HAND TO MOUTH
PERFECT
ROOTING
LONG LATENCY PERIOD SLOW, IMPERFECT
HAND TO MOUTH
BRISK, COMPLETE, DURABLE
COMPLETE
GRASP
FINGER GRASP IS GOOD STRENGTH IS POOR
STRONGER
CAN LIFT BABY OFF BED INVOLVES ARMS
HANDS OPEN
MORO
BARELY APPARENT
WEAK NOT ELICITED EVERY TIME
STRONGER
COMPLETE c̄ ARM EXTENSION OPEN FINGERS, CRY
ARM ADDUCTION ADDED
?BEGINS TO LOSE MORO
CROSSED EXTENSION
FLEXION & EXTENSION IN A RANDOM, PURPOSELESS PATTERN
EXTENSION BUT NO ADDUCTION
STILL INCOMPLETE
EXTENSION ADDUCTION FANNING OF TOES
COMPLETE
AUTOMATIC WALK
MINIMAL
BEGINS TIPTOEING GOOD SUPPORT ON SOLE
FAST TIPTOEING
HEEL-TOE PROGRESSION WHOLE SOLE OF FOOT
A PRE-TERM WHO HAS REACHED 40 WEEKS WALKS ON TOES
?BEGINS TO LOSE AUTOMATIC WALK
PUPILLARY REFLEX
ABSENT
APPEARS
PRESENT
GLABELLAR TAP
ABSENT
APPEARS
PRESENT
TONIC NECK REFLEX
ABSENT
APPEARS
PRESENT
NECK-RIGHTING
ABSENT
APPEARS
PRESENT AFTER 37 WEEKS
POSTURE
RESTING
HYPOTONIC LATERAL DECUBITUS
HYPOTONIC
BEGINNING FLEXION THIGH
STRONGER HIP FLEXION
FROG-LIKE
FLEXION ALL LIMBS
HYPERTONIC
VERY HYPERTONIC
RECOIL - LEG
NO RECOIL
PARTIAL RECOIL
PROMPT RECOIL
ARM
NO RECOIL
BEGIN FLEXION NO RECOIL
PROMPT RECOIL MAY BE INHIBITED
PROMPT RECOIL AFTER 30" INHIBITION
20 21 22 23 24 25 26 27 28 29 30 31 32 33 34 35 36 37 38 39 40 41 42 43 44 45 46 47 48

Fig. 12-1. Brazie and Lubchenco's gestational age inventory. (Adapted from Lubchenco, L. O.: P. Clin. North Am. **17**:125, 1970. In Kempe, C. H., and others, editors: Current pediatric diagnosis and treatment, ed. 4, Los Altos, Calif., 1976, Lange Medical Publications.)

to touch responses, feeding behavior, and posturing patterns. Locomotion can be easily assessed by using the step scale for reciprocal creeping (see boxed material on p. 150).[15]

Finally, the severely injured infant is evaluated according to basic rhythm patterns. Sleep-wake states, spontaneous cry, and spontaneous sucking behavior are recorded on a periodic time chart by the

Table 12-4. Categories of adaptive and maladaptive mothering behaviors*

	Adaptive	Maladaptive
Feeding behaviors	Offers appropriate amounts and/or types of food to infant.	Provides inadequate types or amounts of food for infant.
	Holds infant in comfortable position during feeding.	Does not hold infant, or holds in uncomfortable position during feeding.
	Burps baby during and/or after feeding.	Does not burp infant.
	Prepares food appropriately.	Prepares food inappropriately.
	Offers food at comfortable pace for infant.	Offers food at pace too rapid or slow for infant's comfort.
Infant stimulation	Provides appropriate verbal stimulation for infant during visit.	Provides no or only aggressive verbal stimulation for infant during visit.
	Provides tactile stimulation for infant at times other than during feeding or moving infant away from danger.	Does not provide tactile stimulation or only that of aggressive handling of infant.
	Provides age-appropriate toys.	No evidence of age-appropriate toys.
	Interacts with infant in a way that provides for infant's satisfaction.	Frustrates infant during interactions.
Infant rest	Provides quiet or relaxed environment for infant's rest, including scheduled rest periods.	Does not provide quiet environment or consistent schedule for rest periods.
	Ensures that infant's needs for food, warmth, and/or dryness are met before sleep.	Does not attend to infant's needs for food, warmth, and/or dryness before sleep.
Perception	Demonstrates realistic perception of infant's condition in accordance with medical and/or nursing diagnosis.	Shows unrealistic perception of infant's condition.
	Has realistic expectations of infant.	Demonstrates unrealistic expectations of infant.
	Recognizes infant's unfolding skills or behavior.	Has no awareness of infant's development.
	Shows realistic perception of own mothering behavior.	Shows unrealistic perception of own mothering.
Initiative	Shows initiative in attempts to manage infant's problems, including actively seeking information about infants.	Shows no initiative in attempts to meet infant's needs or to manage problems. Does not follow through with plans.
Recreation	Provides positive outlets for own recreation or relaxation.	Does not provide positive outlets for own recreation or relaxation.
Interaction with other children	Demonstrates positive interaction with other children in home.	Demonstrates hostile-aggressive interaction with other children in home.
Mothering role	Expresses satisfaction with mothering.	Expresses dissatisfaction with mothering.

*Adapted from Harrison, L.: Nursing intervention with the failure-to-thrive family, Am. J. Maternal Child Nurs. 1:111, 1976. Copyright March/April 1976, the American Journal of Nursing Company. Reproduced with permission from MCN, The American Journal of Maternal Child Nursing, vol. 1, No. 2.

mother for 3 or 4 days. The chart is then evaluated for spontaneous rhythmicity patterns that delineate the infant's needs for periodic variations in the sensory environment.

Caregiver-infant interaction

Caregiver-infant behaviors involve the interactions of each. Feeding, a universal event, is an excellent source for data collection (Table 12-4). Mothering behaviors to be evaluated include: sensitivity to stress; satiation cues of the infant; how growth is fostered through visual, tactile, auditory, and kinesthetic stimulation; and how distress is alleviated in the infant. Reciprocal infant behavior can also be easily evaluated (Table 12-5). Infant behaviors to be evaluated include prefeeding arousal level, approach and motor attachment behavior, attentiveness, level of motor activity, cues of satiation or distress, responses to mothering behavior, and success in achieving the task. Attention should also be directed at how the infant and mother "read" each other and who is in charge.

NURSING INTERVENTIONS: PRINCIPLES

A therapeutic program of nursing interventions based on the neurophysiological needs of the individual infant is always developed with the caregivers. Research has proved the value of a multiplicity of approaches. It is evident that certain principles are essential for success. First, the family unit (or primary caregivers) is the most economical and effective agent for fostering and sustaining an infant's neuromotor development.[22] Caregivers serve as motivators, and their responsiveness provides the infant with incentive to develop. More enduring effects are evident when parental involvement occurs in early infancy and before admission in special preschool programs. In addition, parents should participate in the planning of interventions. This promotes parental understanding of the infant's uniqueness and enhances the interactional process.

Second, intervention must be based on the physiological and developmental status of the infant. Piaget has demonstrated that each stage of development is the basis for

Table 12-5. Categories of adaptive and maladaptive infant behaviors*

	Adaptive	Maladaptive
Sleeping behavior	Receives adequate sleep for normal growth—at least 16 hours per day—without restless sleep patterns or prolonged crying at nap or bedtime after other needs have been met.	Receives inadequate sleep for normal growth—less than 16 hours per day. Shows restless sleep patterns and/or prolonged crying at nap or bedtime.
Feeding behavior	Actively seeks food offered. Effectively sucks and swallows food. Demonstrates pleasurable relief after eating.	Resists food offered. Does not suck effectively. Remains fussy after adequate amount of feeding—no pleasurable relief.
Response to environment	Demonstrates active response to environment by exploring or reaching-out behavior.	Seems apathetic to environment.
Vocalizing	Demonstrates vocalizations when alert, if developmentally ready.	Makes infrequent or no vocalizations during visit although developmentally ready.
Smiling	Demonstrates smiling behavior if older than 2 months.	Does not demonstrate smiling behavior during visit.
Cuddling	Cuddles when held.	Resists being held or stiffens when held.

*Adapted from Harrison, L.: Nursing intervention with the failure-to-thrive family, Am. J. Maternal Child Nurs. 1:111, 1976. Copyright March/April 1976, the American Journal of Nursing Company. Reproduced with permission from MCN, The American Journal of Maternal Child Nursing, vol. 1, No. 2.

the next level of development.[45] One must be aware of and utilize behavioral continuums in conjunction with existing infant behaviors to reinforce present appropriate responses and facilitate new behaviors. For instance, vestibular stimulation should be provided for the 28-week-gestational-age infant to enhance neuromuscular integration and limbic system maturation, thus fostering the infant's ability to deal with the earth's gravitational pull.[35] As infants progress to head lifting, they will learn new ways of handling gravity.

Interventions are created with four objectives, which are: to inhibit abnormal patterns of response, to enhance development of neuroassociation circuits, to facilitate appropriate responses for sequential development, and to foster an environment within the infant's sensory threshold tolerance. Examples of each are:

1. To inhibit abnormal patterns, such as inversion until relaxation in the hypertonic infant
2. To enhance development of neuroassociation circuits, such as stimulating sucking activities during gavage feedings
3. To facilitate appropriate responses, such as alerting and toning exercises for hypotonic infants
4. To foster a sensory environment, such as reducing random light touch experiences for preterm infants and providing repetitive, gentle and firm touch experiences

Successful programs also utilize a variety of interventions. In neonatal nurseries, stimulation programs consist of temporally regulated low-frequency repetitive movements[35] and sounds,[43] appropriate visual configurations and colors,[30] animate auditory and visual stimuli when alert,[40] and sensorimotor exercises.[12]

Finally, interventions must demonstrate complete learning loops. Infants are prepared for success, actively participate in the behavior, and are positively reinforced for their accomplishments. For instance, the preterm infant is alerted before responsiveness to visual stimulation can be evaluated. The visual stimulus (such as the caregiver's face) is placed within visual range and then responds to the infant's gaze (such as smiling).

All interventions utilized in the following case study were based on these principles. Many interventions in the study are not discussed. Only those interventions most directly affecting neuromotor facilitation are described. Additional resources may be used for interventions indirectly related to neuromotor development.[20, 21, 25, 28, 31]

CASE PRESENTATION

The assessment data on a client and family are presented to demonstrate an application of the proneness and assessment profiles. Since a proneness profile is the initial basis for assessment, it is incorporated within the data presented.

Perinatal health indicators

Mother. Ms. M. planned her pregnancy with her husband. This pregnancy was their first, and they experienced a normal cognitive style[38] until its interruption at 26 weeks. During her adolescence, Ms. M. frequently baby-sat for neighbors and relatives. Both parents reported affectionate and stable nuclear families. All grandparents provided major emotional support after delivery. Ms. M. was a vegetarian and had a 15-pound weight gain. She took no medications during her pregnancy and did not smoke. Her prenatal physical examination revealed normal physiological findings.

Premature labor lasted 6 hours. No fetal distress was noted during labor, and Ms. M. received no medications. Although both parents expressed shock, apprehension, and grief during the labor and postnatal period, they proceeded through the stages of grief at appropriate time intervals.

Infant. H. M. was delivered at 26 weeks' gestational age, was appropriate weight, and had 1 minute/5 minute Apgar scores of 4/6. H. M. experienced severe hyaline membrane disease and bronchopulmonary dysplasia requiring oxygen, continuous positive airway pressure, and ventilatory support for the first 12 weeks of her life. Surgical repair of patent ductus arteriosus was performed on her third day of life. She had one episode of prolonged hypoglycemia on her first day of life. Her highest arterial oxygen tension was 96 mm Hg, and her lowest was 48 mm Hg. Her lowest arterial pH was 7.08. She received antibiotics for a total of 3 weeks. She demonstrated no seizure activity during hospitalization. She also had hyperbilirubinemia, requiring phototherapy for 8 days. Her highest serum bilirubin level was 14 mg/100 ml.

Home health status. H. M.'s parents lived in a small, well-furnished, and clean six-room home, which they were purchasing. It was located in a small, suburban, middle-class community. Ms. M. was a registered nurse, and Mr. M. was a student in health administration. Both grandfathers were physicians. A separate room for the infant had been planned but not completed at the time of delivery. No equipment had been purchased. Three days after H. M. was removed from oxygen therapy, her parents purchased a crib and clothing. The parents were advised by nurses as to anticipatory home needs, and appropriate home improvements were devised by the parents and grandparents. Although toys were minimal, they were selected according the H. M.'s responsive level. The parents gave H. M. her first toy at the age of 5 weeks and in accordance with her behavioral cues.

Characteristics of caregivers

Mother. Ms. M. had obtained a college degree and worked 2 years as a pediatric nurse. Both parents were relatively calm, affectionate people who faced this crisis by sharing their feelings and supporting each other. Ms. M. had initially expressed her frustration indirectly but became more direct when she felt comfortable. Ms. M. perceived her marriage positively. Both parents felt that this crisis was a growth period in their religious life, requiring patience, trust, and stamina. They sought guidance from their minister as they examined why this had happened to them. They demonstrated positive coping mechanisms during the grief process, and Ms. M. adapted appropriately to an altered maternal role.[39] She was sensitive to her infant's cues and used appropriate methods to alleviate distress.

Father. Mr. M. was studying for a master's degree. He directly expressed his frustration by confrontation and reality validation. Mr. M. struggled longest with adaptation to an altered paternal role and moved more slowly into the acceptance phase of grief. He was equally sensitive to H. M.'s cues. Ms. M. taught him appropriate methods to alleviate distress. Both parents eagerly sought our resources for learning how to promote their child's growth and contributed equally for such provisions.

Characteristics of infant

On the second day of life, H. M. was estimated to be 26 weeks' gestational age by Brazie and Lubchenco scoring. An examination confirmed this age, and no abnormalities were identified at that time. At 10 weeks of chronological age, H. M.'s acute illness problems were resolved, and she was weaned off ambient oxygen. Her only identified chronic problem was bronchopulmonary dysplasia. A complete neurological assessment was performed, and in problem-oriented format the findings included:

Problem: growth and development

S: *Reflexes:* Appropriate—corneal, glabellar, pupillary, hand-mouth reflex of Bakin; abdominal; galant; perez; plantar grasp; standing; walking; placing—assymetrical; neck righting; tonic deviation of head and eyes, nystagmus (fast).

Flexion angles: Popliteal—90; wrist—45; ankle—0.

Motor tone and maturity: Appropriate—heel to ear maneuver; scarf sign; arm recoil (beginning flexion). Inappropriate/absent—neck flexors, neck extensors; body extensors; vertical; horizontal; leg recoil (delayed, asymmetrical); two divergent qualities—little response when moved and hypertonic with handling; much sudden tonus change; cogwheellike jerkiness with overshooting in all states.

Activity and posture: Some flexion; much hand on face with sudden arm and leg extension; with manipulation—separation of arm and leg organization; defensive movement was nonspecific with short latency; great discrepancy between spontaneous and elicited activity; tremulousness in state 4, startles × 3.

Autonomic nervous system (ANS): Sinus bradycardia and apnea with multiple trials of stimulation.

Behavior: Initial state—drowsy; predominate state—drowsy, crying.

ORIENTATION: Variable alerting and habituating responses, seizure activity with first trial of pinprick.

SOCIALIZING: Only response was precarious and to animate auditory.

ALERTNESS: Brief, delayed, difficult to obtain.

EXCITEMENT: Irritable cry × 3.

SELF-CONTROL: Unconsolable with abrupt change, no gradual subsiding of agitation; state changes were inappropriate, abrupt, and unpredictable; no control over terminating stimulation (apnea, cyanosis, random eye movement); three mood swings.

ENDURANCE: Exhausted with orientation; poor color with mottling, no recovery.

ROBUSTNESS: Poor in all states.

O: *Head growth curve:* Consistent with preterm sick infant curve.

A: Preterm infant with poorly organized CNS, unstable autonomic nervous system, variable alerting and habituation, low sensory threshold tolerance, poor socializing, abnormal reflex patterns, poor motor tone and maturity, poor endurance.

P: *Infant stimulation program:* Vestibular stimulation; rocking waterbed asynchronized movement every hour for 1 minute.

Inhibiting stimulation: Music box every hour for 2 minutes; firm touch only.

One week later H. M. had improved in the following:

S: *Reflexes:* Appropriate—rooting (premature pattern); standing.

Motor tone and maturity: Leg recoil (delayed); neck extensors (poor but some increased tone).

Activity and posture: Defensive movements —no tremors; no startles; minimal activity at rest, much elicited; more activity seen in alert state than in crying state.

Autonomic nervous system: No arrhythmias, no bradycardia.

Behavior: Initial state—deep sleep; predominate state—drowsy, crying.

ORIENTATION: Variable alerting; habituation present after 2 or 3 trials, sudden diminution of response.

Socializing: None; resisted being held.

EXCITEMENT: Irritable cry × 10; easily agitated.

SELF-CONTROL: Looked fatigued with orientation; used stimuli briefly to become better organized; no control over terminating stimuli (apnea, cyanosis, random eye movements); nine mood swings.

A: *Some improvements:* Brief CNS organization; stable ANS; less variable alerting; variable socializing; some motor tone improvement.

P: *Continue infant stimulation program:* Discuss with parents.

The next week H. M. was examined with active participation of the parents. The examination process and all findings were discussed, and the following improvements were noted:

S: *Reflexes:* Palmar grasp stronger; walking (premature).

Motor tone and maturity: Neck extensors (holds head up for few seconds); body extensors (straightening of trunk brief); vertical (arms hold baby).

Activity and posture: Defensive movements —nondirected swipes; activity appropriate with state.

Behavior: Initial state—light sleep; predominate state—drowsy, crying.

ORIENTATION: Consistently good alerting response; habituated at right trials.

Socializing: Attentive and responsive to animate auditory and auditory-visual stimuli; participated in cuddling.

ALERTNESS: Brief and somewhat delayed.

EXCITEMENT: Irritable cry × 3; appropriate activity level.

SELF-CONTROL: Consoled with holding and rocking; thirteen mood swings, better organized with stimulation; terminated stimuli × 3.

ENDURANCE: Intermittently exhausted but could refuel self with help.

ROBUSTNESS: State maintenance precarious.

A: *Continued improvement:* CNS organization with stimulation; stable alerting; stable habituation; socializing to animate environment; motor tone improvement; sensory threshold tolerance improved but precarious; endurance improved.

P: *Continue infant stimulation program:* Add parental holding and rocking on all visits with auditory and visual stimulation.

Caregiver—infant interaction
(third-week evaluation)

Mother. Growth was fostered through the use of pacifier and animate auditory-visual stimulation during gavage feeding. Infant distress was alleviated by rocking and holding.

Infant. No prearousal behavior was noted. The infant was briefly attentive to the mother. Motor activity was decreased by the end of the feeding process, and the infant was irritable at times (see behavior evaluation).

SUMMARY

Caution must be exercised by nurses when preparing an intervention program for third and fourth trimester infants. Overzealousness to facilitate neuromotor development can lead to detrimental effects. Creating a therapeutic milieu for these clients demands more investigation by nurses. Certainly nurses need to refine their repertoire of assessment skills. The profession can no longer afford to waste the precious time and potential of its clients.

REFERENCES

1. Ayres, A.: Tactile functions, Am. J. Occup. Ther. **18:**6, 1964.
2. Babson, S., and others: Management of high-risk pregnancy and intensive care of the neonate, St. Louis, 1971, The C. V. Mosby Co., pp. 9-21.
3. Barnard, K.: Important; the first four trimesters of life, paper presented at the University of Washington, Seattle, May 4-6, 1975.
4. Barnes, A. C.: Intra-uterine development, Philadelphia, 1968, Lea & Febiger.
5. Barnett, C., and others: Neonatal separation; the maternal side of interactional deprivation, Pediatrics **45:**197, 1970.
6. Bodemer, C.: Modern embryology, New York, 1968, Holt, Rinehart & Winston.
7. Brand, M., and others: The effects of chronic hypoxia on the neonatal and infantile brain, Brain **92:**233, 1969.
8. Brazelton, T.: Neonatal behavioral assessment scale. In Clinics in developmental medicine, vol. 50, London, 1973, Spastics International Medical Publications.
9. Brazie, J., and Lubchenco, L. O.: The newborn infant (adapted from Lubchenco, L. O.: P. Clin. North Am. **17:**125, 1970). In Kempe, C. H., and others, editors: Current pediatric diagnosis and treatment, ed. 4, Los Altos, Calif., 1976, Lange Medical Publications.
10. Broussard, E., and others: Maternal perception of the neonate as related to development, Child Psychiatry Hum. Dev. **1:**16, 1970.
11. Broussard, E., and Hartner, M. S.: Further considerations regarding maternal perception of the first born. In Hellmuth, J., editor: Exceptional infant, vol. 2, New York, 1971, Brunner/Mazel, Inc., pp. 440-448.
12. Buerger, E. M.: Unpublished data, 1976.
13. Center for Disease Control: Diphtheria, tetanus, and pertussis status report, 1974, Atlanta.
14. Clark A., and others: Childbearing; a nursing perspective, New York, 1976, F. A. Davis Co.
15. Coyner, A.: Unpublished paper, 1971.
16. Desmedt, J.: The somatosensory cerebral evoked potential of the sleeping human newborn. In Clemente, C., and others, editors: Sleep and the maturing nervous system, New York, 1972, Academic Press, Inc., pp. 230-252.
17. Eastman, N., and others: Weight relationship in pregnancy, Obstet. Gynecol. Surv. **23:**1003, 1968.
18. Fanaroff, A., and others: The amazing newborn, a film presented at the University of Southern California Conference on New Vistas in Perinatal Critical Care, Los Angeles, March 1-3, 1976.
19. Frank, L.: Tactile communication, Genet. Psychol. Monogr. **56:**209, 1957.
20. Freeman, J., and others: Project A.D.A.P.T.; a developmental curriculum for infants exhibiting developmental delay, Santa Barbara, Calif., 1975, Tri-Counties Regional Center.
21. Godfrey, A.: Sensori-motor stimulation for slow-to-develop children, Am. J. Nurs. **75:**56, 1975.
22. Gordon, I.: A home learning center approach to early stimulation, Institute for Development of Human Resources, Gainesville, Fla., University of Florida at Gainesville, 1973.
23. Grimwade, J.: Sensory stimulation of the human fetus, Aust. J. Ment. Retard. **2:**63, 1970.
24. Harris, F.: Multiple-loop modulation of motor outflow, Phys. Ther. **51:**391, 1971.
25. Harrison, L.: Nursing intervention with the

failure-to-thrive family, Am. J. Maternal Child Nurs. **1:**111, 1976.

26. Head, H., and others: Studies in neurology, vol. 2, London, 1920, Oxford University Press.

27. Hyden, H., and others: Nuclear RNA changes in nerve cells during a learning experiment with rats, Proc. Natl. Acad. Sci. USA **48:**1366, 1962.

28. Johnson, S.: The premature infant's reflex behavior; effect on maternal-child relationship, J. Obstet. Gynecol. Neonat. Nurs. **4:**15, 1975.

29. Kennedy, J.: The high-risk maternal-infant acquaintance process, Nurs. Clin. North Am. **8:**549, 1973.

30. Kennell, J., and others: Care of the mother of the high-risk infant, Clin. Obstet. Gynecol. **14:**926, 1971.

31. Klaus, M., and others: Human maternal behavior at the first contact with her young, Pediatrics **46:**187, 1970.

32. Levine, S.: Stimulation in infancy, Sci. Am. **202:**81, 1960.

33. Melker, R., and others: Maturational features of neurons and synaptic relations in raphe and reticular nuclei of neonatal kittens, Anat. Rec. **172:**366, 1972.

34. Mountcastle, V.: A study of the functional contributions of the lemniscal and spinothalamic systems to somatic sensibility, Bull. Johns Hopkins Hosp. **106:**316, 1960.

35. Neal, M.: Relationship between vestibular stimulation and the developmental behavior of the premature infant, New York, 1967, New York University, unpublished doctoral dissertation.

36. Norton, Y.: Minimal cerebral dysfunction, Am. J. Occup. Ther. **26:**135, 1972.

37. Rocke, L.: Myelination of the brain in the newborn, Philadelphia, 1969, J. B. Lippincott Co.

38. Rubin, R.: Attainment of the maternal role, parts 1 and 2, Nurs. Res. **16:**237, 1967.

39. Sakalys, J.: States of adaptation to illness and disability; a psychosocial view. In Duffey, M., and others, editors: Current concepts in clinical nursing, vol. III, St. Louis, 1971, The C. V. Mosby Co., pp. 271-290.

40. Scharr, S.: The effects of early stimulation on low birth weight, paper presented at American Public Health Association, Minneapolis, October 14, 1971.

41. Scheibel, M., and others: Maturative processes in dendrites of spinal cord and brain stem in the cat, paper presented at Society for Neuroscience, second annual meeting, Oct. 8-11, 1972.

42. Scheibel, M., and others: Maturation of reticular dendrites, Exp. Neurol. **38:**301, 1973.

43. Segall, M.: Cardiac responsivity of auditory stimulation in premature infants, Nurs. Rev. **21:**15, 1972.

44. Sterman, M.: The basic rest-activity cycle and sleep; developmental considerations in man and cats. In Clemente, C., and others, editors: Sleeping and the maturing nervous system, New York, 1972, Academic Press, Inc., pp. 175-199.

45. Wadsworth, D.: Piaget's theory of cognitive development, New York, 1971, David McKay Co., Inc.

46. Werner, E., and others: The children of Kanai; a longitudinal study from the prenatal period to age ten, Honolulu, 1971, University of Hawaii Press.

47. Willerman, L., and others: Infant development, preschool IQ, and social class, Child Dev. **41:**69, 1970.

48. Witte, J. J.: Recent advances in public health, Am. J. Public Health **64:**939, 1974.

ADDITIONAL READINGS

Katz, V.: Auditory stimulation and developmental behavior of the premature, Nurs. Res. **20:**196, 1971.

Klaus, M., and others: Maternal attachment importance of the first post-partum days, N. Engl. J. Med. **286:**460, 1972.

Purpura, D., and others: Principles of synaptogenesis and their application to ontogenetic studies of mammalian cerebral cortex. In Clemente, C., and others, editors: Sleeping and the maturing nervous system, New York, 1972, Academic Press, Inc., pp. 5-31.

Rubin, R.: Basic maternal behavior, Nurs. Outlook **11:**828, 1963.

Rubin, R.: Maternal touch, Nurs. Outlook **12:**36, 1964.

Rubin, R.: Cognitive style of pregnancy, Am. J. Nurs. **70:**502, 1970.

Scherzer, A. L.: Early diagnosis, management, and treatment of cerebral palsy, Rehabil. Lit. **35:**194, 1974.

CHAPTER 13

Developmental screening

MARCENE POWELL ERICKSON

This chapter is intended to aid nurses and other child care professionals in understanding the need for skilled use of a variety of screening and assessment tools. Traditional developmental screening practices are contrasted with current trends and practices, and the screening process is explained. Certain screening tools are discussed: three popular developmental screening inventories, two instruments used in early case finding and prevention of mental retardation, and one relatively new environmental assessment device used in conjunction with developmental assessment tools. Thorough, accurate developmental assessment is an essential component of early case finding, prevention, and practical management of children with mental retardation.

Although many disciplines are involved in assessing development, the variety of nursing roles demands that nurses be knowledgeable about growth and development, a number of screening tools, and the procedures for administering these tools. Nurses find developmental screenings essential in case finding, planning and implementing programs, and evaluating outcomes of their efforts. All nurses should incorporate developmental screenings into their practice with developmentally disabled children and their families.

CHANGING TRENDS

In the past, child care professionals patterned developmental assessment after a traditional medical model, waiting for gross clinical manifestations to appear before making a diagnosis or initiating a treatment plan. They collected all the developmental screening data on a particular child at one time, using subjective methods. They generalized freely about a child's behaviors and problems, emphasizing negative characteristics by attaching labels. They assessed a child's functional and adaptive levels within the environment but did not assess the environment itself. And, significantly, they focused almost exclusively on the child, overlooking the important role of observation and assessment by parents and other caregivers as agents of change.

As developmental screening practices evolved, professionals changed their orientation. Now they rely more on a developmental model, looking for sequential changes in a child and facilitating early intervention whenever developmental delays are detected. More objective methods of developmental assessment are used by observing a child's simultaneous progress in gross motor skills, fine motor skills, receptive and expressive language skills, personal-social adaptive skills, and preacademic behaviors (such as attention span, problem-solving abilities, and discrimination). Collecting data over a period of time makes it possible for professionals to follow a child's developmental progress and to more adequately plan future intervention. Labels can interfere with individualized approaches to planning intervention goals, set up self-fulfilling prophecies, negate an individual's strengths, and confuse parents and other professionals. A child's environment is examined to determine whether it promotes or impedes the child's development.

Perhaps most important, professionals now increasingly observe how parents interact with a child and respond to developmental changes and whether the parents encourage or hinder change. Professionals share developmental information with parents to help alleviate parental anxieties and to help the family set realistic goals for increasing a child's independent functioning. They no longer dismiss parents with empty phrases, such as "he'll catch up" or "don't worry." Instead, they are beginning to acknowledge the validity of parental concerns by listening carefully to what parents say and asking parents to systematically collect data that set the stage for later intervention. The current aim of nurses and other child care professionals is to help parents feel adequate and to become active, resourceful problem solvers early in the process of planning and decision making.

THE DEVELOPMENTAL SCREENING PROCESS

Developmental screening of any newborn, infant, or child is a process directed at determining a child's level of independent functioning within the environment. The process consists of: (1) preparing the child and parent by helping them establish feelings of security and maximal comfort; (2) observing and recording data, being careful to administer each developmental screening item in the same way; (3) scoring each item by comparing individual data with standardized, normative data; (4) analyzing the child's strengths and weaknesses by interpreting the data; and (5) communicating both results and implications to parents in an appropriate way.

Professionals now rely on a number and variety of standardized tools designed to do a more accurate job of developmental screening and assessment than ever before. For each tool, the screening and assessment protocol is carefully spelled out, the directions for administering developmental items are clear, and the criteria for passing or failing a child are readily available for reference. Carrying out each screening procedure in a standardized way results in valid information about a child's behaviors and removes confusion and guessing about how well the child is doing. There is evidence that screening tests can be useful in secondary prevention of handicapping conditions. The 1951 Commission on Chronic Illness defined screening as:

the presumptive identification of unrecognized disease or defect by the application of tests, examinations, or other procedures which can be applied rapidly. Screening tests sort out apparently well persons who probably have a disease from those who probably do not. A screening test is not intended to be diagnostic. Persons with positive or suspicious findings must be referred to their physicians for diagnosis and necessary treatment.*

Screening tools are intended for assessment of a child's developmental status before intervention and at periodic intervals during intervention. Until carefully conducted longitudinal studies of normal children of different racial, socioeconomic, and educational backgrounds have been completed, the majority of developmental screening inventories popular today cannot be used for predicting a child's future.[23] Developmental screening tools should not be misused. They are not intended to represent or substitute for a full psychometric evaluation. They do not diagnose children.[11] Furthermore, no single standardized developmental screening test will satisfy the needs of all professional disciplines; certain

---

*From Chronic illness in the United States, vol. 1, Prevention of Chronic Illness, Commission on Chronic Illness, Cambridge, 1957, Harvard University Press, p. 45.

tools have benefits for one discipline but only limited usefulness for others.[11]

Nevertheless, when used by an individual well trained in procedures for administering, scoring, and interpreting results, screening tools can produce narrative descriptions that are useful in planning for the needs of a child who is mentally retarded. An individual becomes proficient in using screening tools and maintains proficiency by practicing with a number of children of different ages and levels of development, trying out a variety of screening tools in different environments, and talking with parents who have concerns about their children. Practicing with a new tool in the presence of someone who is already proficient in its use increases systematic objectivity and lessens subjective errors in interpretation.

PARENTAL PERCEPTIONS OF CHILDREN'S DEVELOPMENT

Children with mental retardation may manifest a variety of behaviors that are difficult to interpret and respond to correctly. Mash, Terdal, and Anderson have studied how a child's behaviors affect parental responses and suggest using the Response Class Matrix[20] to help parents modify inappropriate responses to their children.[19] The Response Class Matrix helps child care professionals to systematically record parental behavior classes (commands, command-questions, questions, praise, negative behaviors, interaction, and no response) and the child's antecedent behavior classes (compliance, independent play, competing behavior, negative behavior, verbal or nonverbal interaction, and no response). The objective results may help parents of mentally retarded children improve parent-child interactions.

Despite the fact that parents may be confused when trying to interpret the behavior of a mentally retarded child (who may present a blurred image, so to speak), they are capable of much more uniformly accurate assessments of their children than formerly assumed. In 1945 Rheingold was one of the first to report that parents usually closely estimated their child's level of functioning.[22] Twelve years later, Ewart and Green reported that parents rated boys more accurately than they rated girls and that a serious physical abnormality in a child did not seem to affect the parents' accuracy.[14] Apparently, younger children were more accurately rated than older children, and children were rated more accurately if they were younger when their parents first became concerned about their development. Ewart and Green also found that more accurate ratings were made by mothers who were younger, more highly educated, or of higher occupational status.[14] Soon afterward, Zuk reported that parents consistently rated the abilities of their children higher than a "relatively objective observer." However, according to Zuk, parents of children with motor impairments were more accurate in their ratings of development than were parents of children without motor impairments.[26]

In the middle 1960s, Capobianco and Knox reported that fathers' judgments were not significantly different from their children's test scores but that mothers tended to overestimate to a statistically significant degree. They found an absence of any relationship between parental ability to judge children's IQ scores and the degree of marital integration that existed between the mother and father.[10] Barclay and Vaught also reported that mothers of handicapped children tended to overestimate their child's potential for future achievements. (The average mother's rating was 97.40 points; the average professional's rating was 58.92 points.[2]) Bickley and Martin found that mothers of retarded children significantly overestimated their children's future social adaptation when compared with the preschool teachers' estimates.[4]

The findings of a study done by Kurtz revealed that parents' estimates of children's development correlated most closely with a pediatrician's assessment, next with an intelligence test, and least with a speech pathologist's assessment. Forty-four percent of parental judgments fell within 10 points of an IQ test. Kurtz noted that parental estimates were more accurate for children who were functioning at lower levels of development.[18] At about the same time, Ehlers reported that families with children who were moderately or severely retarded sought and received diagnostic services before the children were 2 years old.[12] In 1967, Gorelick and Sandhu reported that mothers overestimated their children's development by only 7 developmental quotient points.[16] In the same year, Meyerowitz reported that parents of children with mental retardation evaluated their children consistently lower than did parents of a control group.[21]

In 1971, Broussard and Hartner published a study of maternal perceptions of their firstborn. Of the normal 1-month-old infants perceived to be not better than average by their mothers, 40% had sufficient psychopathology to warrant therapeutic intervention at $4^{1}/_{2}$ years of age.[7] Wolfensberger and Kurtz reported that parents demonstrated realism in predicting future developmental attainments in children, especially in academic achievement.[25]

The majority of the above studies included parents of handicapped or mentally retarded children. Controls were generally not well established. Although most were parents of older children, a wide age range of children was represented in these studies. The results show that parents were generally accurate in estimating their children's abilities. When they were incorrect, parents tended to overestimate the child's abilities.

CONSIDERATION OF CHILD AND PARENT NEEDS DURING ASSESSMENT

The most effective way to obtain reliable results with screening and assessment tools is to promote the child's optimal performance through careful consideration of the needs of both the child and the parents. The wise examiner conveys sensitivity to each child's uniqueness, attention to the child's individual ways and rates of responding, and regard for the child's strengths and weaknesses. A child who is mentally retarded is best assessed by an examiner who

can observe and encourage a child's best behavior, no matter how difficult the assessment task. The examiner must have skills beyond those required to screen a well, or normal, child. Not only are observational skills vital, but ability to interpret what the child can or cannot do is important. The examiner must be able to determine and accentuate what the child can do rather than be satisfied with what the child cannot do because what the child can do may be far more important.

An examiner should be continuously sensitive to the variety and number of cues that the child emits in response to the requests being made. Such cues include willingness to perform, ability to separate from a parent, attention to the task at hand, interest in participating, ability to ignore irrelevant stimuli, eagerness to please, and eagerness to succeed. Of course, children need a chance to warm up to a new environment and to the unfamiliar person who will be examining their developmental achievements. Screening should begin only after the child is comfortable and able to perform optimally. The examiner should encourage the child to respond to one request at a time. If stimuli interfere with the child's ability to perform, the child usually attends best to one task when both animate and inanimate stimuli are reduced. However, the examiner can observe the child attending to a number of stimuli in order to get an accurate picture of the child's learning and performance needs. If the child seems overwhelmed, confused, anxious, or becomes withdrawn or increasingly active, the examiner needs to consider the amount of stimuli to which the child is responding as well as how the various stimuli are being presented to the child.

Flexibility in attempting different observational approaches with a child who is exhibiting unusual or bizarre forms of behavior is essential for assessment outcomes. If a child exhibits a variety of confusing behaviors, it is wise to plan for more than one observation session with the child and caregiver. If the child's behaviors are not clear to the observer, specific and discrete portions of selected behaviors should be observed rather than attempting to complete an assessment in one session. The child may do better when the examiner proceeds at a relaxed pace and speaks in an unhurried way, using simple sentences and avoiding long, complex verbal commands. Directions should be simple and must be heard and understood by the child. An examiner has the greatest success when the child is oriented to the task, a format is established, and what is expected of the child is made clear. Children should be allowed to perform at their own rate and should receive feedback on their efforts. The examiner should realize that most children are sensitive to acceptance, approval, indifference, or enthusiasm during a developmental screening session.

Remaining alert and sensitive to the needs of parents during a screening procedure is also very important. The examiner should listen to parents' comments about themselves or about the child's past or current abilities. Parents may be pleased with the developmental achievements their child has made. However, they may be dissatisfied, frustrated, and negative and require additional attention by talking about the child's progress and future plans. All parents, whether their outlook is positive or negative, should be acknowledged for their objective, important observations about the child's performance and for the appropriate encouragement they give.

The child care professional should always be supportive of parents, particularly during the stressful experience of discovering the existence of one or more developmental delays. Parents usually benefit from learning first about the child's strengths, abilities, and positive attributes, and the examiner should ask whether parents agree with these positive observations. Next, the examiner should ask whether they have noted any unusual behavior or observed that one task was not as easy for their child as another task passed with greater ease or facility. If parents have noticed a developmental deficit or unusual behavioral patterns, the examiner should determine how long they have

been aware of it and whether it has been a concern to them. If parents use terms such as "slower than," "behind other children," "different," or "lazy," the examiner should ask them to define precisely their use of these terms and to give examples, if possible. It is important to know whether the parents have been told of a delay and exactly what they were told, when, by whom, and what it meant to them.

Parents' needs for support may be acknowledged by statements such as, "This may not be easy for you to observe or to talk about." The examiner should verbally recognize the frustration that parents may have experienced in not seeing behavioral changes occur and should emphasize that their help will be needed in deciding what they wish to do in the future. Gorham and associates have provided some guidelines for both professionals and parents to follow during and following assessments of children with mental retardation.[17]

Suggestions for professionals:

1. Have the parent(s) involved every step of the way. The dialogue established may be the most important thing you accomplish. If the parent's presence is an obstacle to testing because the child will not cooperate in his presence, the setup should include a complete review of the testing procedure with the parent. (Remote video viewing or one-way windows are great if you are richly endowed.)

2. Make a realistic management plan part and parcel of the assessment outcome. Give the parents suggestions for how to live with the problem on a day-to-day basis, with the needs of the child, the capacities of the family, and the resources of the community all considered. Let the parents know that you will suggest modifications if any aspect of the management plan does not work.

3. Inform yourself about community resources. Give the parents advice on how to go about getting what they need. Steer them to the local parent organization.

4. Wherever possible, make the parent a team member in the actual diagnostic, treatment, or educational procedures. It will give you a chance to observe how the parent and the child interact.

5. Write your reports in clear, understandable, jargon-free language. Professional terminology is

a useful shortcut for your own note-taking; and you can always use it to communicate with others of your discipline. But in situations involving the parent, it operates as an obstacle to understanding. Keep in mind that it is the parent who must live with the child, help him along, shop for services to meet his needs, support his ego, give him guidance. You cannot be there to do it for him. So the parent *must* be as well informed as you can make him. Information that he does not understand is not useful to him. The goal is to "produce" a parent who understands his child well enough to help him handle his problems as he grows up.

6. Give copies of the reports to parents. They will need them to digest and understand the information in them; to share the information with other people close to the child; and to avoid the weeks or months of record-gathering which every application to a new program in the future will otherwise entail.

7. Be sure the parent understands that there is no such thing as a one-shot, final, and unchanging diagnosis. Make sure he understands that whatever label you give his child (if a label must be given) is merely a device for communicating and one which may have all kinds of repercussions, many of them undesirable. Make sure he understands that it says very little about the child at present and even less about the child of the future. Caution him about using that label to "explain" his child's condition to other people.

8. Help the parent to think of life with this child in the same terms as life with his other children. It is an ongoing, problem-solving process. Assure him that he is capable of that problem solving and that you will be there to help him with it.

9. Be sure that he understands his child's abilities and assets as well as his disabilities and deficiencies. What the child *can* do is far more important than what he cannot do, and the parent's goal thereafter is to look for new abilities and to welcome them with joy when they appear. Urge him to be honest and plain speaking with his child. Tell him that the most important job he has is to respect his child, as well as love him, and to help him "feel good about himself." Tell him that blame, either self-blame or blame of the child, has no part in the scene. *It is no one's fault.*

10. Warn the parent about service insufficiencies. Equip him with advice on how to make his way through the system of "helping" services. Warn him that they are not always helpful. Tell him that his child has a *right* to services. Tell him

to insist on being a part of any decision making done about his child.

11. Explain to him that some people with whom he talks (teachers, doctors, professionals of any kind, other parents) may dwell on negatives. Help train the parents not only to think in positives but to teach the other people important in his child's life to think in positives.

Suggestions for parents:

1. You are the primary helper, monitor, coordinator, observer, record keeper, and decision maker for your child. Insist that you be treated as such. It is your *right* to understand your child's diagnoses and the reasons for treatment recommendations and for educational placement. No changes in his treatment or educational placement should take place without previous consultation with you.

2. Your success in getting as well informed as you will need to be to monitor your child's progress depends on your ability to work with the people who work with your child. You may encounter resistance to the idea of including you in the various diagnostic and decision-making processes. The way you handle that resistance is important. Your best tool is not the angry approach. Some of your job will include the gentler art of persuasion. Stay confident and cool about your own abilities and intuitions. You know your child better than anyone else could. You are, obviously, a vital member of the team of experts.

3. Try to find, from among the many people whom you see, a person who can help you coordinate the various diagnostic visits and results. Pick the person with whom you have the best relationship, someone who understands your role as the principal monitor of your child's progress throughout life and who will help you become a good one.

4. Learn to keep records. As soon as you know that you have a child with a problem, start a notebook. Make entries of names, addresses, phone numbers, dates of visits, the persons present during the visits, and as much of what was said as you can remember. Record the questions you asked and the answers you received. Record any recommendations made. Make records of phone calls too; include the dates, the purpose, the result. It is best to make important requests by letter. Keep a copy for your notebook. Such documentation for every step of your efforts to get your child the service he needs can be the evidence which finally persuades a program director to *give* him what he needs. Without con-

cise records of whom you spoke to, when you spoke to him, what he promised, how long you waited between the request and the response, you will be handicapped. No one can ever be held accountable for conversations or meetings with persons whose names and titles you do not remember, on dates you cannot recall, about topics which you cannot clearly discuss.

5. Make sure that you understand the terminology used by the professional. Ask him to translate his terms into lay language. Ask him to give examples of what he means. Do not leave his office until you are sure you understand what he has said so well that you can carry the information to your child's teacher, for instance, and explain it to her in a clear, understandable language. (Write down the professional terms too. Knowing them might come in handy some time.)

6. Ask for copies of your child's records. You probably will not get them, but you *could* ask that a tape recording be made of any "interpretive" conference. It is very hard to remember what was said in such conferences.

7. Read. Learn as much as you can about your child's problem. But do not swallow whole what you read. Books are like people. They might be offering only one side of the story.

8. Talk freely and openly with as many professionals as you can. Talk with other parents. Join a parent organization. By talking with people who "have been through it already," you can gain a perspective on your particular problems. Besides, you will receive moral support and will not feel quite so alone. Get information from parent organizations about services available, about their quality. But bear in mind that a particular program might not help your child even though it has proved helpful for another child. Visit programs if you have the time and energy to do so. There is no substitute for firsthand views.

9. Stay in close touch with your child's teacher. Make sure you know what she is doing in the classroom so that, with her help, you can follow through at home. Share what you have read with her. Ask her for advice and suggestions. Get across the idea that the two of you are a team, working for the same goals. Make your child a part of that team whenever possible. He might have some great ideas.

10. Listen to your child. It is *his* point of view that he is giving you, and on that he is an expert.

11. Work hard at living the idea that differentness is just fine—not bad. Your child will learn most from your example. Help him to think of problems as things that can be solved if people work at them together. *

SCREENING TOOLS

A number of developmental assessment or screening tools are available for use with children and their families. The following sections present six screening and assessment tools that are becoming integrated into the nursing assessment of the child with developmental disabilities.

The Washington Guide to Promoting Development in the Young Child (1 to 52 months)

The Washington Guide to Promoting Development in the Young Child was constructed and revised in 1969 to assist child care professionals, particularly nurses, to be more effective in assessing and preventing handicapping conditions in children.[3] The tool is used by a variety of nurse clinicians in a number of settings: community health nurses; nurses in day care centers, residential schools, maternity and infant care projects, and institutions for children with handicapping conditions; and nurses in general pediatric settings.

The Washington Guide is constructed to encourage direct observations of the child's activities of daily living; it relies on parents' descriptions of the child's behaviors less than other tools. Developmental items in the guide are arranged from simple to more advanced tasks, reminding the examiner of the progressive tasks a child masters with increasing chronological age. Scoring consists of indicating the developmental items that the child is observed to perform. The remaining items, the developmental tasks that the child is not currently performing, provide clues to priorities for intervention.

The Washington Guide has certain inherent limitations. The most obvious is that it was not standardized on a large number of children in different age groups from birth to

---

*From Gorham, K. and others: Effect on parents. In Hobbs, N. J., editor: Issues in the classification of children, vol. 2, San Francisco, 1975, Jossey-Bass Publishers, pp. 183-186.

52 months; however, valid developmental norms for assessment purposes are used. In addition, it does not emphasize clearly defined, uniform directions for observing an individual child perform each developmental task. However, direct observations of the child carrying out individual tasks are an advantage for the observer. The observer does not rely on verbal reports alone but obtains a picture of the child's strengths and adaptive behaviors as well as behavioral deficits and behaviors that require attention for more appropriate functioning within the environment.

Nevertheless, the guide is appealing because it does not require elaborate testing equipment. The nurse relies on what is available in the child's learning environment: toys, feeding equipment, and other items that affect developmental progress. Another unique feature is that information accompanying every set of developmental norms suggests ways to promote development if the child has not yet achieved the proper age-related norms. Therefore, the Washington Guide is increasingly being used in combination with other screening tools as a reference for suggestions on ways to promote development when deficits are discovered.

Like other assessment tools, the Washington Guide is best used on a serial basis for planning and changing intervention approaches as a child develops. The tool was not designed to produce numbers or scores but to systematically focus on a child's strengths and adaptive abilities within the environment.

The Denver Developmental Screening Test

The Denver Developmental Screening Test (DDST) helps screen a child's performance in four categories: personal-social skills, fine motor achievements, receptive and expressive language abilities, and gross motor tasks.[15] The DDST is not considered an IQ test. It simply helps determine a child's progress with tasks that all children of similar ages are attempting to accomplish.

Researchers designed the DDST by testing more than 1,000 infants and children under identical conditions. Because the test is standardized, it serves as a valuable frame of reference. It assesses the progress an individual child makes from one time period to another and compares a child's abilities with those of other children the same age. The DDST manual includes instructions for preparing the parents and child, administering test items, and scoring. Each child is asked to perform an item in the same way, using the same test materials, and each child is given the same number of opportunities to successfully complete the task. Scoring is done in terms of the ages at which 25%, 50%, 75% and 90% of the standardization population could perform a particular test item. In addition, the test form provides space to note the child's general attitude, compliance levels, cooperativeness, general adjustment to screening, and specific interpersonal interactions between the child and the examiner or parent.

Results of the DDST should be presented to parents in a positive manner and in a way that encourages them to participate by asking questions and sharing observations. First, the child's strengths, skills, and appealing behaviors are discussed with parents. The examiner then moves on to areas that were not "as easy" or were more frustrating for the child to perform with success. Specific examples of tasks that were not as easy can be compared with those items that the child readily passed. The examiner should also offer parents opportunities to discuss their own observations. Parents may benefit from the knowledge that children simply do not learn everything at once but that they learn and proceed according to their own rate, needs, and previous successes with other skills. The examiner should emphasize the beginnings a child is making.

The DDST is an ideal screening tool to use in combination with the Washington Guide to Promoting Development in the Young Child. Results from the DDST provide information regarding the child's developmental achievements; the Washington Guide simultaneously suggests activities for promoting the child's development.

The Developmental Profile

The Developmental Profile was standardized on 3,008 infants and children in 1972.[1] It consists of 217 items divided into five scales measuring physical abilities, self-help skills, social behaviors, academic skills, and both receptive and expressive communication skills. Each scale is arranged according to age levels (6-month intervals from birth to $3^{1}/_{2}$ years, and yearly intervals thereafter).

In contrast to other screening tools, the Developmental Profile relies largely on verbal responses to questionnaire items. Observations of the child's behavior are also encouraged. The parent or another individual who is well acquainted with the child being screened gives information about whether the child "does" or "can do" each item listed in the inventory. For purposes of accurate scoring, parents can furnish additional descriptions of the child's behavior or the child can be asked to perform certain tasks. It is important that questions be presented to the parent in the prescribed order set forth in the manual, without any changes in the content. For example, the examiner must be sure that a child does every one of a series of items if the word "and" is used; the child must do one of several items if the word "or" is used.

The examiner should tell parents ahead of time that the questions will begin in an area where the child is likely to be having success and will progress to items that are advanced for the child's age level. The parents must be aware that the child is not expected to pass all items. The examiner should tell them that it may seem like the same question is being asked more than once; however, the examiner is just getting into more complex questions about a particular set of behaviors. The examiner should also assure parents that the results will be shared with them and that they are welcome to ask questions and to use all the time they need for answering a question.

Administering the Developmental Profile has been shown to be an efficient means of eliciting accurate and valid developmental information from people who know the child best. It is vital that child care professionals remember that parents' perceptions of their children and their functioning is critical to development. The Developmental Profile provides a structured way for nurses to listen to what parents are saying about their children. By listening actively and purposefully, the nurse can often help parents get their concerns out in the open. Expressing and discussing concerns are often the parents' first step toward changing their expectations to a more realistic level (either higher or lower) commensurate with the child's functional abilities. Sharing the results of the Developmental Profile with parents should be done positively; the examiner should concentrate first on the child's strengths and then on areas that were not as easy for the child. It is not considered helpful to simply give parents numbers for developmental results. An age level may indicate that the child is functioning within his chronological age, but it does not begin to clarify or reinforce strengths or developmental achievements.

The Developmental Profile has advantages over tools that require direct observation. It can be used with children who are ill and cannot currently perform tasks in an optimal way. It can be used with parents of children with acoustical impairments, sensory-motor disorders, emotional disturbances, and intellectual deficits. It can be used in a highly effective manner in a hospital setting to help formulate the child's daily nursing care plan. In all such cases, the Developmental Profile can provide important information about a child as well as give the reassurance that most parents need but do not consistently and uniformly obtain.

The Neonatal Behavioral Assessment Scale

Among the most exciting and revolutionary data to emerge in the infant and early childhood assessment field are T. Berry Brazelton's findings, which show that a 1-day-old infant is far from being a passive recipient of its environmental stimuli.[5] Child care professionals and others now know that neonates can shut out noxious sounds and other stimuli they do not like; they can maintain attention for relatively long periods of time; they can coordinate certain motor movements; they can initiate activity and readily adapt to most situations; they can quiet and console themselves in a stressful environment; and they sense their needs and try their best to communicate them.

The Neonatal Behavioral Assessment Scale developed by Brazelton and his associates over the past 20 years is the first major tool of its kind to focus on the newborn.[5] Brazelton, a pediatrician and practitioner in normal child development, searched in the early 1950s for a tool to assess newborn behavior. He looked for a means of determining how the environment shaped the child and of documenting the observable individual differences in neonates. However, after years of study, Dr. Brazelton became convinced that neonates shaped their environment much more than the environment shaped them. The implications of such a finding should ideally have tremendous impact on the quality of care the neonate receives and the interactions among neonates, their care providers, and their parents.[13] The Neonatal Behavioral Assessment Scale is recognized as the best available means of assessing the subtler behavioral responses of neonates as they adjust to and shape their environment, gain mastery over themselves, and enter the critically important formative period of cognitive and emotional development during infancy.

The Neonatal Behavioral Assessment Scale measures a total of twenty-seven behavioral responses, including the neonate's inherent neurological capacities, as well as responses to certain sets of stimuli. Each item is repeated several times, and neonates are rated on their best, not average, performance.

The items are divided into six categories: (1) habituation—how soon the neonate diminishes responses to specific stimuli; (2) orientation—how much and when the neonate attends to auditory and visual stimuli; (3) motor maturity—how well the neonate coordinates and controls motor activities; (4) variation—how often the neonate exhibits alertness, state changes, color changes, activity, and peaks of excitement; (5) self-quieting abilities—how much, how soon, and how effectively infants can use their own resources to quiet and console themselves when upset or distressed; and (6) social behaviors—how often and how much the neonate smiles and cuddles. (See p. 150 for a summary of scoring.)

Serial use of the scale is of considerably more value than just one assessment.[21] Repeated assessments through the first month can yield information about the various mechanisms infants are developing to adapt optimally to their own needs and to the conditions of their particular environment.

Findings from a study conducted by Tronick and Brazelton suggest that the Neonatal Behavioral Assessment Scale is an excellent predictor and a sensitive instrument for discriminating between normal and abnormal or suspect infants.[24] Used in its entirety, the Neonatal Behavioral Assessment Scale has greater predictive value than if only certain parts of the scale are employed, in which case the instrument has diminishing predictive value.

Examiners using the scale should be trained in the proper administration of test items and should also be familiar with special considerations regarding assessment of an infant. An examiner must practice testing at least ten infants before reliable independent ratings can be assured.*

The Neonatal Behavioral Assessment Scale is a valuable resource and guideline for teaching parents about their newborn's individual state changes, temperament, and behavioral patterns. Parents can learn, for example, when to present stimuli to their infants and when to pick up and console them. They can also learn the most effective and easiest ways to interact with and adjust to their infant.[13]

---

* A list of trained examiners who can teach others may be obtained by writing directly to Dr. T. Berry Brazelton.

The Neonatal Perception Inventory

The Neonatal Perception Inventory (NPI) is used to assess maternal perceptions of infants, with the aim of both promoting the mental health of the newborn and mother and serving as an early case-finding tool.[6,7]

Dr. Elsie Broussard, who developed the NPI, became convinced after years of experience in observing mothers and children that infants who are not perceived as better than average by their mothers may be at risk in their future development. She and her associate, Dr. M. S. Hartner, completed a longitudinal study in 1967 for the purpose of identifying the interrelationship between the first-time mother's initial perceptions of her infant and the infant's developmental profile at age 4 1/2 years.

As part of her doctoral dissertation, Dr. Broussard developed the "your baby inventory" and the "average baby perception inventory," designed to measure the mother's perceptions of her infant as compared with her concept of the average infant with regard to crying, spitting, feeding, elimination, sleeping, and predictability.[7] Each behavioral item is scored on a scale ranging from 5 ("a great deal") to 1 ("none"). The score for the "your baby inventory" is subtracted from the score for the "average baby perception inventory." The difference is the neonatal perception inventory score. A positive score indicates a favorable perception of the infant; zero and minus scores indicate a less favorable maternal perception. (See pp. 147-148 for the NPI tables.)

Broussard asked 318 primiparae who had delivered normal, full-term infants to complete the two inventories at 1 or 2 days' postpartum and again 1 month later. The total scores for the 318 "your baby" and "average baby" perception inventories were examined to determine if the mother rated her infant as better than, less than, or the same as the average infant. At the first rating during the first or second postpartum day, it was found that 46.5% of the mothers rated their infants as better than average.[6] The second rating by the mother took place at 1 month of age. It was found that of the 318

women, 61.2% of the mothers rated their infants as better than average. Of the remainder, 13.2% rated their infants as equal to the average, and 25.6% rated their infants as less than the average baby.[6]

To test the hypothesis that the mother's perception of her 1-month-old infant was associated with the child's subsequent emotional development, Broussard divided the original sample into two groups of "high-risk" and "low-risk" infants. The low-risk infants were those whose mothers had rated them as better than average at the end of 1 month. Those infants who had not been rated as better than average at 1 month comprised the sample who were at high risk for their later emotional development. Findings from the study suggest that almost 40% of the mothers had probably commenced unsatisfactory interactions with their infants that might lead to subsequent emotional problems as the infants grew older.[6] The hypothesis that the mother's perception of her 1-month-old infant was associated with the child's emotional development was first tested when 85 of the original population of firstborns were assessed at 4 1/2 years of age. When the 85 children were assessed independently by a clinician who did not know the original ratings of the child, 60.0% were diagnosed as having healthy responses.[6] It is notable that 66% of the children originally rated as high risk were evaluated as needing intervention, whereas 20.4% of the children originally rated as low risk were found to be in need of therapy. The proportion of children judged to be high risk (not rated as better than average) in the original study and the 4 1/2 year follow-up study were almost identical.[6] The study documented that the mother's perception of an infant at 1 month of age is important for the child's future development.

When the NPI has shown that a mother does not rate her infant as better than average, prompt intervention should occur. Ongoing intervention that focuses on the mother's needs and helps her interact with her infant may reduce stress and disturbances in parent-infant interactions, whereas failure to intervene may result in irreversible damage to the child. Parents usually know when problems exist between them and their infants, but they need professional support to seek help so that the situation can be resolved.

The nurse should turn the mother's attention to the infant's unique strengths in an empathetic and supportive way while helping the mother sort out her concerns about herself and the infant. It is crucial that the mother begin to experience a positive orientation and to express positive feelings about the infant's unique features and behaviors.[13] The nurse should reinforce and accentuate any positive features of the infant that are pointed out by the mother. A mother who does not view her infant as better than average may herself be vulnerable. The nurse might need to reassure her that her infant really does like her, as is evident from the many positive ways the baby responds to her. The mother may need to hear many favorable comments about her infant before she attains a positive perspective. She may also need reassurance from one or several persons on a continuing basis that the behaviors she considers most negative are temporary and will be repeated only until the infant has adapted in a better way to the new environment. In an unpublished study, Dr. Broussard selected another population of 281 full-term, normal, healthy, firstborn infants. Based on the administration of the NPI, she identified a population of infants at high risk and developed a pilot preventive program for them. On the basis of her intensive clinical work with this population, she reports that "the mothers of infants at high risk seem to have very low self-esteem, lack confidence in themselves as individuals and as mothers, and have difficulty in understanding the infant's cues and responding to the infant's needs."[8]

Broussard's findings suggest that nurses and other professionals need to be sensitive to what mothers are experiencing and remain in tune with the way they are receiving professional input. A nonjudgmental attitude on the part of the professional is critical if change in a mother's perception about her infant is to occur.

Because the NPI is a significant instrument of prevention and prediction, all child care professionals face the exciting possibility of being able to diagnose potential problems and work to prevent them, thus assuring more children of their right to healthy development.

Home Observation and Measurement of the Environment

A new trend in assessment is emerging, focusing not only on a child's development but also on the environment in which development is occurring. Child care professionals are becoming more sensitive to the need for assessing how an environment either promotes or negates each child's development. Measuring an environment to determine its strengths or deficits allows professionals to capitalize on strengths and to plan with parents in order to eliminate deficits. The Home Observation Measurement of the Environment (HOME) was developed by Dr. Bettye Caldwell and goes hand in hand with developmental screening tools in producing the most comprehensive picture of a child's levels of development and whether the environment (the home environment or any other significant environment) is enhancing or hindering developmental change.[9]

HOME consists of two inventories that measure the subtle aspects of a young child's environment that are most likely to influence development.[9] The first inventory (birth to 3 years) measures: the emotional and verbal responsivity of the mother, avoidance of restriction and punishment, organization of the physical and temporal environment, provision of appropriate play materials, maternal involvement with the child, and opportunities for variety in daily stimulation. The second inventory (3 to 6 years) measures: provision of stimulation through equipment, toys, and experiences; stimulation of mature behavior; provision of stimulating physical and language environment; avoidance of restriction and punishment; pride, affection, and thoughtfulness; masculine stimulation; and independence from parental control.

Using the two inventories, professionals can provide feedback to parents about ways to regulate environmental changes to best facilitate their child's development. Such feedback also helps parents meet their own needs for assuring their child an appropriate environment at different stages of development. A child's development depends on both the quality and quantity of kinesthetic, auditory, visual, and other sensory inputs received. Children need appropriate amounts of novelty, consistency, trust, dependability, and organization of their environment. An adequate environment will influence the extent to which children gain mastery of themselves and their environment as well as their progress in fine motor, gross motor, personal-social, and language skills.

In discussing HOME results with parents of children with mental retardation, the nurse should naturally describe the strengths of the environment first.[13] Parents should be asked if they have any questions or concerns or if they have thought about the way they select toys, provide opportunities for variety, or respond consistently when their child initiates a conversation with them. The parents' observations of the environment can be a significant point of reference for discussion purposes. The nurse should compare parental observations with what the assessment guide revealed.

A unique facet of HOME is that the observer rates the interactions seen. Judgments are not made about the observer's interactions with a child or mother, but judgments are made about the interactions occurring between mother and child as well as those that are reported. Like other assessment tools, HOME produces accurate results only if interrater reliability is established. Caldwell suggests that observers work in pairs on the first twelve home visits to increase objectivity of assessment and to decrease subjective interpretations. One HOME assessment alone can never be con-

sidered sufficient to determine the adequacy of an environment. Using HOME on a serial basis allows professionals to observe environmental changes in a systematic manner, to offer parents objective feedback, and to help parents see the changes they were able to implement.

HOME is relied on as a sensitive indicator of the appropriate kinds and amounts of animate-inanimate stimulation of infant or child needs.[13] It offers a valid way of observing environmental structure and consistency of stimuli, gives a profile of the organization of a typical day, and presents objective information about who helps with selected aspects of caregiving. Therefore, it serves as a basis for meaningful intervention. This inventory is particularly helpful in determining intervention and ways to meet the unique needs of the child with mental retardation.

SUMMARY

New trends in developmental screening practices and the careful sensitive use of the screening tools discussed here are greatly aiding child care professionals in early case finding, prevention, and management of mental retardation in children. Nurses, in particular, should be involved in performing developmental assessments and using screening tools to guide their practice with developmentally delayed children and their families.

REFERENCES

1. Alpern, G. D., and Boll, T. J.: Developmental profile manual, Aspen, Colorado, 1972, Psychological Development Publications.
2. Barclay, A., and Vaught, G.: Maternal estimates of future achievement in cerebral palsied children, Am. J. Ment. Defic. **69:**76, 1964.
3. Barnard, K., and Erickson, M.: Teaching children with developmental problems; a family care approach, ed. 2, St. Louis, 1976, The C. V. Mosby Co.
4. Bickley, J. C., and Martin, D. J.: A comparative study of mothers' and teachers' estimates of the future social adaptation of preschool retarded children, Boston, 1967, Boston University, unpublished master's thesis.
5. Brazelton, T. B.: The neonatal behavioral assessment scale, Philadelphia, 1973, J. B. Lippincott Co.
6. Broussard, E., and Hartner, M. S.: Maternal per-

ception of the neonate as related to development, Child Psychiatry Hum. Dev. **1:**16, 1970.

7. Broussard, E., and Hartner, M. S.: Further considerations regarding maternal perceptions of the first born. In Hellmuth, J., editor: Exceptional infant; studies in abnormalities, vol. 2, New York, 1971, Brunner/Mazel, Inc., pp. 432-449.

8. Broussard, E.: Personal communication, 1976.

9. Caldwell, B.: Home observation and measurement of the environment; birth to three and three to six, 1976, Little Rock, Ark., unpublished manuals.

10. Capobianco, R. J., and Knox, S.: IQ estimates and the index of marital integration, Am. J. Ment. Defic. **68:**718, 1974.

11. Capute, A. J., and Biehl, R. F.: Functional developmental evaluation prerequisite to habilitation, Pediatr. Clin. North Am. **20:**3, 1973.

12. Ehlers, W. H.: The moderately and severely retarded child; maternal perceptions of retardation and subsequent seeking and using services rendered by a community agency, Am. J. Ment. Defic. **68:**660, 1964.

13. Erickson, M.: Assessment and management of developmental changes in children, St. Louis, 1976, The C. V. Mosby Co.

14. Ewart, J. D., and Green, M. W.: Conditions associated with the mother's estimate of the ability of her retarded child, Am. J. Ment. Defic. **62:**521, 1957.

15. Frankenburg, W., Dodds, J., and Fandal, A. W.: Denver developmental screening test manual, 1970 edition, University of Colorado Medical Center, 1970.

16. Gorelick, M. D., and Sandhu, M.: Parent perception of retarded child's intelligence, Person. Guid. J. **46:**382, 1967.

17. Gorham, K., and others: Effect on parents. In Hobbs, N. J., editor: Issues in the classification of children, vol. 2, San Francisco, 1975, Jossey-Bass, Inc., Publishers, pp. 183-186.

18. Kurtz, R. A.: Comparative evaluations of suspected retardates, Am. J. Dis. Child. **109:**58, 1965.

19. Mash, E. J., Terdal, L., and Anderson, K.: The response-class matrix; a procedure for recording parent-child interactions, Eugene, Ore., 1970, University of Oregon Medical School, unpublished manuscript.

20. Mash, E. J., Terdal, L., and Anderson, K.: The response-class matrix; a procedure for recording parent-child interactions, J. Consult. Clin. Psychol. **40:**163, 1973.

21. Meyerowitz, J.: Parental awareness of retardation, Am. J. Ment. Defic. **71:**1971.

22. Rheingold, H. L.: Interpreting mental retardation to parents, J. Consult. Clin. Psychol. **9:**142, 1945.

23. Thorpe, H. S., and Werner, E. E.: Developmental screening of preschool children; a critical review of inventories used in health and educational programs, Pediatrics **53:**362, 1974.

24. Tronick, E., and Brazelton, T. B.: Clinical uses of the Brazelton neonatal assessment. In Friedlander, E. Z., editor: Exceptional infant; assessment and intervention, vol. 3, New York, 1975, Brunner/Mazel, Inc.

25. Wolfensberger, W., and Kurtz, R. A.: Measurements of parents perceptions of their children's development, Genet. Psychol. Monogr. **83:**3, 1971.

26. Zuk, G. H.: Autistic distortions in parents of retarded children, J. Consult. Clin. Psychol. **23:**171, 1959.

CHAPTER 14

Identification of the visible child in the community

SANDRA ERICKSON OEHRTMAN

Every family that conceives a child knows the hopes and fears of the ensuing waiting period. Morning sickness, the first movement, hopes, expectations, and plans fill the time. Occasionally there is the pushed-aside thought, or moment of tears, when fears surface that all may not be as planned for the "perfect" baby. Usually all is well, and a healthy child is delivered. For some 3% of American families, however, the child's birthday is not a joyous occasion. They become grieving families when their children are born defective.

For a pediatric clinical nurse specialist working in a public health nursing agency, this situation is unfortunately familiar. Such families are to be found throughout the wide array of community settings. As a helping professional familiar with the community's particular mores and culture, the nurse is frequently one of the few professionals to initiate and maintain contact with these families.

CONCEPT OF VISIBILITY

The family of a defective child is a system within the community that is particularly vulnerable to threats on its integrity. Each family system has particular processes by which it deals with threats. Sometimes these processes break down or are ineffective, and

the family is unable to resolve its problems or maintain its integrity. The family is then in a crisis state and as a nonorganized system is visible to the community. The community identifies the family system in a crisis state as visible because it utilizes societal cues in ways other than those that society expects. Societal cues are not utilized normatively due to the family system's disorganized reception or perception of societal cues, because its integrity is not maintained.

Society deems certain ways of functioning as appropriate. Most people utilize societal cues and function in those certain normative societal patterns; they are therefore basically invisible. There are other creative, highly intelligent people who are visible on an above-normal basis. They fail to use, or they use uniquely, societal cues as a condition necessary for their creative survival. The defective child is also visible but on a destructive level. The child fails to utilize societal cues due to receptive, cognitive, or perceptual problems, and society frowns on the child's behavior. The parents are told to do something about their child. Society deems it appropriate to deal with destructive visibility. Consequently, institutional placement or referral to a social agency may be initiated.

The concept of visibility is particularly

useful to the nurse working in the community setting. As the professional who often identifies a deviant child, the nurse's assessment alone is usually not enough to diagnose a child as being mentally retarded, developmentally disabled, behaviorally disturbed, or minimally brain damaged. Rather, these types of diagnoses come from the assessments of an interdisciplinary team of professionals. The nurse, however, should assess the child or family as visibly defective and initiate intervention. The nurse should perform this function before the community at large has identified the child as deviant and demanded action from the family.

A FRAMEWORK FOR ACTION

The community nurse needs to utilize a particular set of cognitive skills to help families with defective children reduce their visibility to society. The individual child, the family and, on occasion, the community become the major concern. All of these are open, living systems, affecting themselves and each other. As open, living systems, they are characterized by a continuous interchange of material and energy with the environment moving in the direction of increasing order and complexity in an organized pattern.

Process is also a characteristic of open systems. Through particular processes, activities of each system are mediated towards identifiable goals. Process is a term denoting the change that occurs through a set of sequential, interdependent activities toward an identifiable end.

In order to provide services to children, families, and communities, the nurse needs to function within a systematic, scientific framework. Nursing process, which is the same type of process that other open systems utilize, fulfills that need for a scientific framework. Turner agrees with the concept of nursing process as a systematic method of interacting with clients.[3] Individuals and groups of individuals are recognized as open systems that affect and are affected by internal and external environments. The nursing process serves as a guiding framework for the actions of nurses with and for their clients.

Nursing process may be divided into three major components: assessment, intervention, and evaluation. By using the nursing process, nurses can intervene to help families and children reduce destructive community visibility.

FROM THEORY INTO PRACTICE

With recent trends of early hospital discharge for mother and newborn, increased case finding of children deviating from normal growth and development patterns has become the community nurse's responsibility. Subtle variations from normal often escape detection during the newborn hospital period or become apparent only at later stages of development.

Parents often express their denial of the child's visibility by failing to seek usual well-child care or by covering up their child's inadequacies for long periods of time. The following clinical examples help to explore a few of the many ways the community nurse identifies the deviant child and within the systematic framework of nursing process endeavors to help the family reduce their child's visibility.

The process of nursing assessment begins with a detailed history of the child's growth and development, health care, perinatal events, present concerns about the child, and a general family health history. The C. family serves as an illustration of how a nurse can utilize the assessment process, and a discussion of the intervention and evaluation process follows.

Willie C., a 3-year-old and the youngest of the six children of a single parent was the child identified as visible. Ms. C. initially reported an uneventful pregnancy and delivery with Willie. He had an uneventful newborn period. All other children in the C. family were healthy and doing well in school. Willie had received episodic health care and was hospitalized at 2 years of age for cellulitis of the knee. His general growth and development were slower than that of his siblings. Motor development included sitting alone at 7 months, walking at over 12 months, and accomplishing toilet training between 2 and 3 years of age. His first word was "ma-ma," spoken around 12 months. Ms. C. sought services at a community child health clinic because she was concerned with Willie's speech. He rarely combined more than two words.

During Willie's clinic visit, the DDST was administered. Arrangements were made for screenings by the physician, nutritionist, speech and hearing specialist, and social worker to collect additional data. Willie's physical exam was essentially negative, his nutrition was found to be adequate, and nothing remarkable was noted by social services. The speech and hearing therapist found a language delay but normal hearing. The DDST administered by the nurse revealed normal personal-social and fine motor areas, multiple refusals in the gross motor area, and multiple failures in the language area. Willie was easily distracted, had difficulty establishing eye contact, and frequently seemed to misunderstand verbal instructions. The clinic team felt further referral was necessary, most likely to the developmental disabilities clinic of a nearby children's hospital. The nurse shared the team's assessment of Willie with Ms. C. and began the intervention step of the nursing process.

Ms. C. had already defined Willie as deviating from the norm. The clinic assessment verified her concerns about Willie's delay in language development. The nurse reviewed the assessment findings carefully with Ms. C., being certain to stress positive points, such as no physical problems, normal hearing, and normal development in fine motor and personal-social areas. A more complete evaluation at the developmental disabilities clinic was suggested. Ms. C. readily agreed. Ms. C. also agreed to the nurse's recommendation to enroll Willie in a Head Start program for additional stimulation in all areas of his development. Ms. C. contacted the Head Start program and was able to enroll Willie at a center within walking distance of their home. Subsequent evaluation at the developmental disabilities clinic revealed a diagnosis of delayed language development, and weekly individual speech therapy was initiated. No specific reason for an associated developmental lag was found.

Assessment, intervention, and evaluation repeat themselves in a spiraling, continuous fashion because they are all a part of non-static human systems. The nurse's assessment of the C. family continued. It was discovered that Ms. C's prenatal history was eventful; she had been x-rayed and medicated for gallstones early in her pregnancy with Willie. Assessment of Willie also continued by periodic updates of developmental screenings administered by the nurse. In this manner, it was possible for the nurse to monitor Willie's progress and provide information to the C. family. Intervention with the Head Start teachers involved classroom observation of Willie with his peers and recommendations regarding particular ways to stimulate him according to his developmental level. Intervention with Ms. C. included providing information about transportation available from the welfare department to get Willie to his speech therapy sessions.

Evaluation occurs at every step in the nursing process. Termination of this process will most likely occur when evaluation reveals that the C. family returns to a "level which allows self-resolution of problems and maintenance of maximum integrity."[3] This point may occur when Willie develops normal language with subsequent reduced visibility. It is more likely that this will occur when the cause of Willie's lag is diagnosed, and the C. family is comfortable with the diagnosis and interventions.

Clinics are only one of the many places where the community health nurse can detect the defective, visible child. When nurses serve as consultants to local Head Start programs for enrolled children with handicaps, they also have an additional opportunity to identify visible children. On occasion, deviant children have been enrolled in the Head Start program with no noted problems. When such a child enters the classroom, it becomes obvious to the teaching staff that the particular child is different from most of his peers; the child becomes visible. The nurse provides the staff with confirmation of their observations and intervenes with particular skills to reduce the child's visibility. The S. family serves as an illustration.

Tanya S., a 4-year-old, was enrolled in a Head Start program without any mention of particular problems. Staff observations of Tanya included problems at mealtimes, frequent wetting and soiling, staring at the ceiling while uttering the same word over and over, inability to sit still long enough to complete simple activities, and biting other children to gain attention. The initial nursing assessment confirmed the teaching staff's observations. Developmental screenings were attempted but not completed. The nurse conferred with the staff and agreed that Tanya's behaviors needed to be discussed with Ms. S. immediately. A teacher who had a particularly warm relationship with the mother was selected as the best person to talk with her. At this time, the nurse did not directly intervene with the parent but assisted the teacher in planning intervention. The conference with Ms. S. revealed that Tanya was the only child of a single parent. In order for Ms. S. to finish trade school, she had entrusted most of Tanya's care to a grandmother for her first year of life. Since that time, Ms. S. had enrolled Tanya in a variety of nursery and day care centers in order to maintain employment. Each facility had asked Ms. S. to remove Tanya from their program because her care was too difficult. Therefore, Ms. S. did not tell Head Start of Tanya's difficulties for fear she would not be enrolled in the program.

Tanya's medical care had been episodic. One physician had diagnosed Tanya as hyperactive after a cursory exam and prescribed methylphenidate (Ritalin). After several months of medication, Ms. S. withheld the Ritalin because it made Tanya extremely lethargic. Ms. S. stated that she did

not know where else to seek help. During a follow-up staff conference, it was agreed to keep Tanya in the Head Start program. The nurse would seek appropriate diagnosis and intervention for Tanya. When the medical history from Ms. S. and the nurse's observations of Tanya were considered, several ways to help orient Tanya in the classroom and to decrease excess stimulation were suggested. Tanya would be excluded from any situation where hard-rock music was played; her teacher was to orient her with tactile facial contact as necessary; Tanya was to be given many opportunities for finger painting, sand play, and other messy play with individual guidance; and teaching staff were helped to realistically evaluate their expectations of Tanya. Meanwhile, Ms. S. explored possibilities of a variety of available diagnostic centers with the nurse. Agreement was reached on referral to a local pediatrician knowledgeable about such problems. At this point, a professional from the diagnostic center became the main intervenor in Tanya's case. Ms. S. and the nurse agreed to terminate their relationship. Nursing had fulfilled the immediate needs of Ms. S. by acting at a critical time when Tanya presented day care problems and by pointing the way to resolution of those problems. Intervention had included providing information, support, and referral to an appropriate agency.

Public health nurses have the opportunity to case find while on their home visits. Occasionally, they require the assistance of nursing specialists, such as pediatric clinical nurse specialists. Although such specialists may not be involved in case finding, they can assist the community nurse in identifying and working with defective children.

The public health nurse routinely receives notice of hospital discharges of mothers and their newborn infants. Also, they are typically the professional contacted at the birth of a child because a neighbor felt the nurse's services were valuable when her own baby was new. Opportunities for case finding are many in this type of home visitation program. During an initial visit with a new postpartum mother, the visiting nurse frequently gives a bath demonstration and appraises the infant simultaneously. A useful approach for infant appraisal during the bathing demonstration is outlined by Haynes in *A Developmental Approach to Casefinding*.[1] Nurses will find this reference informative and useful. The entire bath demonstration and infant appraisal should be done with the parent present. This experience allows an opportunity for the nurse to include parents in future planning if a deviation from normal is suspected.

During some visits, the nurse may have a reason to suspect problems with other children in the home. The DDST is invaluable in assessing the young child's developmental

level before entry into school. Toddlers and preschoolers frequently receive only episodic health care. Because they are often not enrolled in a formal school setting, their handicaps may remain invisible or may be easily concealed by family and friends.

A checklist of typical developmental tasks that should be accomplished by a certain age child, including suggestions to further present and future development, is one tool that may be useful to public health nurses (Table 14-1). This form allows the nurse to assess and guide the child's development on every home visit even if time does not permit a complete formal developmental assessment.[2]

Table 14-1. Infant and child growth and development assessment and guidance*

Age	Assessment	Date	Date	Anticipatory guidance
1 Month	Eyes follow to midline			Encourage eye contact with bright object
	Regards face			Talking, pictures on side of crib
	Lifts head when prone			Put in prone position with family
	Responds to sounds			Talking, singing, radio
2 Months	Vocalizes			Responding to sounds of baby
	Smiles responsively			Mirror, touch, smile, laugh
	Follows past midline			Crib gym, bright object on side of crib
3 Months	Stomach head up 90°			Prone position in crib and encourage to lift head
	Laughs			Talk, laugh, touch
4 months	Squeals			Repeat sounds
	Sits with head steady			Infant seat, prop up with pillow
	Eyes follow 180°			Mobile, active environment, bright colors
	Grasps rattle or household objects			Encourage grasp, try to pull rattle away

*Adapted from Jones, K., and Oehrtman, S.: Infant and child growth and development assessment and guidance, Columbus, Ohio, 1974, Community Health Care and Nursing Service, unpublished form.   *Continued.*

Table 14-1. Infant and child growth and development assessment and guidance—cont'd

Age	Assessment	Date	Date	Anticipatory guidance
5 Months	Smiles spontaneously			Mirror play
	Rolls back to front and vice versa			Blanket on floor with toys out of reach
	Reaches for object			Blanket on floor with toys, mobiles
6 Months	Pull to sit without head lag			Encourage at bath time, diapering, dressing
	Beginning to bear weight on legs			Encourage at bath time, diapering, dressing
	Turns toward sounds			Musical toys, television, radio
8 to 9 Months	Sits alone			Put on firm surface
	Looks after fallen object			Play game to encourage this, bait casting
	Transfers object from one hand to another			Blocks, rattle, spoon, plastic cups
	Feeds self cracker			Encourage finger foods
	Plays peek-a-boo			Put toy under blanket and encourage baby to find it
	Rakes and attains raisin			
10 Months	Pulls self to standing			Give opportunity, safety
	Stands holding on to solid object			Give opportunity
	Says "da-da" or "ma-ma"			Encourage "ah" sounds, encourage baby to imitate sounds
	Initially shy with strangers			Normal, games such as hide and seek
	Resists toy pull			Games, such as tug of war, bait casting, pull toys
12 Months	Cruises-walks holding on to furniture			Give opportunity out of crib and pen
	Stands alone			Encourage and praise
	Bangs two cubes held in hands			Block play, noise-making toys
	Thumb-finger grasp, beginning pincer grasp			Put objects in empty oatmeal box and in matchbox, finger feed

Table 14-1. Infant and child growth and development assessment and guidance—cont'd

Age	Assessment	Date	Date	Anticipatory guidance
18 Months	Walks well			Give opportunity out of crib and playpen
	Stoops and recovers toys on floor			Action songs, pull toys
	Drinks from cup			Give opportunity
	Indicates wants (not cry)			Talk to child, encourage verbalization
	Pincer grasp			Same as thumb-finger grasp
	Beginning to scribble			Help with simple household chores
	Puts one block on another			Block play
2 years	Feeds self with spoon			Give opportunity
	Tower of two to four blocks			Block play
	Three words other than "ma-ma" and "da-da"			Imitate familiar sounds, such as "planes," talk, sing-read magazines and books, point out "dog," and so forth
	Scribbles spontaneously			Finger painting
	Dumps small objects out of bottle after demonstration			Water play; put toys into basket and encourage child to dump out and put it in again
	Kicks ball forward			Kick balloons and balls
	Walks backward			Pull toys
3 years	Pedals tricycle			Pedal toys
	Uses plurals			Look at books, picture cards, magazines
	Knows first name			Use child's name in conversation
	Washes and dries hands			Demonstrate how (step stool to stand on)
	Jumps in place			Jumping games, follow the leader
	Copies circle			Demonstrate (show pictures, point out round objects)
	Can follow two commands, involving "on," "under," and "behind"			Talk with child while going through day's routine, games

Continued.

Table 14-1. Infant and child growth and development assessment and guidance—cont'd

Age	Assessment	Date	Date	Anticipatory guidance
4 years	Builds bridge of three blocks after demonstration			Demonstrate
	Copies cross (+)			Demonstrate (point out objects in environment, such as traffic signs, telephone poles)
	Identifies longer of two lines			Talk about concept
	Knows first and last names			Address child, label child's room and belongings with name
	Comprehends "cold," "tired," and "hungry"			Talk regarding these concepts, such as cold, ice, hot coffee
	Beginning to separate from mother easily			Play hide and seek, blind man's bluff
	Plays interactive games with other children, tag			Allow experience to play with other children, tag, imaginative play
	Dresses with supervision			Give opportunity to play "dress up," allow to help select own clothing, give praise for accomplishment
5 years	Hop on one foot			Games, such as hopscotch, jump rope, and imaginative games, such as hop like a bunny
	Catches bounced ball thrown 3 feet			Games with a ball
	Dresses without supervision			Give opportunity (see above)
	Draws man three parts			Look in mirror, ask child to draw what he sees, also from snapshot
	Recognizes colors (three out of four)			Point out colors in environment, such as blue shirt, red car
	Heel to toe walk (two out of three tries)			Give opportunity to walk on boards on floor

SUMMARY

Opportunities for case finding and prevention are many for the community nurse. Often as the first professional involved, it is the community nurse with unique skills who identifies the visible, defective child. Then, within the nursing process framework, the nurse begins to assess, intervene, and evaluate the child, the family, and their particular needs. Visible children are identified by the nurse in a variety of settings and at every age. Several case examples have been presented to outline how and where these children are detected and to outline the processes of assessment, intervention, and evaluation.

REFERENCES

1. Haynes, U.: A developmental approach to casefinding, Washington, D.C., 1969, Public Health Service publication No. 2017, U.S. Department of Health, Education, and Welfare.
2. Jones, K., and Oehrtman, S.: Infant and child growth and development assessment and guidance, Columbus, Ohio, 1974, Community Health Care and Nursing Service, unpublished form.
3. Turner, M. N.: Nursing process; an operational framework for nursing practice. In Hall, J., and Weaver, B., editors: Nursing of families in crisis, Philadelphia, 1974, J. B. Lippincott Co.

ADDITIONAL READINGS

Frankenburg, W., and others: Denver developmental screening test manual, 1970 edition, Denver, University of Colorado Medical Center.
Leland, H., and Smith, D.: Mental retardation; present and future perspectives, Worthington, Ohio, 1974, Charles A. Jones Publications.
Thorpe, H. S.: The Thorpe developmental inventory, Los Angeles, 1973, University of California.
von Berttanffy, L.: General system theory; foundations, development, and application, New York, 1968, George Barziller, Inc.

CHAPTER 15

Maximizing services for a mentally retarded child: coordinated efforts

MARILYN KRAJICEK, F. BRUCE ANDERSON, and WILLIAM JOSEPH BURNS

Let each become all that he was created capable of being; expand, if possible, to this full growth, and show himself at length in his own escape and stature, be these what they may.*

This chapter presents a case study about Tammy F., a young adolescent with severe developmental delays. The efforts made by parents and professionals to offer Tammy the opportunity to make the most of her abilities are discussed. There are thousands of children like Tammy whose intellectual impairment precludes their normal progress in development. Treatment programs for the mentally retarded child are often very inadequate because of the lack of funds and personnel to provide high-quality rehabilitative programs.[2]

A unique set of circumstances is presented in which personnel from different helping agencies cooperated to work and plan for Tammy's future. It is hoped that the sharing of staff experiences with Tammy may assist other health personnel in their work with children and families.

The theoretical frameworks that are utilized for purposes of this case study include crisis proneness and coping mechanisms. These frameworks are defined elsewhere in the chapter. Also stressed is the need for early intervention as well as cooperative, working relationships between the agencies that are involved in providing services to mentally retarded children and their families.

CASE STUDY

Tammy F. was 6 years old when she was first seen at the Child Development Center* in 1970 for a complete developmental evaluation. The results of the evaluation indicated that she was functioning in the moderate range of mental retardation with an emotional disorder of a reactive nature. She had multiple congenital anomalies, including cleft lip and palate, congenital heart defect, short and thickened hands and feet, and an abnormal EEG. Although she reacted violently at times to environmental stresses, her limited ability to communicate might have accounted for some of her extreme behavioral reactions. Tammy was the third of four children and required much attention. Her siblings had difficulty understanding and coping with her behaviors.

Tammy had been in Colorado with her family for a year when she came to the Child Development Center. She was also enrolled in a community center school for

---

*From Carlyle, T.: Past and present 1843, Hughes, A.M. D., editor, by permission of the Oxford University Press.

*The John F. Kennedy Child Development Center, University of Colorado Medical Center, Denver, Colo.

trainable children, which had requested consultation concerning the management of her behavior. Her teachers felt that she was regressing academically and emotionally. She had frequent temper tantrums and appeared to lack the inner controls necessary to turn off her own responses once a tantrum began.

There were many inconsistencies in Tammy's behavior management at home. Mr. F. complained that his wife, who was of Hispanic background, was too lenient with Tammy, contradicting her strong disciplinary role with the other children. Mrs. F. complained that her husband used only verbal threats without placing any consequences on misbehavior. At the time of Tammy's diagnostic evaluation, her parents had separated for a short period of time. Following the father's return to the home, the parents became involved in marital counseling for a short time. The question of whether or not the parents had coped with Tammy's mental retardation was raised.

Following Tammy's evaluation, a graduate nursing student was assigned to follow the family for two semesters on an intensive basis. She made weekly home and agency visits and assumed the role of liaison and coordinator for the case as a representative from the Child Development Center. Soon after the student became involved with the family, Tammy refused to ride the school bus and later kicked out a bus window. The family was informed that they would have to make other arrangements for her transportation to and from school. Mr. F. responded to this restriction by complaining that no outside agency had helped the family with their problems.

At this time, Mrs. F. became pregnant with her fifth child. Placement of Tammy in a foster home or a state institution for temporary care was discussed but never materialized during the pregnancy. Both parents were opposed to outside placement at that time. In October, 1971, baby Tina was born via cesarean section; she

was a healthy infant. Mr. F., after having been out of work for several months, completed a drafting course and gained employment.

Conferences continued among the family, school, and Child Development Center during this time. Tammy was placed in a behavior modification program at school and in the home with some success. In addition, Tammy was on a variety of medications in an attempt to control her behavior. The family also faced many financial problems. The second oldest son had behavioral and academic problems in school. The family was unable to plan ahead or problem solve but rather responded only to crises.

In January, 1972, Tina was found dead in her crib. The death was diagnosed 6 days later as sudden infant death syndrome. Mrs. F. was hospitalized and had a hysterectomy. She received much support from the graduate nursing student during these times. Upon returning home from the hospital, she was in a depressed state and found it difficult to go into the baby's room. The family sold their home because they found the memory of the baby's death too painful. They purchased a home in another county.

Due to problems at the community center school, the family terminated Tammy's enrollment and placed her in a preschool program where she progressed in several self-help tasks. There were few behavior problems during this period. Tammy was the oldest child in the program and was frequently given the role of teacher's helper, which she enjoyed. The family was not in contact with the Child Development Center during the period that Tammy was in the preschool.

In November, 1974, Mrs. F. made her first contact with Oak Creek, the community center school serving their new residential county. The F. family found the cost for continuing Tammy's education at the preschool overwhelming, especially while they were trying to save money for a cosmetic operation for

Tammy's cleft lip. In addition, the director of the preschool had expressed concern that their program was not adequate for a 10-year-old, retarded girl. The parents would have preferred to keep Tammy in the preschool program if money had been available for this. They agreed to transfer Tammy to a different school only as a second choice. They were reluctant to consider another community center school because of their disappointing experiences with the first program and also because Tammy had had no major problems during a year at the preschool.

As with other shifts of services for Tammy, the effort required to change her program was almost an overwhelming task for this family, particularly for Mrs. F. Although they were fearful of the move to Oak Creek, the family soon adapted well to the new school. Both parents responded to requests made by the school, although Mrs. F. later reported that her husband had not followed through with school recommendations. Both parents attended several school staffings regarding Tammy. Because these staffings usually dealt with bus or school behaviors, the parents expressed fear that the school would terminate Tammy from the program. However, Mrs. F. supported the school's action when her neighbor complained to her about the way school personnel disciplined Tammy on the bus. Mrs. F. also served as a PTA officer for 1 year, and the two oldest children participated in a teen-aged sibling group for 3 months.

The primary educational service provided for Tammy at Oak Creek was a basic program for trainable mentally retarded children and consisted of preacademic and academic subjects, speech and perceptual-motor therapy, and recreational activities. From the beginning, Tammy demonstrated aggressive behavior toward the staff and classmates by throwing books and chairs. Her frequent outbursts of screaming, shouting, and crying were disruptive. She demonstrated self-abusive and self-destructive behaviors, such as head banging, hand biting, abuse of her body, and frequent attempts to throw herself out of the bus. Several school staff meetings were held to discuss efforts to bring the behaviors under control. Various behavior modification programs were designed by a consulting specialist and implemented in the classroom, the school, and on the bus. All were ineffective after a few days. Tammy was at one time placed in a special classroom where one teacher worked with three emotionally disturbed, retarded children. A bus aide was hired specifically to control Tammy. When the aide was absent, a car was sent from the school to pick up Tammy at home.

The school social worker functioned as case manager from the time of Tammy's entry throughout her enrollment at the Oak Creek Community center school. It was his role to serve as a communication link between the various facilities dealing with Tammy and with her home. He attempted short-term counseling with the parents to work toward more consistency in behavioral management of Tammy in the home. He later assisted the family in the selection of a residential placement.

The Child Development Center was instrumental in Oak Creek's attempts to implement programs for Tammy. During the fall of 1974 when individual play therapy as a possible mode of intervention was being considered, Tammy took an overdose of medication at school. This incident influenced the agencies to press for immediate initiation of individual psychotherapy with the goal of accelerating Tammy's social development. Traditional, weekly play therapy was implemented. A nurse at the Child Development Center provided parent counseling, and meetings were arranged to coordinate efforts with the school.

From November, 1974, through July, 1975, Tammy attended twenty-nine weekly sessions of play therapy with a postdoctoral fellow in child psychology at the Child Development Center. During those months of individual therapy, Tammy made significant progress. Initially, Tammy was careless and often destructive with the therapy room property. She bent pieces of a puzzle in putting them together, threw toys when angry, and refused to help straighten the playroom at the end of each session. Gradually she became concerned with fixing broken toys and cleaning up the playroom before leaving.

During the initial therapy hours, Tammy had two ways of relating to her therapist. Sometimes she passively allowed the therapist to structure her time. At other times, she became demanding. When her demands were not met, she exploded in a tantrum. In later sessions she was willing to negotiate for privileges and spontaneously structured at least a part of the hour's activity for herself and the therapist.

Her mode of expressing anger changed over the 9 months from a quiet resistance in the first sessions, to uncontrolled tantrums in middle sessions, and then to symbolic puppet fighting and verbal expression of anger at the time of termination. These areas of progress seemed to partially fulfill the goal of increasing Tammy's social responsibility.

The therapy method during quiet play sessions was similar to the child-centered approach described by Axline.[1] However, a great amount of structure and activity, following the guidelines suggested by Leland and Smith for play therapy with retarded children, was often contributed by the therapist.[6] Intrinsic and extrinsic reinforcers were identified by the nurse or another observer who recorded behaviors through a one-way mirror. This recorded information was used to plan the therapeutic tactics for subsequent sessions. Social reinforcement in the form of praise ("I like to see you playing quietly") was given frequently during times of socially appropriate behavior. When Tammy's behavior was deemed to

be inappropriate, the therapist turned his back for 1 minute. If her behavior became physically assaultive or dangerous to her own person, some of the more confrontive techniques described by Redl and Wineman were used.[8] During severely destructive tantrums, the therapist physically restrained her until she was calm. At first Tammy's response to physical restraint was anger. Later the length of tantrum time was reduced. As she learned to substitute more appropriate ways of expressing anger, tantrums occurred rarely and were of short duration.

A staff meeting at the school was held in January, 1975, to evaluate Tammy's progress. Although she had made some minimal gains academically, her social behavior at school had not improved significantly. Intervention in the home had produced negligible effects. Therefore, residential placement was suggested as a means of providing more consistent supervision on a 24-hour basis.

Residential placement was discussed during a home visit by the school social worker in February, 1975. The parents admitted having mentioned this idea briefly in the past but felt it was unnecessary, "as long as they could handle her." Mrs. F. stated that her need to have Tammy at home was so great that it would be difficult for her to separate and to look at Tammy's needs independently and objectively. She associated Tammy's leaving home with Tina's death. Mr. F. agreed to consider placement of Tammy and offered to visit the recommended residential facility with the social worker.

Shortly thereafter, Mr. F., Tammy's teacher, and the social worker visited the residential facility. The father appeared more concerned with the day-to-day routines of the children there than with the facility's services for his daughter. However, the parents decided to apply for her admission. Because Mr. F. was unemployed at the time, the county social services department agreed to pay for the residential costs, and the community center agreed to pay for the educational costs.

After referral was made to the private residential facility in February, 1975, the personnel responded positively. They stated that a new girls' residence was to be opened as soon as there were enough applicants to make it financially feasible. The intake procedure required that various educational and psychological evaluations be performed by the residential staff, despite the availability of recent evaluation results and the additional expense to the F. family. Mr. and Mrs. F. were concerned that their application interview seemed superficial and that the interviewers did not appear to grasp the full significance of Tammy's history or the extent of their present problems. This concern was confirmed at the admission conference held by this facility and attended by the Oak Creek social worker. The various evaluators reported that Tammy had been a delightful and humorous child, and they all recommended her highly for their residential and educational programs. The intake worker put little emphasis on Tammy's history of negative behavior reported by other agencies. Tammy was easily approved for admission in April, 1975.

Following the application approval, the school social worker made a home visit to discuss Tammy's pending entry. The possibility of Tammy's immediate admission produced much anxiety in Mrs. F. She became depressed, expressing sorrow about the need to place Tammy outside of the home. After making the referral for residential placement, Mrs. F. expressed appreciation of Tammy's presence in the home. The thought of Tammy actually moving out created much anticipatory anxiety. Mr. F. exhibited no ambivalence toward the placement or understanding of what Mrs. F. was experiencing. Rather he compared Tammy's placement with "sending her off to summer camp."

Due to an insufficient number of applicants, the new residential unit was not opened by the beginning of the September school term. Therefore, the residential staff suggested that Tammy begin attending their day training school program. The staff felt this arrangement would facilitate a quicker and easier transition into the dorm when it opened. Mrs. F. agreed to this arrangement.

About this time, Mrs. F. separated from her husband and filed for divorce. Tammy's behavior became worse after her father left the home. Due to Tammy's behavior problems and the support given by Oak Creek and the Child Development Center for the new placement, this transition was less difficult for Mrs. F. than previous changes in schools.

Although Tammy's behavior remained unchanged with the move to the new school, Mrs. F.'s main concern with the facility was the lack of communication between the residential staff and herself. The staff members were reluctant to share with Mrs. F. the difficulties they were experiencing with Tammy, and they were generally unresponsive to her inquiries regarding her child's program. After 8 weeks in the program, an evaluation of academic and speech areas was conducted. The residential staff concluded that Tammy's behavior would have to improve before she could enter the residential unit.

By the end of this 8-week period, the projected date for the opening of the new girls' residence had been delayed several times. This was discouraging and frustrating to Mrs. F. Her job was already in jeopardy due to special arrangements that had allowed her to deliver Tammy to school and arrive at work late. Her employer was unwilling to let this arrangement continue indefinitely. In November, 1975, Mrs. F. asked for a meeting with the director and intake worker of the residential facility to explain her frustration and to get a commitment for an entry date. Her earlier suspicions of a hasty approval by the facility were confirmed. Tammy's problems were presented as though the staff had been unaware that she had previously exhibited negative behaviors. It was then stated for the first time that the girls' residence had already opened but that Tammy could not enter until her behavior in the day program was under better control. No definition was given for "better control." Although Mrs. F. pointed out that perhaps Tammy needed the consistency of a 24-hour program before improvement could be expected, the position of the staff remained firm.

The meeting was unproductive from the standpoint that an entry date was not secured; however, Mrs. F. was able to express herself directly and appropriately. She concluded from this meeting that the facility was stalling and did not want Tammy to enter. Mrs. F. then requested that the school worker investigate other alternatives for placement.

An alternative placement was subsequently located approximately 200 miles away. Although Mrs. F. had not seen the facility, she spoke by telephone to its director. Because she was given additional encouragement by the staff members of the Child Development Center and Oak Creek, she decided to enroll Tammy in this facility.

In January, 1976, Tammy was admitted. The school social worker offered to drive, due to concern about Tammy's behavior in the car. The maternal grandmother, who had flown from California for this purpose, and a friend of Mrs. F. accompanied Tammy and her mother on the trip. Upon arrival, Mrs. F. appeared quite pleased with the facility and made an effort to learn the other residents' names. She did not get to say good-bye to Tammy, who had a tantrum as the family prepared to leave. After returning home, Mrs. F. discussed her feelings and thoughts about the placement. She mentioned that upon arrival at the residence, she had immediately begun looking for things she could criticize. She felt this was an attempt to assure herself that the

new residence was not superior to the family home in all aspects and that the residence was not perfect. She experienced guilt and asked how she could ever again justify sharing happiness and love with the other children without Tammy in the home. She became very sad and began to remember her baby daughter, who had died 3 years ago to the week that Tammy was placed. She stated that she grieved for both of them.

DISCUSSION
Crisis proneness

Many of this family's actions and reactions may be understood in a crisis framework. Crisis theory has major implications for viewing the families of handicapped children. The concept of crisis proneness, a part of crisis theory, is particularly useful in this case. As viewed in the literature, the crisis proneness of a family is largely determined by its crisis-meeting resources and by its definition of the stressful event.[5] It was pointed out in this case study that the F. family responded to such events in a reactive manner rather than attempting to plan ahead. For instance, changes in the services offered by agencies became crises for them. It was difficult for the family to plan for and deal with crises effectively. Their inability to cope with change was related to the two factors needed to meet crises—family adaptability and family integration. Adaptability refers to the ability to meet obstacles and make needed changes, whereas integration is the solidarity and bonds of unity within the family.[5]

The lack of adaptability within the F. home was apparent at the time Tammy was awaiting admission to the residential facility. The parents appeared to be aware that shifts within the family structure were likely to upset the already delicate balance in which they existed. Roles in the family were distinct and rigid, generally allowing for less adaptation within the structure. These factors suggested a need to maintain the status quo and a reluctance to adapt to the challenges at hand.

This family's integration was also insufficient to adequately deal with crises. In recent years, there were few issues on which the F. family had been united, rather, there was always conflict. Discipline in the home was an issue that was never resolved. Communication between the parents was often argumentative or involved game playing. The family shared few common goals or activities.

The second consideration in crisis proneness is the definition the family gives to the stressful event. This is influenced by their values, prior crisis experiences, and cultural considerations.[5] The F. family did not consider itself capable of coping with crises due to poor resolution of previous crisis experiences. This pessimistic outlook had an influence on the family's crisis definition and on the level of motivation they brought into the present situation. Mrs. F. was also influenced by her Hispanic background, even though she would have liked to discount this factor. Due to this cultural consideration, Mrs. F. experienced demoralization when she had to request outside intervention and placement of her child.

Coping process

According to Olshansky, it is a natural response for most parents of handicapped children to experience chronic sorrow throughout their lives, whether the child is kept at home or placed in a residential facility. Factors such as parents' personality, ethnic group, religion, and social class influence the intensity of the sorrow experienced by the family. This varies from time to time for the same person, from situation to situation, and from one family member to another.[7] The reaction of sorrow is significant and must be considered by professionals in order to be effective in working with families of handicapped individuals.

In addition to an appreciation of the chronic sorrow phenomenon, a look at various coping mechanisms used by the F. family might also help to understand their behavior. Parents of a mentally retarded child typically experience feelings of denial,

anger, guilt, and bargaining. Each is a means of coping with various situations and demands placed on the parent at any given moment. The problem-solving process is also a coping skill and may be employed by parents in some situations. Parents should receive support for their use of these various mechanisms, all of which carry many strong feelings from the individual's past. A lack of support from the marriage partner might offer a partial explanation for Mr. and Mrs. F.'s marital conflict and eventual breakdown. When the F. family was first known to the Child Development Center, both parents employed denial and anger as their primary coping mechanisms. Over a period of 4 years, however, Mrs. F. appeared to develop more positive coping abilities in relation to Tammy, whereas Mr. F. continued to use denial and anger. When they moved from similar coping processes into a sphere where they shared few of the same attitudes about Tammy, the conflict between them increased.

The ability and need of a parent to use a wide range of coping mechanisms were exemplified in the dialogue of Mrs. F. on the return trip from placing Tammy in the residential home. Mrs. F. was able to verbalize her feelings of acceptance for Tammy and her problems. However, she had previously denied the significance and severity of the problem and wished to take Tammy home. Stating that "no child could ever be happy in a residence," she felt guilty about the placement. At the same time that she verbalized relief that Tammy was out of the home setting, she also verbalized guilt feelings for experiencing this relief. These examples show how persons move in and out of the various coping mechanisms, based on their needs at that moment.

Early intervention

What would Tammy's situation be if she had been placed in an early infant program before the age of 4 years? Since 1973, many programs have developed with the philosophy that intervention is more effective in assisting parents in their adjustment when the child is younger. Parental involvement is necessarily a strong component of these programs. Another vital part of any program is interagency cooperation. One program implementing these components was developed in 1975 by the Community Center and the Child Development Center.

Some preliminary data collected by the Delayed Developmental Project have demonstrated that a special effort consisting of a home program (for children birth to 18 months) and a school program (18 months to 3 years) has been helpful to both the parents and the handicapped child.[3] Parents in an experimental group of this project have demonstrated significant differences in attitudes. They seem more realistic, optimistic, and confident. The staffs of community agencies have observed that the children and their parents in the Delayed Developmental Project who move into other programs have demonstrated a higher level of readiness than previously noted. In summary, the project has indicated the following[3]:

1. There is a desire and need for services by parents of handicapped children at the earliest possible date.
2. Services can have a significant impact on the child at crucial developmental periods.
3. The parents are helped in ways that result in improved family functioning.

At the end of the Delayed Developmental Project's first year of operation, the available data strengthen the above conclusions relative to early intervention. We can only speculate that, had a program of this nature been available to the F. family, Tammy's progress would have improved, and her life would have been different.

Need for interagency relationships

Tammy has lifelong supervisory needs. Mrs. F. anticipates Tammy's return home at some point in the future when her behavior is under self-control. If she could return home during her teen-age years, it would still appear appropriate to consider an adult residential placement. Her minimal needs would include sheltered housing and workshop employment. If behavioral improvement is not achieved during the current placement, residential treatment might continue to be necessary.

According to Wolfensberger, retarded persons should not be placed with other adults whose disabilities are different. Inappropriate placement may prevent individuals in each group from successful rehabilitation.[9] Due to the current critical shortage of community facilities, this appears to be an unrealistic expectation. Hence, there is need to compromise concerning the appropriateness of placement.

In a summary of the interagency relationships in this case study, the necessity of cooperation becomes obvious. The staff of the first community center involved with Tammy and her family was reluctant to cooperate in a joint effort with other involved agencies. The case coordinator from that agency found it difficult to deal with the family. She also experienced problems in maintaining communication with her own staff. Although it was not apparent at the time, the family situation was too overwhelming for one individual to coordinate effectively.

In contrast to the first placement, Oak Creek offered a strong support system for its staff. Following a policy that no child could be terminated unless a better program was available, Oak Creek developed strategies to assist the staff in coping with such a demanding child. The team approach appeared successful in meeting this challenge, with the support of the community center's administrative staff. When it appeared that there was no funding for the second residential placement, the administrators from this agency volunteered money from their own budgets to finance Tammy until the next fiscal year.

The interagency relationship in this case resulted in better services through coordination and cooperation. It also confirmed the idea that there must be a belief in the positive value of the interagency relationship. Such an attitude was shared by the Oak Creek and the Child Development Center staffs. The working relationship between these agencies included consulting, planning, and defining individual and joint responsibilities.

A cooperative attitude was not shared by the first private residential facility that had offered minimal services. The relationship among the agencies was superficial and consisted only of acquaintance and information sharing. The attitude seemed to be one of isolation and defensiveness toward the other agencies. One explanation for such inflexibility within an agency may be that as it grows and achieves strength, it tends to turn toward the needs of its own structure rather than the needs of the community.[4]

On the other hand, several accomplishments may be attributed to the cooperative relationship between Oak Creek and the Child Development Center. Better communication of information regarding the client, family, problems, and services was achieved through consultation. The relationship stimulated planning and strengthened the work of both agencies by joint interpretation of problems, goals, and strategies. As problems and solutions extended beyond the two agencies, cooperative efforts were successful in soliciting other needed services. Finally, such an effort served to strengthen the available community services.

SUMMARY

The agencies involved in this case had an open-door policy for the F. family. This is expected to continue until the family is comfortable with and trusts the new agency and its personnel. There is often a tendency for agency personnel to foster dependency on the part of the client. This may occur when much time has been invested in an individual or family. Therefore, it is important that the existing agencies continue to support the family in its movement towards independence in working with new systems and agencies.

There is an obligation for the agencies that have cooperated for the benefit of the child and family to continue to work with the residential facility currently responsible for providing services. The necessity for linkage of services must be stressed in order to maximize effective programming in the lifelong care for a mentally retarded individual such as Tammy. Families having retarded members may need assistance in periods of crisis. Professionals also need to be aware of the various coping mechanisms that may be utilized by such families and to offer their support accordingly.

REFERENCES

1. Axline, V.: Play therapy, Boston, 1969, Houghton Mifflin Co.
2. Coleman, J. C.: Abnormal psychology and modern life, ed. 5, Glenview, Ill., 1976, Scott, Foresman & Co.
3. Delayed Development Project, Stockton Unified School District, Walton Developmental Center, Delayed Development Unit, Stockton, Calif., 1973.
4. DeMarche, D. F., and Johns, R. E.: Community organization and agency responsibility, New York, 1951, Association Press.
5. Hill, R.: Generic features of families under stress. In Parad, H. J., editor: Crisis intervention; selected readings, New York, 1971, Family Service Association of America.
6. Leland, H., and Smith, D.: Play therapy with mentally subnormal children, New York, 1965, Grune & Stratton, Inc.
7. Olshansky, S.: Chronic sorrow; a response to having a mentally defective child, Soc. Casework, **43:**191, 1962.
8. Redl, F., and Wineman, D.: Controls from within, New York, 1952, Macmillan, Inc.
9. Wolfensberger, W.: The principle of normalization in human services, Toronto, 1972, National Institute on Mental Retardation.

CHAPTER 16

Factors influencing outcomes of behavioral home management programs

SARAH S. STRAUSS and JUDITH A. BUMBALO

Since 1965, nurses have developed increasingly more sophisticated skills in utilizing behavioral approaches* and behavioral modification techniques to intervene with developmentally disabled children and their families.[1, 6] As a result of familiarity with and mastery of these techniques, there now appears to be an effort to reevaluate the effectiveness of these methodologies and to redirect energies toward new strategies.[3] Review of the literature and of experiences of professional practitioners illustrates the success of many behavioral home management programs. When the expectation is that behavior will change and family and professional goals will be accomplished, the occasional failure of an attempt to utilize behavioral approaches demands examination

---

*For the purposes of this chapter, *behavioral approach* is defined as a method of intervention that utilizes principles of behavioral psychology to help parents manage or modify a child's behaviors. This method focuses on establishing, changing, or eliminating behavior by systematically determining its component parts and consequent events. This process requires precise observation and documentation of behavior. Intervention may utilize techniques such as positive reinforcement, negative reinforcement, punishment, fading, and shaping. For further descriptions and discussion of this approach, see O'Neil, S., Knapp, M. and McLaughlin, B.: Behavioral approaches to children with developmental delays, St. Louis, 1977, The C. V. Mosby Co.

and explanation. The objective of this chapter is to analyze selected variables operating in "failure" situations in an effort to determine the appropriateness of behavioral intervention.

The primary factors that influence the outcome of home-based behavioral intervention with handicapped children can be grouped into two categories. First, a program using a behavioral approach may be hindered by professional inability to offer services in the most appropriate manner. Second, ineffective functioning of the family due to deficiencies in its structure may prohibit successful outcomes of such programming, despite the best intentions and efforts of the professional. In the following pages, consideration is given to both factors, and illustrative situations are used to identify cues for potential success versus failure. Suggestions for alternative intervention are also discussed.

FACTORS AFFECTING PROFESSIONAL EFFECTIVENESS

The ability of the nurse to offer service depends on a philosophical comfort with, and commitment to, the operant learning principles that are critical to successful behavioral programs. For example, a nurse holding a basic belief that sibling rivalry is inevitable and is the reason for all excessive fighting between school-age brothers would have difficulty analyzing specific antecedent and consequent behaviors and designing an extinction program to eliminate them. Similarly, a person who views positive reinforcement as "offering a bribe" would most likely be very uncomfortable using a token reward system to elicit behavior change. Perhaps most important is the persuasion factor. If a practitioner does not really believe in the potential for success inherent in behavioral programming, parents will be quick to recognize such doubts. In such situations, hesitancy and inconsistency on the part of both nurse and parents are common results.

A sound knowledge base and competency in initiating, maintaining, and evaluating behaviorally based interventions are other crucial variables that influence effectiveness. Improperly planned or executed programs can result in no behavior change or unwanted new behaviors that may add to the family's problems. Literature is replete with examples of injustices done to individuals in the name of behavior modification. Nurses in the field of developmental disabilities must guard against unprofessional or unethical practice that can be the result of an insufficient or improperly applied theoretical framework.

When a behavioral home management program is initiated, consideration must be given to both time and resources available. Successful intervention demands a great number of professional hours. At times, daily telephone or personal contact with parents is necessary. The use of audiovisual equipment or other data-collecting materials may be important. It is also helpful to employ a cotherapist or supervisor to assist in managing a particularly difficult situation. If appropriate support is not available, it may be preferable to postpone intervention until more adequate time and technical advice is obtainable.

FACTORS AFFECTING FAMILY FUNCTIONING

It is not unusual for a skillful and committed nurse to spend hours developing a program for toilet training or remedying sleep disturbances only to find that the plan fails or undergoes numerous revisions. Even when parents participate in every step of planning, a successful program for a specific behavioral problem is not guaranteed. Internal family functioning that is related to an inability to participate or follow through with behavioral programming is an important variable to consider.

The model presented by Satir provides one functional framework for assessing families' receptivity and readiness for a behavioral approach in home program planning. Her summary of important factors that affect family functioning includes: (1) the actual experience of conception, (2) pregnancy and birth, (3) individual circumstances of the family at or immediately after birth, (4) ongoing circumstances or family condition, (5) the relationship of the marital pair, (6) relationship of the grandparents, (7) the adults' level of knowledge, (8) their ways of communicating, and (9) their philosophy of child rearing.[5] Although more than one of these factors may influence a particular situation, each is worthy of examination as an isolated variable.

The experiences of conception, pregnancy, and birth

Ross emphasizes the loss and grief inherent in the birth of a handicapped child.[4] It is hypothesized that loss of the expected perfect child has a profound effect on the establishment of parental attachment patterns. If the birth of such a child is also overshadowed by problems surrounding conception, pregnancy, and the birth experience, such negative events can influence interventions for years. When the nurse is aware of such influences, the inability of a parent to change an interaction pattern can be better understood. Consider the case of the N. family:

A review of the hospital record revealed that Mrs. N. experienced pernicious vomiting throughout her pregnancy with Steven. The immediate postpartum period was complicated by hemorrhage and shock which necessitated an extended hospitalization. When Steven was 3 years old, attempts to help

Mrs. N. deal with his destructive and aggressive behavior through the use of time-out failed. Mrs. N. reported, "I just can't put him in that empty room all by himself. The neighbors must think I'm killing him." Two years later, Mrs. N. revealed to the nurse that her pregnancy with Steven was the result of an adulterous relationship.

The experience of the N. family is contrasted with that of Mr. and Mrs. Y.:

Kim's birth was eagerly anticipated and prepared for by Mr. and Mrs. Y. They had been married for 3 years, were financially secure, and each of them had fulfilling careers. The couple enrolled in a course on natural childbirth, and Mr. Y. was in the delivery room when the infant was born. It was immediately obvious that Kim had Down's syndrome. From the beginning, the family utilized professional guidance and input from other parents in their approach to child rearing. At 3 years of age, Kim's social and self-help skills were at her age level, and she attended a preschool for normal children.

Family circumstances

Consideration of the family's specific circumstances at the time of proposed behavioral intervention can identify crucial variables affecting intended outcomes. If lack of resources and power is such that basic needs are not being met, attempts to focus on child-centered problems will probably be futile.

Mrs. C. had been separated from her husband for 3 months when she first requested help in toilet training her 2^1/$_2$-year-old son, Jimmy. Her primary source of support was from public assistance funds, and by the last week of the month her resources totaled $1.30. She was worried about being evicted from her apartment because of the behavior of her two children. During the course of a ^{1}/$_2$-hour discussion on a strategy for toilet training, she more than once commented, "If only my husband would come back, everything would be okay."

Appropriate timing and a supportive environment can result in behavior change that has previously been thought impossible.

The M. family had recently moved to a new home with comfortable living space. Each of the four adolescent daughters was successful in social and academic spheres. Although Mr. and Mrs. M. were accepting of 7-year-old Amy's profound deafness, they had not previously focused on her overall delay

or lagging socialization skills. The first time Amy slept in a room next to her parents' bedroom rather than in her sister's, she began a nightly ritual of awakening them after wetting the bed. At this time, Mr. and Mrs. M. expressed interest in a behavioral program for toilet training.

Condition of the infant

When infants are born prematurely or demonstrate obvious physical and mental deficits in the neonatal period, such problems may abrogate further development in the eyes of the parents. For example, parental perception of the defective infant becoming a multiply handicapped adolescent makes attainment of change virtually impossible. Consider the case of the B. family:

Margaret, a 12-year-old cerebral palsied child who attended a day care facility, experienced the onset of menstruation. A collaborative nurse/teacher home visit revealed that the mother allowed little independence in physical care activity and frequently referred to her daughter as "our baby." Although this girl possessed sufficient communication skills to make her needs known and to attain some measure of self-care, family and school efforts to establish a program for menstrual hygiene were not successful. Contingencies had minimal effect on Margaret's inclination to request help with or manage changes of sanitary napkins. She appeared content to wait for her mother to provide help.

In contrast to the example cited above, Mr. and Mrs. Y. were quick to recognize developmental changes and growth in their child who was born without arms and legs.

Six-month-old Jennifer received care in a congenital defects clinic. From the beginning of intervention, the parents showed pleasure in her attainment of both physical and social milestones. They are presently involved in a program to maximize trunk control, which is crucial to further rehabilitative efforts. Using a sequential behavioral model, Mr. and Mrs. Y. have facilitated Jennifer's sitting upright in a specially designed prosthesis.

The relationship of the marital pair

Satir emphasizes that two people living together as one unit is difficult at best.[5] This is especially true in a society that bases the marital relationship almost completely on love and imposes demands that love can never solely fulfill. Farber documents that the birth of a handicapped child places further stress on a tenuous, diadic relationship.[2] Many intervention efforts are sabotaged by basic disturbances in the husband-wife relationship that predate, or are exacerbated by, the arrival of a handicapped child.

Mrs. S. felt the entire burden and responsibility for implementing the behavioral program for toilet training her moderately retarded 3-year-old. She expressed ambivalence regarding her relationship with her husband, such as, "I don't really think he cares about me . . . I have the burden of Alice alone . . . I guess he's busy with work, but sometimes I wonder." As the relationship became more sterile and lifeless, Mrs. S. resorted more and more to communicating with her husband by calling him during work hours. Her hysterical recitals of Alice's latest misbehavior were obviously a desperate attempt to establish a basis for interaction in a disintegrating marriage.

The sexual relationship between a couple can also provide clues to the status of the marriage. Often, serious difficulties in sexual adjustment exist concomitant with an inability to deal with the demands of parenting.

Mrs. N. called the clinic requesting assistance in dealing with the behavior of her 4-year-old son. "You've got to help me before he destroys my house . . . my home . . . my marriage." Attempts to find effective behavioral intervention for dealing with the child's destructiveness proved futile. Further exploration by the nurse revealed that Mr. and Mrs. N. had not engaged in sexual intercourse for 3 months.

In contrast to the S. and N. families, in situations where behavioral intervention has proved effective, mutual concern and esteem are evidenced between the marital pair. Such feelings are frequently translated into a willingness by both partners to share responsibility for implementing a behavioral program.

Mrs. Q. complained about an inability to wean her severely allergic 2-year-old from breast-feeding. The nurse held a conference with both parents and devised a plan that required the husband to offer a glass of milk in place of the usual 5:00 AM nursing session. Mr. Q. commented, "My wife just can't go on like this."

The relationship to the grandparents

Frequently, little attention is paid by professionals to intergenerational influences operating in families with a handicapped child. The magnitude of this factor varies with cultural values. However, many husbands and wives remain relatively dependent (financially, socially, or emotionally) on their families of origin. Young parents may themselves still be in the process of resolving the developmental tasks of adolescence, that is, selecting and preparing for an occupation and achieving emotional independence from parents. The birth of a handicapped child superimposes a situational crisis on yet unresolved aspects of the adolescent developmental crisis. The result is increased difficulty in accomplishing normal developmental tasks.

Grandparents, too, have problems when grandchildren begin to arrive. Many are in the midst of the developmental crisis of middle age. It is difficult for some of them to relinquish old patterns of relating with children who have become adults. This is particularly true when a situational crisis, such as having a handicapped grandchild, causes their child (parent) to regress to old dependency patterns that invite judgments and advice regarding child rearing.

Mr. and Mrs. S. lived in a duplex apartment. Mr. S. had recently assumed the responsibility of the family business. Because the office of the business was located in the parents' home, Mr. S. spent most evenings working there while Mrs. S. remained in their apartment with Alice. Alice obtained attention from her mother during this time by having tantrums.

Mrs. S. reported that the paternal grandparents insisted that Alice was "all right" and that their son had demonstrated comparable behaviors at the same age. Thus, the grandparents' opinion was that specific interventions were unnecessary. By perpetuating the financial and social dependence of their son, they passively encouraged his nonparticipation in programs designed to eliminate Alice's tantrums.

Methods of communication

According to Satir, families with low self-esteem demonstrate numerous communication problems.[5] A common threat with communication difficulties is double-level messages, that is, sending a message in which words are asynchronous with tone of voice and body language. The combination of low self-worth and the double-level communication patterns results in confusion and lack of clarity within the family. It also causes confusion and lack of clarity between the nurse and the family about the purpose, plan, and goals of a home program utilizing the behavioral approach. This sets the stage for the family to fail to follow through with implementation.

Satir further describes four patterns of communication that have relevance for analyzing and predicting behaviors of families unable to implement programs designed to change the behavior of a handicapped member.[5] One aberrant communication mode is referred to as placating. The placator uses verbal messages that convey "I agree" but sends body language that communicates, "I'm helpless." These individuals have internalized feelings of worthlessness. They agree with any criticism of themselves and take responsibility for anything that goes wrong.

In explaining Alice's continuing tantrum behavior to the nurse, Mrs. S. stated, "I guess I'm just a weak person," or "I know I'm wishy-washy." She alternated this explanation for lack of progress in limit setting with frequent verbalizations about Alice ". . . holding a grudge against me."

Mrs. S. was using placation to evoke guilt in the nurse and to prevent her own low self-image from being further eroded.

Another aberrant mode of communication is called computing. In this mode, the individual sends abstract verbal messages that sound very reasonable, but the timbre of the voice may be a dry, cracking monotone. The body stance is relaxed, thus conveying a calm attitude. This communication pattern serves as a defense against feelings of vulnerability, but it is also used to evoke envy in others. Individuals may exhibit all or only some of these characteristics.

Mrs. N. kept herself and her children impeccably groomed and dressed. A similar concern for orderliness was reflected in her immaculate and tastefully decorated home. She readily agreed to a program utilizing a behavioral method in managing her 3-year-old retarded son. She evidenced understanding of the underlying principles of this method by correctly identifying reinforcers in the environment. During home visits, a typical comment from Mrs. N. was "Do you think we should change the reinforcement schedule? Perhaps we should use both primary and secondary reinforcers with him."

The parent using such a sophisticated communication pattern is frequently assumed to be an optimal candidate for participation in a structured program of intervention using behavioral methods. This individual may be verbally articulate, demonstrate understanding of a contingency model, and readily enter into a contract situation; however, a facade serves as a cover for low self-esteem. The problem becomes evident when the terms of the contract are consistently broken. Professionals are frequently entrapped by the initial assessment. They tend to blame themselves or their methods for the failure of the program because the parent is obviously extremely competent. With the passage of time and close examination of the situation, the "computer's" main objective becomes apparent: to have the nurse as an ally rather than to focus on the child's problem.

Another aberrant communication mode is blaming. The "blamer" uses verbal messages that convey "I disagree" and exhibits body language that communicates, "I am the boss!" This individual has internalized feelings of loneliness and lack of success, resulting in a poor self-image. Through fault finding, the blamer seeks to enhance feelings of superiority, thus inhibiting comprehension of the true basis of a presenting problem. The function of blaming is to evoke fear in the hope of obtaining obedience. This person frequently blames failure to accomplish specified developmental goals on the methodology or professional incompetence.

Mrs. N. blamed, in succession, the school, the foster parents, and the institution where her son was eventually placed, for his lack of progress. By accusing sources supposedly outside of her control, she relieved herself of direct responsibility and left open the possibility that someone might obey her directives, thus reaffirming her self-worth.

The last aberrant mode of communication is labeled distracting. The person uses irrelevant words that make no sense. A concise response to a question is impossible. The body movement may be excessive; the singsong voice may be out of tune with the words spoken. The internal feeling is one of dizziness, resulting in a "dizzy" self-image. This individual experiences intense loneliness and a lack of purpose.

Mrs. S. described her frustration with her husband's nonparticipation in child rearing and Alice's behaviors with a placid facial expression and pleasant voice. During home visits, she frequently referred to herself as a "basket case." When questioned as to causes for this state, she would repeatedly relate catastrophic events within the extended family demonstrating the same placid affect. Attempts were made to focus the long tangential monologues, such as:

Nurse: "What did you do when Alice screamed and kicked when you put her to bed?"

Mrs. S.: "She got up and came into the living room where I was watching TV. She just loves the TV, especially the commercials [laughs]. She sings along with them. . . . Do you know that commercial. . . ."

This pattern of communication can readily be identified when the interview extends beyond the specified time, but specific topics related to the parent-nurse contract have rarely been discussed despite the best intention and efforts of the nurse. Obviously, this individual uses professional interest and assistance as means of allaying loneliness. The purposelessness of this person can soon permeate the total interaction pattern with the professional. Plans and contracts become purposeless.

Level of knowledge

The level of understanding of mental retardation and other handicapping conditions and the general versus specific implications generated by those problems have a profound influence on any attempts to use behavioral methodology in the home. Since experiences with handicapped individuals

before those with their own child are usually minimal, many parents relate to their child in terms of stereotyped beliefs or myths about handicapped persons. The stereotype does not usually attribute emotional needs or potential for developmental change to the retarded person. Parents may fall into a cycle of believing the behavior of retarded children cannot be changed; therefore, any attempts to change behavior will be systematically ineffective.

Part of Mrs. S.'s failure to consistently follow through with suggestions related to limit setting can be attributed to her beliefs that the hitting, screaming, and kicking behaviors exhibited when Alice was put to bed, placed on the toilet, or dressed, were inherently related to her moderate mental retardation. That Alice was fully capable of learning to participate in these tasks willingly and that she would respond to the same expectations and contingencies as other children were incomprehensible to Mrs. S. She seemed unable to identify with the nurses' success in teaching Alice to hang up her coat.

Contrast this with Mrs. M., who demonstrated her comprehension of her daughter's developmental deficits as well as her need for emotional security through appropriate limit setting:

During a telephone conversation, Mrs. M. discussed problems encountered in a brief respite placement in a foster home. "I told them Susan functioned at a 2- to 3-year-old level and that her pesky behaviors were typical of that age group. We deal with her aggravating us at home by sending her to her room. If she doesn't get the message, sometimes I have to swat her behind. It seems actions speak louder than words!"

Philosophy of care

Parents' philosophy of child care is related to their understanding of mental retardation. Our culture is filled with folk sayings related to child rearing; some are based on truths and some on fallacies. For example, a parent who believes in immediate corporal punishment for misconduct ("spare the rod and spoil the child") may have difficulty realizing such punishment is one form of attention. Ignoring undesirable behavior may be impossible for them.

Parents with rigid belief systems about children may desire short-term results for their efforts. A behavioral program that demands perseverance and long-term commitment may be difficult for them, especially if such a program conflicts with preexisting belief systems. Magical thinking may also be evidenced by parents holding rigid beliefs and desiring short-term results, as the following example illustrates:

Mrs. G. took Debbie, her 4-year-old moderately retarded daughter, to the chiropractor for "neck adjustments." The child's many undesirable behaviors were attributed by her mother to her "neck being out and pinching a nerve." Mrs. G., however, willingly brought Debbie to the child development clinic for assistance in behavior management.

It is also common for parents who have successfully reared older children to rely on past experiences and information that may not always be transferable to a retarded child.

The M. family expressed reluctance to get Susan up during the night for toileting to solve the problem of 7 years of bed-wetting. Mrs. M. told the nurse that her pediatrician had advised against this if nighttime bladder control was ever to be achieved. Further exploration of this subject revealed the suggestion had been made for the older normal daughters in the M. family when they were toddlers.

ALTERNATIVE SUGGESTIONS FOR INTERVENTION

When careful analysis and reassessment lead to the conclusion that implementing a program of behavioral management will not be successful, other alternatives for intervention must be considered. Since communication failure has already been defined as a potent variable in families unable to follow through with home programs, an effort to improve communication patterns would seem appropriate. Family therapy with a competent therapist before or concomitant with planning or implementing a program with the child is the optimal alternative. The primary goal of the nurse becomes helping the family to recognize the need for therapy. In such situations, an extensive repertoire of communication skills is needed by the professional. The nurse must be able to consistently clarify and refocus on the primary problems that must be resolved before any program using behavioral methodology can commence.

Families may require time before they can accept the contingencies of a behavioral program or the alternative of family therapy. The extent of nursing involvement during this interim period depends on personal philosophies of care, the range of clinical competencies, and demands on time. One factor the nurse may wish to evaluate before determining the level of continued involvement is the family's access to community support systems and ability to use them. Relationships from which some support can be derived may exist in the form of family, neighbors, and various health and social agencies. If support does not exist within traditional systems, such as personal relationships, nontraditional supports, such as healers, may be sought. Such relationships may help families to cope at times when they are unable to benefit from professional intervention.

When alternatives are considered, it is important to remember that nurses have traditionally accepted the dependence of people with physical impairments. Allowing temporary dependence of people with behavioral and communicative impairments may be equally acceptable. A family unable to carry through with a behavioral program or unwilling to seek therapy may be able to participate in a maintenance program, provided that someone else assumes responsibility for changing the behavior of the child. This might be accomplished by temporary residential placement of the child for the specific purpose of facilitating developmental change in an environment where contingencies can be planned and controlled by professionals. It can also provide respite time for the family, which may be essential to regaining coping mechanisms. When such a program is undertaken by professionals, concomitant efforts should focus on strengthening the skills and self-esteem of the parents. Parents must realize that their participation in a maintenance program, once behavior change has been achieved, is a valuable contribution to the child's growth and development.

SUMMARY

Working with retarded and handicapped children and their families necessitates careful analysis in order to determine priorities and methodologies for intervention. It is an undisputable fact that the behavioral approach is a valuable method for dealing with the problems presented by many children. However, the approach most suitable for treating the child may not be the best approach when both professional expertise and the total family are taken into account. Before undertaking a behavioral program, the nurse should first consider the skills, resources, and commitment (professional and family) that will be necessary. Consideration should also be given to the fact that the complexities of many family situations permit successful behavioral programming only when intervention also focuses on the total environment in which the child resides. It is naive to expect parents to use be-havior modification techniques to toilet train a child or eliminate tantrums when overall family functioning demands that their priorities be placed elsewhere. In situations such as these, the nurse must recognize and accept the fact that a behaviorally based home management program is not appropriate. When the family functioning permits, a behavioral management program can be successful. Timing is an important key.

REFERENCES
1. Amundson, M. D.: Nurses as group leaders of behavior management classes for parents, Nurs. Clin. North Am. **10:**319, 1975.
2. Farber, B.: Effects of a severely retarded child on family integration, Monogr. Soc. Res. Child Dev. **24:**2, 1959.
3. O'Neil, S. M.: Behavior modification, toward a human experience, Nurs. Clin. North Am. **10:**373, 1975.
4. Ross, A. O.: The exceptional child in the family; helping parents of exceptional children, ed. 2, New York, 1968, Grune & Stratton, Inc.
5. Satir, V.: Peoplemaking, Palo Alto, Calif., 1972, Science and Behavior Books, Inc.
6. Whitney, L., and Barnard, K.: Implication of operant learning theory of nursing care of the retarded child, Ment. Retard. **4:**26, 1966.

CHAPTER 17

Community mental health and mental retardation

WILMA LUTZ

Many resources and agencies are available to assist families with a mentally retarded member. The services available to families overlap and are duplicated in some resources and agencies; however, a variety of services are available to help meet the needs of the family and the mentally retarded member. Briefly, some of these services include special education, counseling, respite care, diagnostic evaluations, and home management.

One of these resources available to help families with a mentally retarded member, especially with counseling, is the community mental health center. Knowledge and previous experience in mental retardation are substantial assets to the counselor or therapist, particularly when needs are identified and when counseling and intervention strategies are selected or adapted to foster maximum growth or change in the family or the mentally retarded individual. In a discussion on the preparation of nurse specialists for children, Florence Erickson outlines the need for knowledge and experience. The specialist's knowledge base should include an understanding of growth and development, family dynamics, the effects of illness, and the vulnerable physical and emotional periods for children at each age level. A pediatric nurse specialist should have experience in communicating with children, families, and professionals as well as expertise in collecting and analyzing data related to the care of children. Furthermore, the nurse specialist is capable of adapting care to ill and handicapped children.[2] This chapter focuses on the nursing management and intervention used with one family that has a mentally retarded adolescent. This case study serves as a partial illustration of the role of a nurse specialist in mental retardation in a children's mental health center.

CASE STUDY

Referrals for assistance with behavior problems in children and youth are frequently seen in a children's mental health center. R. T., a 14-year-old girl, was referred by her mother in October due to behavior problems at home and at school. Throughout her schooling, R. had been placed in specialized classes and programs for children with mental retardation. Currently, she is enrolled in a curriculum that is designed to prepare her for independent living. She attends classes in remedial English and mathematics, cooking, and other homemaking skills. In her fourth year of this program, she may select and learn a vocational skill, such as typing or food preparation. In the referral, her mother also indicated that R. had been hospitalized recently for ingesting twenty to thirty minor tranquilizers.

During the assessment phase, the intent was primarily twofold. It was necessary to obtain a comprehensive composite of R. and her family and to establish rapport with R., her family, and community professionals assisting the family. Assessment information was gathered pertaining to health and developmental status, family pattern and relationships, and school-community relationships. A variety of sources was utilized to assist with this assessment, including sequential observations and interviews with R. and her family, collateral contacts with school and community persons, and medical and psychological evaluations. Following this, problem areas were identified and priorities established.

Sequential observations and interviews revealed valuable data concerning R.'s development and health status as well as family interactions and relationships. In the initial interview, R. repeatedly made statements about her appearance. She pointed out her new coat and dislike for her hairstyle and clothing and indicated her greatest concern about her height and appetite. Physically, she was developing secondary sexual characteristics. Menarche was at age 12, and menses were regular. Height and weight were within normal limits for adolescent girls. Her long, light brown hair was dirty and uncombed but contained no lice. Her skin was clear and clean but appeared dry. Her nails were dirty and showed signs of being bitten. She slept approximately 8 hours each night without apparent disturbance or difficulties. She realized that her purpose in coming to the center was for school and home problems; however, she emphatically stated, "I don't care what happens to me—nobody else does!" In general, R. showed signs of normal physical development in adolescence but indicated problems in self-concept and identity.

Special attention was given to the method of questioning. A minimal number of open-ended questions were used. Questions and statements tended to be specific and direct with regard to use and meaning of words. Words that R. may not have understood were avoided, and the nurse directly clarified any doubts or misunderstood words that were used.

The family unit consisted of the mother, R., and two younger sisters (aged 5 and 7). R.'s father was deceased, and her mother was divorced from the younger siblings' father. Culturally and geographically, the family originated from and had resided in several Appalachian states. They had lived in their present neighborhood for 2 years but had moved to three or four different houses. The family was involved with a social service agency that assisted them in obtaining welfare payments, food stamps, adequate housing, clothing, and medical services. With written permission from Mrs. T., the nurse maintained contact with this agency to share pertinent information and avoid referrals that duplicated services for the family.

Mrs. T., a 40-year-old woman, reported in the initial interview that the family ate meals together and regularly visited grandparents. Other activities as a family unit were limited by finances. The entire family had frequent colds. Nutritional information indicated that the family received a balanced diet. No abnormalities were observed in the health and developmental status of the younger siblings. In this family, R. was identified as the "problem" child and the ill child. The mother frequently took R. to a physician for her numerous complaints of aches, pains, nausea, and fatigue. Mrs. T. stated, "She's always complaining about something!" R.'s medical reports indicated normal blood values and a normal physical examination and suggested that her complaints were psychophysiological in nature.

Mrs. T. expressed greatest concern regarding R.'s behavior at home and at school. Lately, R. had become more profane, refused to do chores, intentionally aggravated her sisters and mother, and frequently was out of the home 1 or 2 hours past the legal curfew time. Discipline was inconsistent for all of the children. Mrs. T. threatened to spank the children or to deny privileges but did not follow through with action.

R. had several responsibilities at home. Frequently, she baby-sat for her sisters. She also cleaned the house and washed dishes both at home and at her grandparents home. She worked every Saturday morning in a bakery to earn spending money. She had a boyfriend whom she was allowed to see in her home but not to date. She had only one girl friend with whom she associated in and out of the school setting. Furthermore, her two sisters constantly teased her about her personal appearance.

While the nurse was observing the family interactions, R. directly stated to Mrs. T. and her sisters, "You know you don't give a damn about me!" Despite the attempts of the mother and sisters to express concern for R., she replied, "No, you don't." R. perceived her ingestion of tranquilizers as a mere accident without intent to harm herself. She took two pills because her sisters irritated her. When the initial dose did not work within 5 minutes, she took more pills. The mother also perceived this event as an accident; however, she now locks all medicine in a cabinet. In brief, the family patterns and interactions indicated that R. was identified as the "problem" child, that there was inconsistent discipline, and that there were frequent arguments and disagreements among the family members. Also, although the mother perceived and verbally expressed a family concern for R., R. did not perceive or feel such a concern.

According to school psychological reports, R.'s skills in mathematics, language usage, and reading comprehension were at first- and second-grade levels. The reports also indicated immature social behaviors. She was absent 20 days out of the first 35 days of school and was tardy ten times. The numerous absences and tardiness in previous years were seen again throughout her attendance record.

During a meeting with school personnel, R.'s problems at school were more specifically defined. R. continually disrupted class by talking out of turn, swearing, hit-ting, and pushing classmates. If a classmate returned a hit, pushed, or argued with her, R. began to whine and cry. Class assignments were rarely finished. According to the school nurse, R. had attempted to avoid gym class by feigning illness on several occasions. She also went to great lengths in her attempts to avoid school for the entire day. On one occasion, she gagged herself until a clear emesis was produced. The principal stated that R. had few friends at school. She interacted with only one classmate at recess. Contacts with other peers usually ended in a fight. R. had been suspended for 1 day for fighting during the current school year. Unless R. began to change her behavior, it would be necessary to suspend or expel her for a longer time. The school personnel identified R.'s fighting as the most disruptive and immediate problem at school. They provided additional information about R.'s attempts to avoid school activities with illness and more specific information about her interactions and relationships with peers.

This composite of R. and her family identified the following areas in need of nursing intervention: (1) acceptable behaviors (that is, no fighting or swearing) at home and at school, (2) numerous bodily concerns and complaints, (3) self-concept and identity, and (4) family interaction patterns.

Three primary factors were considered in establishing priorities for the problem areas. A very important and immediate factor was that R. was near suspension and possible expulsion from school because of her behaviors. A second factor was the availability of resources within the center, such as adolescent groups or parent groups. A new group for retarded adolescents was being formed with the focus on home and school problems and on improving social interaction skills. The third factor involved Brammer's statements on helping, which are defined as a dynamic process that enables persons to grow in a direction of their choice.[1] The person being helped learns how to deal effectively with feelings and environmental demands and how to resolve problems. Another part of this process allows for changes to occur within the helper, such as realizing that the client does not always overtly state the desired direction of growth. R. gave only behavioral clues to her desired direction of growth, which included self-concept, identity, and knowledge of socially appropriate behaviors.

The initial nursing goals were to prevent R.'s suspension from school and to reduce conflicts at home. A more specific goal was to establish a reward system for appropriate behaviors in both environments. At school, R. was praised by her teachers and the principal for completing assignments, for not fighting during recess, for having a clean and neat appearance, and for arriving at school on time. R. was allowed to leave school early on Fridays according to the following schedule. She was allotted 1 hour for not fighting during the week; 45 minutes if only one incident occurred, $1/2$ hour for two incidents, and only 15 minutes for three incidents. Next, R. began to participate in the group sessions at the center. Although the nurse was not directly involved in these sessions, communication was maintained with the group leaders and R. to monitor progress.

After 1 month, a parent group was formed to assist with management of problem behaviors at home. Mrs. T. expressed interest in attending the eight group sessions. However, Mrs. T. missed three sessions due to illness, so assistance was provided on a one-to-one basis. Mrs. T. first identified that she wanted R. to decrease or stop swearing, especially in front of her younger sisters. Next, Mrs. T. kept a record for 1 week of the number of times R. used profanity between arriving home from school and bedtime. Mrs. T. informed R. of the record and of exactly what was being recorded. This data showed that R.'s use of profanity drastically decreased toward the end of the first week. She stated that R. expressed a dislike of the record. After the baseline data were obtained, a reward system was established. If R. had five or fewer swearing incidents, she was permitted to go skating or to a movie with her boyfriend or girl friend. Consis-

tency was firmly stressed. Concurrently, the nurse and Mrs. T. discussed the physical changes that occur during adolescence as well as ways to handle the fighting and arguments among the children.

These initial strategies appeared to be successful. R. was not suspended or expelled from school for fighting. However, she was suspended for 1 day for smoking on school grounds. The teachers and the principal reported less fighting and noticed more attempts by R. to finish her work. Mrs. T. stated that the use of profanity over a 4- to 5-month period was nearly eliminated. R. began to do her chores, and Mrs. T. reported fewer conflicts within the family. Small changes were also noted in R. after she completed the group sessions. She began to interact positively with other adolescents in the center and with her classmates.

The remaining problem areas involved long-range nursing goals. These goals included promoting and developing a positive self-concept and reducing bodily concerns. The results of psychological tests at the center supported the fact that R.'s concept of herself was negative and that her self-esteem was low. Also, there were indications in the report that she was unsuccessfully coping with an unresolved conflict.

Self-drawings were utilized to begin achieving these long-range goals. In her first session, R. drew two pictures of herself, one at 9 years and the other at 14 years of age. The self-drawing at 9 years of age was a stick figure with a dress, curly hair, and a smile. Arms, legs, and trunk were proportionate. She talked about how happy and pretty she was then. The drawing at 14 years of age was a strikingly different stick figure. This figure had disproportionately longer legs and arms, wore pants, and had straight hair. Interestingly, R. also drew breasts and a frown on the figure. She described herself as being sad and ugly.

Developmentally, her drawings did not compare with expected adolescent self-portraits.[3] However, the drawings assisted in identifying that R. was concerned about her sudden growth and secondary sexual changes. While drawing, she further correlated her present sadness to the time when her father had died. Later, Mrs. T. related that R.'s father had suffered considerable pain and had been confined to bed during a long illness. The family had given him much physical care and attention during that time. R. was 9 years old when her father died, but she still cries when looking at his picture.

In subsequent contacts with R., the sessions focused on teaching her about normal adolescent growth and sexual changes. On each visit, the nurse mentioned one positive aspect about R.'s appearance, such as neat or clean hair, pressed clothes, or clean hands and nails. The sessions were also geared to help her resolve the remaining grief from her father's death. Role playing was used to allow opportunities to learn and practice new ways to handle teasing about her growth and ways to handle her anger. Later, this strategy was used to further assist her in developing peer interaction skills.

By the end of the school year, R. had made definite changes in her behavior. Fighting and tardiness had decreased markedly, and more assignments were completed. There were fewer confrontations between mother and children as well as among the siblings. During the last month of school, R. was present every day and did not feign illness to get out of school. The mother also reported fewer physical complaints from R. The greatest measure of success, in the nurse's opinion, occurred when R. called to request an earlier appointment time because she wanted to discuss quitting school and going to work. Between the phone call and the appointment time the next day, R. had decided *on her own* that quitting school was not the best solution for her. She was beginning to deal with and resolve her own problems.

Counseling continues with R. and her family to reinforce the changed behaviors. Also, concerns relating to self-concept and identity are being resolved, such as appropriate behaviors in heterosexual relationships and personal grooming.

SUMMARY

This case study partially illustrates the counseling role of a nurse specialist in mental retardation within a community mental health setting. Other roles mentioned include involvement with individual parents, and parent groups and communication and collaboration with community agencies and professionals.

REFERENCES

1. Brammer, L. M.: The helping relationship; process and skills, Englewood Cliffs, N.J., 1973, Prentice-Hall, Inc.
2. Erickson, F.: Nurse specialist for children, Nurs. Outlook **16:**34, 1968.
3. Murray, R., and Zentner, J.: Nursing assessment and health promotion through the life span, Englewood Cliffs, N.J., 1973, Prentice-Hall, Inc.

CHAPTER 18

Developing sexuality among people who are retarded

ANN WIZINSKY PATTULLO

The last decade has forcefully brought to the attention of nurses, other professionals, paraprofessionals, and the general public many issues regarding human sexuality. A positive trend toward more openness and honesty is reflected not only in human behavior and lay publications but also in the professional literature of the health services and educational systems. Lief states that society's definition of what is normal has undergone change in that the former emphasis on reproductive sex has shifted to relational sex.[12] He also recognizes the trend toward the sanctioning of recreational sex.

A concurrent and related trend has been the proliferation of approaches in the "growth of self," or "human fulfillment," movement. Striving for self-actualization and for optimally enriching relationships with others are processes whereby one's life experiences, including sexual expression, become more fulfilling.

Many factors influence the lifelong developmental process of being sexual. The degree to which each human being reaches fulfillment in any aspect of personhood varies according to the nature and quality of life

This chapter was supported by a grant from the U.S. Department of Health, Education, and Welfare, Public Health Services, and Mental Health Administration, Maternal and Child Health Services, Project No. 923.

experiences and emotional, physical, and cognitive developmental processes.

Within the past 10 years there has been increased awareness that the multifactorial interactive nature of human sexual development applies also to people who are retarded. The aspiration for human fulfillment, including sexual fulfillment, for these people is an acknowledged goal reflected in much of the literature. The emphasis has been on adolescence and adulthood. This chapter examines the factors that impact on the achievement of this goal, with an emphasis on the early phases of fulfilling sociosexual development for these people. The nursing role in facilitating this process is explored.

CURRENT PERSPECTIVES

The goal of full appreciation of the uniquely human individuality and sexuality of people who are retarded has not yet been achieved. The use of the term "retardates" does not convey the concept of unique personhood. The current use of this term in the literature in reference to people who have retardation as one of their characteristics strongly implies that there are some professionals in the field who, at some emotional level, have retained a dehumanizing perspective of the people who are supposed to benefit from their interventions.

Sweden has strongly influenced the life-styles of people who are retarded and of people who influence their development. It is in large part due to the leadership demonstrated in Sweden that normalization and humanization have become increasingly evident in the linguistic and behavioral repertoires of professionals in the United States. Grunewald has described the guiding philosophy of normalization; it does not deny the existence of the retardation but does exploit the other mental and physical characteristics of each individual so that the handicap is less pronounced.[7] When the uniquely human individuality of people who are retarded is accepted, it follows that they have the same human rights and responsibilities as any other person insofar as they demonstrate capability. The right to human fulfillment to the highest degree possible is at the basis of accepting the right to expression of sexuality to the highest degree possible. The two are inextricably interwoven.

CURRENT KNOWLEDGE

Sexuality in some form begins to be an integral part of the human personality in infancy. Growth of love for oneself and for others begins then through being held closely and caressed in the many ways that express love and tenderness. The infant learns that the body is both a receiver of and a source for pleasurable, sensuous experiences. These may have an erotic component. Eroticism can occur during childhood; masturbation in infancy has been documented.[2]

It is generally accepted that nonerotic factors are of greater importance to the very early development of fulfilling sexuality. These include the development of a positive body image and gender identity, feelings of self-worth and mastery of the environment, effective communication with others and relating in other ways that result in the expression and reception of caring.

Children who are retarded frequently are deprived of many experiences that would enhance their human fulfillment. Too frequently they are not taught or even permit-ted to master their environment and themselves. They often reach adulthood lacking the basic skills that lead to the strategy of making choices. They also have little experience in appropriately expressing feelings and in experiencing their bodies as sources of pleasure for themselves and for others.

Morganstern's studies of children and young adults, aged 7 through 20 years, provide the only research data available regarding youthful psychosexual development of people who are mentally retarded. The methodology required that the subjects exercise choices. His work led him to infer that people who are retarded are deficient in sensitivity, do not form personal relationships, and are unable to comprehend both the reception and expression of love in relation to themselves. Morganstern revealed his own uncertainities about the validity of these inferences by suggesting that his readers apply caution in reaching conclusions about the emotional development of those who are retarded. Many unknowns, including those within the context of the environment, influence the behavior of this population. The personal and relational sexual self is subject to modification through environmental experience.[14]

Mattinson's work with adults revealed that mental retardation did not in itself preclude the formation of love relationships. She interviewed thirty-two married couples who had been institutionalized and was impressed with the quality of the relationships she saw. Approximately 60% of these couples had an affectionate and supportive relationship. They were indeed sensitive to their own and each other's needs. One partner compensated for the other when necessary.[13] They had positive life experiences in marriage that helped them to attain a degree of fulfillment that could not have been predicted when they were tested, labeled, and placed in institutions.

Within the past several years, the aspect of mental retardation and relational sexuality has been broached in America. Perske has been the earliest and most explicit in describing the similarities between the needs of the person who is retarded and others, particularly in regard to risk taking, sensuality development, and the concept of interdependence in their relationships with each other and with others in their environment.[17, 18]

In order to prevent loneliness (one of the greatest problems of people who are mentally retarded), Katz recommends that relationships be facilitated. Opportunities for the formation of relationships with persons of the opposite sex can change the meaning of life, whether the contacts result in sexual relationships or in warm friendships.[10] Signs of caring and wanting to be together should be evidenced by a couple before their pairing is facilitated. Perske warns against manipulating young people through undesired and unnecessary pressure to become intimate.[18]

NEED TO REORIENT PARENTAL AND PROFESSIONAL ATTITUDES
Deinstitutionalization

Increased numbers of people who were formerly segregated from mainstream contact are now living in communities. Some have come into the community after years of institutional living, and others have not been accepted by institutions that have recently restricted their populations. These changes have impacted on communities in many ways. Professionals, other service providers in the community, parents, and citizens with no former real experience with retarded individuals are being required not only to expand and improve services but also to reexamine their attitudes toward these people and their capabilities.

Attitude reassessment

Major conceptual areas. Attitude reassessment needs to occur at both the emotional and intellectual levels of those responsible for the socialization of people who are retarded if these persons are to become as fully human and as sexually fulfilled as possible.

Major conceptual areas that need to be examined occur within the framework of the idea of the unique personhood of both the people who are retarded and of those who influence their development. Knowledge regarding adaptation to change needs to be applied to both, especially at the present time because of the change from institutional to community living. Of paramount importance is the idea that feeling good about oneself is vital to a healthy adaptation to a new life-style. The activities involved in facilitating fulfilling expressiveness constitute a new life-style for people who are retarded and a new life–professional style for those who assist them in their development.

A common stereotype that interferes with the promotion of a positive self-concept among people who are retarded is that of the weak ego status, often viewed as inherent in the condition. The ego of people who are retarded is in large part dependent on the nature and quality of the life experience of these persons, just as it is for any other person. Unfortunately, the people who influence their development contribute to the "weak ego" theory through the way they interact with them. When expectations for behavior are unrealistically high or insultingly low, the person develops a poor self-perception.

As the ego develops, most people, including children, will usually try to fulfill expectations that are reasonably realistic and clearly communicated. This pattern of response, when positively reinforced, is likely to continue to adulthood. I have observed this phenomenon even when the change in some interpersonal relationships occurred following institutionalization and after the person had reached adulthood. One of the more remarkable examples is that of an obese woman, Janet, who needed both touch and verbal support to respond to questions during group counseling sessions. Janet decided to lose weight so that she would be more attractive. Because she was able to help herself at meal times, she ate less. Also, during this time, she was socially reinforced as it became evident that she was indeed losing weight. Janet became more vocal within the group. A year after the counseling sessions had ended, Janet was in a dental clinic waiting room when I entered and did not recognize the slim young woman who sat across the room. Janet, initiating a conversation, demonstrated no shy or withdrawn behaviors as she animatedly described how she had met her boyfriend in a sheltered workshop.

People with retardation generally are not expected to be able to conceptualize in abstract terms. Yet, I vividly recall an experience as a public health nurse serving a school for retarded students. A 17-year-old young man, who was enrolled in this special education program and interested in music, was asked to write a song about how he felt about growing up. The final line in his song was, ''And I gave my love a plastic ring.'' His lyric was a symbolic abstraction of the expectation that he would never be able to experience a fulfilling marriage. Given the opportunity to do something that was not a ''retarded'' activity, he clearly revealed that he was able to communicate his needs in a way that was on a higher level than that expected of a person who is labeled retarded.

The nature of the sexuality of people who are mentally retarded has been the subject of mythology that is untrue and often contradictory. These people have been described as oversexed, undersexed, asexual, late in maturing, and infertile when their retardation is severe.[8] The mythology is pervasive, in spite of concrete evidence to the contrary. The truth is that their sexual experience, particularly in relationship to physical development, impulses felt, and potential for optimally fulfilling expression, rarely differs from that of people who are not retarded.

Interpersonal influences. Among the factors that contribute to attitude reorientation are the interdependent, interpersonal influences of basically three groups of people: (1) those who are retarded, (2) their parents, and (3) the professionals who intervene with these two. The degree of sexual fulfillment actualized is a function of the interaction

between these persons with their unique characteristics and reactions.

People who are retarded. When children who are retarded begin to show signs of maturing, their emotional climate often becomes one of internal conflict and turmoil. In this, they are not unlike many of their normal peers; however, they often have less accurate knowledge about what is happening so that understanding and accepting the change is difficult.

Maturation and erotic impulses introduce factors into conduct that are too complex to be left to instinct or to be ignored. These people may behave in ways that produce social distance and reinforce stereotyped myths. False information and inattention to their social coping skills often result in behavior that is childish when their bodies are not. Two examples are offered to illustrate what can happen.

One young man who had moved into a community group home was convinced that he would damage his genitals if he masturbated. A physician in the institution had told him this activity would cause ''blue balls.'' The need for sexual expression was a major problem for him since he was not homosexually active, and heterosexual intimacy in the institution was severely punished. The move to the community exacerbated his problems; sexual stimuli increased, and young women in revealing dress provided the impetus for increased preoccupation with sexual fantasies. A house staff member observed him following girls and asked him what he was doing. He revealed that he fantasized about having intercourse and was planning to stop a girl and say, ''Hello, do you want to fuck?''

Another young man, who was usually modest and sensitive, upon learning that his house parents in a community living home were leaving, could not verbalize his feelings so he dropped his pants at the sheltered workshop. This act brought immediate punishment, but more important, attention to his cry for help. His house parents were informed of the incident. They were able to talk with him about his feelings and helped him to verbalize them. He still was apprehensive, disappointed, and worried, but he eventually learned that one of the realities of life in the community is that of change and that lost relationships can be replaced so that anxieties and sadness disappear.

Parents of people who are retarded. Many factors influence how parents react to the sexuality of their children. Hall has paraphrased Tarjan in describing how parents whose intelligence quotients are close to their adolescent child's usually accept their adolescent's expression of sexuality, whereas more intelligent parents tend to ignore and try to conceal or suppress evidence about maturation and its sexual implications.[8] It is my experience that the most influential parental characteristic is not intelligence but the degree of parental comfort in discussing sexuality. This may be a function of how they are currently experiencing their own sexuality.

Those who are comfortable with their sexual selves are more likely to perceive their child's sexuality in its widest and most positive dimension. Less secure parents may exhibit a very restricted and negative view of the implications of sexual development in their children. The parents' problems in handling the sexual development of their children may arise from a number of sources. Parents may want to avoid being confronted with a reawakening of those feelings that occurred during their own traumatic entry into puberty. Religious proscriptions may be in conflict with newer societal views regarding sexual expression.

Some parents may never have resolved the dynamic conflict of having a child who is retarded. Resolution may have been delayed by professional advice that they should not look to the future since their child would never mature.[8] Well-established, overprotective, and infantilizing practices often are maintained and rationalized as expressions of caring for the dependent child. Such caring prevents the child from taking any risks that might result in the pain of failure. This deprives the child of the pleasure of eventually achieving mastery through practice.

When the child reaches adolescence, the need to establish interpersonal relationships outside the home may be thwarted. Any activity that could be viewed as possibly developing into a love relationship is especially threatening. Being involved in a love relationship puts the adolescent or adult at risk of experiencing the trauma that occurs if the relationship ends. Focusing on the possible trauma, overprotective parents have difficulty in seeing the benefits to be gained. There is much joy and pride in oneself during the life of a caring relationship. The pain resulting from the loss of a love object can be overcome. When a new relationship is developed, self-growth and reaffirmation of self-worth occur. This is true for all people, retarded or not.

Denial of sexual maturation may result in the continuation of infantilizing caring practices. Fathers may continue to help bathe and dress their daughters. Mothers may select clothing that is unattractive and purposefully designed to hide breasts and hips. The need for a deodorant may go ignored. Sensuously pleasant experiences and articles, such as attractive hairstyles and body scents, may be seen as unnecessary and even dangerous.

Many parents may lack accurate knowledge about what to expect regarding their maturing adolescent's body and behavior. It is not unusual for them to have received no support and guidance regarding preparation of their children for maturity.[9] Common parental fears include inability of daughters to handle menses, public exposure of the genitals, vulnerability to sexual exploitation, public masturbation, pregnancy, and socially disapproved ways of handling sexual curiosity. Ways of handling these fears are offered later in the chapter.

Professionals. This section refers to all persons who are responsible for providing care and guidance, from the direct service provider to the administrator. As with parents, professionals who have not resolved their own sexual problems only contribute to those of the people who seek their guidance. Such professionals exacerbate problems for their clients out of their own confusions and needs. When their own sexual needs are not adequately met, they may act out of their own needs rather than those of the people who are retarded. This may take a number of forms. The two polarities will be identified. Adolescents and young adults may be pushed into intimacies for which they are not ready and that they may not want. At the other extreme, any approximation to sexual activity may be suppressed or severely punished. This may be due to a combination of envy and a dehumanizing view of people who are retarded, resulting in the thought, "If I can't have it, why should it be available to them?" Suppressive tactics may be the result of threats of personal retribution against institutional staff and group home managers if any residents in their charge become pregnant.

Some professionals in the community deny the value of parent or parent surrogate involvement in sex education programs for people who are retarded, even at the level of sanctioning the program. The professional who does this sabotages the program by not giving enough credit to the influence of the parents on the sexual development of their children and by making assumptions about how the parents will react. Discussing the need for guided sex education may be a first step in helping the parents to overcome denial when it does exist. Most parents welcome the opportunity for personal growth for themselves and for their children through involvement in appropriately guided experiences to enhance the self-perception and relational skills of their children. Parents who are excluded from involvement, especially if denying the sexuality of their child, may be afraid that if the child finds out about sex, ideas that never occurred to the child before may be stimulated. This reaction is heightened when the child is an adult and physically equipped to act on these "stimulating ideas." An example describes possible results. A professional decided that the adults in a rehabilitation program were of legal age; therefore, they would be treated as adults and be permitted to decide for themselves if they wanted to become involved in a sex education program. Some of these persons lived at home, others in a group home. One client misconstrued the implications of what he had learned and announced that he had been told to have intercourse with girls. His horrified mother withdrew him from the program and brought the matter before the local parents' association. Other students dropped out of the program. Many meetings were held to explain the purposes of the program and to assist the parents in understanding the need for the program before it was resumed. Considerable confusion, defensive feelings and reactions, and delay could have been prevented.

Other professionals may not have accurate knowledge about sex. Ignorance can contribute to the professional's own sexual dilemma, and confusion is compounded when this is reflected in communications with those seeking knowledge. False information can be particularly destructive because people who are retarded often do not question the validity of information given to them.

THE NURSING ROLE: A PREVENTIVE COUNSELING APPROACH

The goal of a preventive approach is to facilitate optimal sociosexual development through early intervention and anticipatory guidance. In a previous publication, I cited these two processes as particularly applicable in nursing interventions with persons who are retarded and their families.[16] Both of these processes involve counseling. Their application early in the life of the child who is handicapped could greatly ameliorate or prevent many of the problems and conflicts that arise when physical indices of maturation and the concomitant need to deal with expression of sexual impulses occur.

Nursing assets and opportunities

The nursing processes of both anticipatory guidance and early intervention have as underlying concepts the developmental quality of life and the prevention of problems. This is not to imply that only nurses can facilitate human fulfillment, including the sexual aspects of personal fulfillment. However, nurses do have knowledge regarding both physical and emotional development and related problems. They also possess skills that assist families to cope with or prevent those life experiences that impede the optimal physical and emotional health of persons. The combination of knowledge, skills, goals, and opportunities in many settings does place the nurse in a critical position to be a "fulfillment facilitator." I choose to use this descriptor rather than "caretaker," "direct service provider," or "helper." The words "fulfillment facilitator" are used to describe the role of professionals who impact on the lives of persons who are retarded because these terms challenge professionals to realize how much their interactions with these persons influence their self-concept.

Nurses are present when a baby is born and for the several days that the infant and mother remain hospitalized. Hospital nurses are in a position to hear the concerns of the parents and to help them begin to sort out their feelings about having a baby who is identified as having a syndrome characteristic of mental retardation. These nurses can identify resources in the community available to help the parents. With the parents' consent, a referral to a public health nurse should be made before the mother and infant leave the hospital. Public health nurses have knowledge regarding both physical and emotional development and related problems. They also possess the skills needed to assist families to prevent or cope with those life experiences that impede the optimal physical and emotional health of the whole family and particularly that of the child who is retarded. Public health nurses provide preventive guidance and intervene when crises arise. They also know how to refer a client when the therapeutic process requires skills they do not possess.

Public health nurses, on receipt of a newborn referral, have an opportunity for early intervention that benefits the developing sexuality of the child who is retarded. During these early contacts, the nurse has opportunities to counsel the parents in areas that relate directly and indirectly to the future sexual expression of the child. Such intervention gives permission to the parents to discuss their sexual concerns early and creates a climate that is conducive to the parents' handling of sexual issues as a normal and natural component of parenting.

The nurse in any setting should have a "third ear" tuned in for any sexual concerns. I recall visiting a mother of a 4-year-old boy who had Down's syndrome. The mother's primary concern was related to toilet training. During one visit the mother, a nurse and wife of a physician, requested help in preparing a daughter for menarche. After the request was filled, I recognized that there were many resources this mother could have used, including her own knowledge. The possibility that she might actually have been asking for help in relation to her concerns about her son's sexuality was considered. She was asked if she ever thought about the sexuality of her son. The mother looked relieved and revealed she had indeed been concerned since the time she held him as an infant. She worried about how her upper middle-class neighborhood would react if her son innocently lifted a girl's skirt out of curiosity or exposed himself. She was afraid these situations would occur when he was an adolescent. This mother was advised that the whole family could teach him about privacy through role modeling. His curiosity could be satisfied by viewing naked infants and pictures of children of both sexes and by having experiences in nonsegregated peer toileting, as are provided in many nursery schools and Head Start programs.

Frequently, parents of children who are retarded do not have any opportunity to express concerns they might have about their child's sexuality, unless signs of maturation are present. Since much information relative to sexuality is acquired before the age of school entry, it is imperative that parents be sensitized and educated regarding the sexual needs of their child.[20] As previously stated, this is best done through inclusion of the area of sexuality as a component of the early intervention process beginning in infancy. If this has not been done, it can be accomplished when the nurse includes sexuality while ascertaining the health history of the child in providing anticipatory guidance.

I have made it a practice to incorporate an opportunity for parents to discuss their concerns about their child's sexuality in assessment interviews. This is done with parents of children with developmental disability and without discrimination as to age and type of problem. When such acceptance is communicated, parents are relieved, particularly when sexual concerns are uppermost in their minds. For example, David, a 7-year-old, was referred to the clinic because he was not achieving to the level of his potential. His father was an educational administrator, and his mother was a nurse. The parents were informed that part of the nursing assessment would provide for an exploration of David's abilities to label and handle feelings. They were also told that they would have the opportunity to discuss any concerns they had regarding his sexuality. David's mother was surprised and pleased to have this opportunity to discuss sexual concerns. She stated that these were of highest importance to her. In spite of this, she did not reveal such concerns to anyone until the area was identified as appropriate for discussion during the nursing assessment process.

The subject of feelings was brought up by presenting several pictures when David was experiencing difficulties during another nursing assessment task. He first picked happy expressions. These were not accepted as real, since his face and body indicated tense anxiety. He then picked a picture of a person worrying but quickly discarded it to pick another happy photograph. There was a long, uncomfortable silence when David was asked if it was difficult to talk about how he felt.

David was more comfortable in discussing anger. He was able to describe occurrences in his own life that made him angry. In this assessment situation, he was fluent. When his mother asked him why he did not express such feelings at home, he said that he was embarrassed. He also felt that talking about his feelings would be ignored, whereas "screaming," "yelling," and "hitting," brought immediate attention. It subsequently became apparent that David's opportunities to observe verbalization of feelings were limited.

David was not present during the discussion regarding sexual concerns. His mother was in conflict about expressing affection physically with David. She felt she might be acting more out of her own needs than David's. This remark initiated a conversation between the parents about their sexual activity. David's father explained in detail how he had come to be reserved in expressing affection. His wife's background had included verbal and physical expressions of positive feelings. Other evaluations were in agreement with my evaluations. Family therapy that would include the opportunity for the family to engage in continued discussion of their feelings around the area of their sexual styles was recommended.

Early intervention

Early in the previous section, it was stated that nurses have opportunities for guiding parents in assisting in the development of processes that occur early in life. Some of these early interventions may not appear to relate directly to the expression of sexuality itself, but they do impact on the way adolescents who are retarded behave as social and sexual persons. It is critical that the problems of adolescents described earlier in this chapter be prevented through consciously structuring for children's learning in the areas of appreciating their bodies as capable of gratifying sensual needs, developing a positive body image and gender identity, expressing feelings, and making choices. Intervention related to these developmental tasks should occur long before physical indices of maturation become apparent. Our knowledge of social learning theory must be applied to children who are retarded and should be done in a positive fashion early in their lives.

Major sources of early socialization are parents, pictures, and most significantly, peer modeling and television. Baran reviewed the literature regarding the effects of television on the social learning of children who were institutionalized.[3] He concluded that television has at least the same, if not greater, impact on their socialization as it does on normal children. He related most of the findings to the fact that the institutionalized children depended on others for their very existence and to the fact that contacts with appropriate persons who are aware that they are modeling social behaviors are relatively rare and brief.[3] In a subsequent study of children who were retarded and living in the community, he concluded that peer modeling and television outranked parental influences on socialization.[4] From Baran's work, it can be surmised that today's parents of children who are retarded could relinquish their control over the major sources of stimulation that influence the knowledge their children obtain concerning socialization and sexuality. For this reason, they must consciously guide their children beginning in earliest infancy in order to control the nature of television viewing and peer modeling of behaviors.

The earliest experiences of oneself as a sexual being occur in infancy. The process of learning that the body is good and pleasure giving begins even before infants learn to differentiate themselves from others. Soon after birth, infants experience being held closely and caressed gently. They learn through experience how all the body's senses are used to produce good feelings about oneself as well as benefiting cognitively and socially from the interpersonal contact. They are offered experiences in sensuous pleasuring that involve the eyes, ears, nose, mouth, and skin. These sensuous experiences of pleasure are often excluded from or diminished in the developmental process of children and adults who are retarded. The sensuous pleasuring loss that

results may have its effect even in infancy. A public health nurse reported that on making a first visit to a mother whose newborn had Down's syndrome, the mother apologized for the infant's plain dress. Bringing out a beautiful dress, she said, "I just couldn't put this on her. She's not the baby of my dreams." The dress was symbolic of the loss of a perfect baby. Its substitute by a plain dress was a denial of the infant's sensuous pleasuring, which the grieving mother was not ready to give to her imperfect baby. It can be assumed that her other interactions with the infant also communicated her feelings of disappointment and rejection. To help this mother reach the place where she could give her daughter a positive message about her body, much counseling was needed to help her work through the feelings she was bringing to the attention of the nurse.

Children who are handicapped physically in addition to being retarded often get proprioceptive feedback that gives them the message that their bodies are not good. A colleague who was not retarded but who had one leg shorter than the other said she remembered differences in the way that leg was handled. The message she got was that part of her body was repulsive. Children who are retarded may not be able to speak so eloquently for themselves, but there is no doubt that they are able to feel and react to differential handling of their bodies and to carry these feelings throughout their lives.

During a recent visit to an institution in Sweden, I was deeply moved by a staff activity that recognized the human need for sensual pleasuring of a young couple who were so physically handicapped and profoundly retarded that they required assistance to get into their separate beds. Over time, it became evident that this man and woman enjoyed being near each other. Recognizing the development of a caring relationship, the staff helped them into the same bed. In bed together, they touched each other. Sensual pleasuring through touch was the level of sexual expression that was within their capabilities. The human need for sexual experience at the highest achievable level was facilitated. This was not an isolated incident. The contrast to staff handling of residents *of all ages* in American institutions does not require elaboration.

Many early intervention stimulation techniques are sensual in nature and promote a feeling of well-being for the child while increasing psychosocial and cognitive skills. These techniques also teach the infant and child which sensory input and body receptors produce pleasurable and sensuous feelings. Stroking the infant or child with the hands and with materials of varying texture while verbalizing the names of body parts helps in promoting an awareness of body image in addition to other learnings. Producing various sounds that serve to elicit many kinds of responses and providing differing olfactory and taste experiences are only two of the techniques used. As children learn to discriminate among those sensory inputs that produce sensuous pleasuring, they behave in ways that serve to maintain them. Thus, children who receive such sensory stimulation learn that they can exert control over their environment to promote pleasant experiences with their bodies. They also learn about those body parts that hold the greatest sensual gratification.

As children mature, they become aware of erogenous areas and ways to stimulate pleasurable gratification themselves. Masturbation, if not punished and if practiced in privacy, can be a source of comfort and sensual growth. A 4-year-old girl who was severely retarded soothed herself to sleep after an exhausting day by masturbating. Her parents viewed this as adaptive and were concerned only that she use this technique to relax in a private place.

Infants learn about their bodies in a number of ways, including exploration with their hands and mouths. Older children learn about similarities and differences between themselves and others through satisfying curiosity by observation of family members, peers, and pictures. Children in some Head Start programs can casually observe each other's physical and functional differences and similarities without incident. Some children have this opportunity to see differences among children and adults when the whole family bathes together or when the child is able to observe parents or siblings toileting or dressing. The child has an opportunity to satisfy curiosity about sex at a young age when there are no guests in the home. This practice can occur very casually with parents who are mentally healthy. The child has the opportunity to observe at will and is not pushed into the situation. Usually, curiosity is satisfied long before puberty.

Wilbur and Aug have addressed themselves to the differences in form and content of the information sought and needed by normal children as they mature.[20] It is significant that they identify indirect learning as likely to have an impact more on sexuality than on any other area of development. Of relevance to mental retardation, adults' emotional reactions of disgust, anger, and revulsion may prevent the child from integrating knowledge about sexuality and may interfere with learning in general.

Early life experiences related to feelings, including parental modeling, influence how children learn to express their feelings in addition to teaching feelings about sexual expression. Verbal identification of feelings can begin in infancy. Some parents do this automatically when attending to the infant's physical needs. How often have we heard parents say "you are really happy" when an infant laughs or "you really are unhappy" when an infant cries? Talking to infants occurs even when it is obvious that the infant does not understand the words. This kind of process should be continued throughout the childhood and adolescence of children who are retarded to help them learn to label their feelings as early as possible. This beginning step in learning to handle feelings prevents the development and use of social distancing behaviors to express feelings.

Children need to learn that they are not held responsible for the feelings they have in a given situation but that the behaviors they use to express these feelings are subject to social sanction. There is a large vocabulary available for children to learn. They do not need to be restricted to the use of "love," "hate," and "mad." They will decrease the frequency of their maladaptive, acting-out behavior during adolescence and adulthood if they are taught the names of feelings by having the adults who interact with them verbally identify the name of the feeling at the time it is occurring and by modeling verbalization of their feelings.

It is also helpful to have photographs of people expressing disappointment, loneliness, frustration, anger, fear, happiness, surprise, embarrassment, and the many other ways of communicating sadness, happiness, and love. The photographs can be shown to children when the feelings are being experienced. The photographs could also be used in a game in which children are rewarded each time they correctly identify the feeling being portrayed in the photograph. Photographs can be cut out of magazines or purchased. Some photographs that may be used for this purpose are manufactured by the Instructo Corporation in Paoli, Pennsylvania, and are called Understanding Our Feelings, No. 1215.

Another area of early intervention involves the experiences needed to develop the skill of making simple choices so that eventually the strategy of decision making can be acquired. This involves simple, concrete, two-option choices as the first approximation to the development of the complex strategy of making decisions with an awareness of possible or real contingencies.

Two-year-old children are more likely to be cooperative when a choice is offered rather than an action demanded. Simple choices teach children that (1) they can learn to discriminate between two objects and that (2) they can act on their environment. At first, children may not be aware they *are* choosing, but through repeated opportunities they learn that they can be instrumental in determining what happens to them. Certain sensory experi-

ences become associated with specific objects. This process is enhanced when the sensory possibilities are verbally described. Gradually, the complexity of the task is increased through offering more objects from which to choose and by decreasing the concreteness of cues. Children are asked to choose between two activities. The contingencies can be verbalized, but they are not as obvious as in the more simple task of choosing between two objects. The complexity of the task is increased in approximations of the degree of difficulty at which the person is able to learn. This process continues through adolescence and even into adulthood. Many women, and some men, will need the strategy of making decisions to help them make a truly informed consent about having sterilization.

Anticipatory guidance

Parents may seek assistance regarding preparation for maturation on their own, on referral, or it may occur as one of the components of the total assessment process. Ideally, early pubertal children and adolescents, both boys and girls, and their parents should be seen for a maturation assessment. This should be done whether or not a concern regarding sexuality is expressed.

The initial step in anticipatory guidance is the assessment interview, which should begin with preparation of the parents and the child for the experience. It is essentially an information-gathering process regarding maturation, or "growing up." The parents are always interviewed before the child. This is done so that the parents can participate and contribute in the following ways:

1. Contribute significant data, either observable or historical, regarding factors that may be influencing the child's behavior.
2. Legitimate the assessment process.
3. Approve the content areas and view and approve of the visual aids used in information gathering.
4. Become aware of the extent and nature of their child's learning needs.

5. Assist in interpreting or obtaining responses from their child.

The process not only serves to de-escalate feelings of anxiety but also adds to the parents' own self-esteem through active participation in facilitating the development of their child. Many parents prefer to be present when their sons or daughters are interviewed. Adolescents who are more severely retarded and prepubescent children who are physically precocious usually accept the option of having their parents included.

The objectives of the assessment or information-gathering process are:

1. To ascertain how the child and parents view and react to the child's maturation.
2. To observe how all members of the family interact during the process.
3. To explore both the parents' and the child's goals in relation to vocation, independent living, and expression of sexuality.
4. To become familiar with what is currently occurring to achieve those goals.
5. To identify strengths and concerns of each family member to help in determining if follow-up counseling is advisable.

Feelings regarding the expression of sexuality may be de-escalated when put within the framework of other aspects of maturation. This is carried out by systematically exploring the areas of vocation and independent living first. When a typical day's activities are reviewed, knowledge is often obtained that can be concretely examined by both the parents and the counselor to see what is being done to teach the described goals. Ways of expressing feelings, comfort and confidence in making choices, and ability to assume responsibility are also ascertained.

Following this, concerns and goals regarding sexuality are explored. Again, current experiences and other influences that contribute to the achievement of the goals are ascertained. Decisions are made with the parents regarding the content area to be discussed. Visual aids, such as booklets, pictures, and dolls with genitalia, are shown to the parents for their approval. Their reactions during this process and the feelings they express are observed.

Occasionally, attempts to approach sexuality within the total framework of growing up are quickly dismissed by the parents in order to have their very high concerns regarding sexuality handled. Mothers most frequently cite masturbation and the onset of menstruation as major concerns. Some fathers express anxiety about how to discuss nocturnal emissions. It is extremely rare for fathers to express concern about masturbation if it occurs privately. This may reflect the traditional double standard. Occasionally, one parent will initially deny any need to discuss sexuality further because the adolescent has seen a film at school or has heard older siblings talk about their dating experiences.

The parents' desire to remain during the interview with their young or severely retarded son or daughter is frequently an indicator of their willingness to become involved in subsequent counseling as well as a function of the age and cognitive ability of their child. A major value of having parents remain is that they frequently become aware of the nature and extent of the learning needs of their child. It also provides the interviewer with an opportunity to assess the degree of comfort of the parents in handling sexual discussions with their child. Rarely does the presence of the parents inhibit the responses of those children who choose to have them present. Occasionally, a child will glance at a parent to seek permission before responding. This may also occur in response to questions regarding future goals for vocation and living situation.

Some attention has been given to the need for children who are retarded to learn about the physical differentiation between the sexes and the functions of sexual organs, as a popular manual for interviewing these children demonstrates.[5] A useful technique for eliciting knowledge and feelings in relation to the individual's sexuality is the use of visual aids. The interviewer should ask the child to "tell me about this picture." Helpful assessment aids include books and booklets,[5, 1, 11, 19] male and female dolls, menstrual grooming materials, and Renwal's Visible Woman with interchangeable breast and abdomen plates and pregnant and non-pregnant uteri.

Usually, differentiation between sexes and ages and identification of the one most like the person being interviewed are ascertained first. A comfortable entry for discussion around explicit sexual behavior is the section on dogs in *How Babies Are Made.*[1] Children are familiar with animals, and some have seen dogs mate. Talking about dogs also provides an opportunity to learn what the child knows about the similarities and differences in relationships between humans and those between animals, particularly in regard to parenting behaviors and responsibilities.

Pictures and other visual aids provide for discussion of pregnancy, birth, menstruation, mature male and female genitalia, masturbation, affectionate heterosexual behavior, and intercourse under bed covers. Pictures of the latter activity are provided in two of the available booklets.[1, 5] When viewing *How Babies Are Made,* many children indicate that they know what is happening by flipping back to the picture of the dogs mating. Diffuse, arousallike feelings in the genitals may already be present. Masturbatory activity, sometimes to orgasm, as well as nocturnal emissions may also be occurring. Usually the parents are aware of this.

The assessment interviews may reveal that the parents need only guidelines to help them do the counseling themselves. Other parents may wish continued help with the counseling process.

Individual counseling

The parents are seen first to ascertain their priorities in presenting their concerns. Sometimes more history is added at this time. One mother who wanted help in dealing with the implications of physical changes was asked how she explained the development of breasts to her daughter who was severely retarded but well-developed physically. The mother had told her the breasts were to feed a baby. Not until she responded to the question did the mother realize she was implicitly telling her daughter that she could rear babies.

Usually, only one or two concepts can be learned in one session by the younger or more limited child or adolescent. The parents are then assigned responsibility for providing learning experiences to reinforce the concepts. Occasionally, an uncomfortable parent chooses to leave during the counseling session. Parental discomfort is nonverbally communicated to the child, who then typically refuses to cooperate. If the parent has absented herself or himself, the child is requested to tell the parent what was learned when the group reconvenes. Whenever parents have absented themselves, it has usually been for only one or two sessions.

The child who is uncomfortable may giggle, be silent, cry, or quickly lift a shoulder and say, "I dunno." The latter should not always be taken literally. Frequently, the adolescent or child is using an avoidance technique and has more to say. It is often helpful for counselors to encourage a verbal response by explaining that they want to help but cannot do so unless the client takes the time to think about the idea.

The next session begins with the parents' report of how learning reinforcement experiences were carried out and what the results were. In relation to preparation for menarche, I learned from experienced mothers that if their daughters had seen someone else menstruate and change a sanitary pad, the daughters very readily learned how to do so. This exposure communicated that menstruation is a universal female experience and reduced their anxieties and confusion so that learning could occur. Why this modeling is so important is perhaps explained by the work of Gellert, who studied children's conceptions of the content and function of the human body. All of her hospitalized, intellectually normal subjects below the age of 11 years considered blood to be indispensible to life.[6] Daughters who have had changing a pad modeled for them did not see menstruation as a function of their particular handicap, nor did they believe that bleeding from the vagina could lead to their death. So that their sons would not think that nocturnal emission is a function of their handicap, fathers are urged to discuss wet dreams as a male experience.

Inappropriate childish behavior may be a parental concern. These parents are urged to reinforce the identification of secondary sex physical changes that have occurred within themselves and to emphasize that this happens to everyone by identifying changes in adolescents that the prepubescent child can see; diagrams also help. Once physical changes are accepted as real, more mature behaviors that are modeled are more readily learned. Occasionally, the denial underlying the problem takes many sessions to ascertain. One young girl did not accept maturational indices as proof that she was growing up. Her refusal to accept the need for changed behaviors was understandable because she persistently denied the concrete evidence of her development. It was later found that the girl friend of her 17-year-old brother was going to have a baby, and this was causing the whole family to be sad and worried. It was no wonder that this girl refused to acknowledge that she was physically growing in the image of her brother's girl friend.

Erotic sensations and masturbation are discussed so that these universal experiences are communicated and accepted. It is important to teach that masturbation is normal, is not harmful, and must occur in a private space. If parents are to teach their sons and daughters to masturbate in a private place, the parents must respect the private space and always knock on closed doors before entering. An apology is due the son or daughter if the parents open the door before hearing a response indicating permission to enter. Safe masturbatory techniques may need to be taught so that bodily injury does not occur through the use of objects that are unyieldingly abrasive or breakable, could cut, or otherwise traumatize the vagina or penis.

Occasionally during counseling, the real concern is not communicated until trust has been well established. One mother of a 12-year-old girl who was severely retarded asked for help in preparing her daughter for menarche. Other frequent concerns were brought up. Finally, the mother said that her daughter had been raped. She wondered how her daughter would react if approached again. The daughter was nonverbal, so the counselor asked the mother's permission to touch the daughter's breast. The mother gave permission and when the touching was done, the daughter immediately recoiled and went toward her mother. This was a reassuring experience for the mother.

Parents often express concern about their adolescent's vulnerability to sexual exploitation. Explicit rules regarding behavior must be learned as part of the change in behavior that physical maturation requires. As children, adolescents had learned about the dangers of being around hot stoves and on streets. The same explicitness and consistency are required for the rules of the new behaviors of puberty. These rules are more readily learned when they are modeled by family members. Examples are: zippers on pants and buttons on blouses are kept fastened except in privacy; young couples do not wander away from the group during playground activities and picnics; bedroom and bathroom doors are kept closed during private activities, such as toileting, bathing, dressing, and masturbating; permission from parents is required before any plans for activities are changed when away from home or school; and candy and rides in automobiles are not accepted from strangers. Parents should monitor their child's activities at least periodically to see if the rules are followed.

Parents may request counseling for themselves. This is particularly true when their concern has to do with sterilization of their daughter. Sterilization has many negative connotations, primarily due to the way in which it has been historically abused. Murdock completed a thorough review of the literature and concluded that the law, "At least in many instances, should maximize personal choice and recognize the capability of many retarded persons to decide for themselves whether or not they want to be sterilized, rather than seeking to extend the scope of involuntary sterilization."[15]

However, Hall has stated well the quandary that the obtaining of truly informed consent often presents. "The same behavioral characteristics which suggest the necessity for permanent birth control probably obviate the possibility of informed consent."[8] She paraphrases Tarjan regarding the problems of consent for sterilization:

1. Since the mentally retarded are not sufficiently competent to authorize surgical procedures and since they are highly suggestible and easily influenced by authoritative figures, *their* consent cannot be considered as truly informed;

2. *Parents* are too emotionally involved with the topic of sexuality in their adolescents to reach an objective decision on sterilization; and,

3. *Arbiters* and/or *guardians* may not be able to rationally decide what is best, based on symptomatology present today in the adolescent but which might not be present at a later date.*

I have observed adults who left institutions without experiences in exercising choices but who subsequently were taught the skills and demonstrated them in major areas in their lives. Attention to the development of this skill is mandatory before one expects the person who is retarded to make the informed, irreversible choice of sterilization. In many instances, these per-

---

*From Hall, E.: Sexuality in mental retardation. In Green, R., editor: Human sexuality, a health practitioner's text, Baltimore, 1975, The Williams & Wilkins Co., pp. 185-189.

sons can reflect informed consideration of the alternative contingencies. If basic skills or capabilities are present, those who seek permanent termination of any possibility of pregnancy, as well as those who do not, should receive training in child care and testing of their desire and ability to rear children. This would provide a significant piece of data for an informed choice.

I have had some experience with the quandary described by Hall.[8] In contradiction to Tarjan's second point, older parents have asked if their adult daughters who still function cognitively at the preschool or early school-age level should be sterilized so that they could marry the men with whom they had caring relationships. It is my belief that if the possibility of pregnancy is all that is keeping such a couple from experiencing a fulfilling relationship, then sterilization should be done. Parents have been supported in this decision.

The ability of people who are retarded to develop skills over time is the basic thesis of this chapter. No suppressive measure, especially sterilization, should be administered before the person has had an opportunity to demonstrate the ability to grow under optimal learning conditions. Parents who seek sterilization for daughters who have never had the opportunity to learn the skills necessary for decision making and child care should be counseled regarding the need to test their child's ability to learn these skills. They also need counseling and support in providing for temporary contraceptive methods for their daughters. Under optimal conditions, child rearing can be learned by many people who are mildly retarded. Usually, support for the parents is necessary from a community agency to provide early intervention and anticipatory guidance as well as the development of skills to cope with the problems that occasionally arise in almost all young families. Support and guidance are often provided by public health nurses. Knowledge of such support helps to reassure parents.

Some adolescents and adults who are still

living at home while receiving counseling do not want to have their parents involved. A number of factors must be considered in relation to the issue of confidentiality in such cases. Crises that are occurring in the home or school need to be known, since they frequently influence the behavior of the client. Consistency between messages given by the counselor and those given by the parent reduces client confusion. Discrepancies between client and family sexual values need to be known. If clients are unable to communicate relevant aspects of their past and current lives, the counselor should attempt to negotiate a contract with them. The contract will specifically state the questions that will be asked of the parents. It should also provide for the possibility of communication regarding problem areas which the parents can ameliorate or prevent.

Group counseling

If counseling is undertaken in a group, it is best to limit the group size to four. This allows opportunities for each group member to be actively involved in questioning and providing feedback. It is often necessary to go over a particular topic repeatedly until each group member demonstrates understanding.

Mixed group counseling is advantageous with adults in both institutions and community settings. Before counseling, strategies should be developed with those who have primary responsibility for the care of the retarded individuals. Curriculum, methodology, and a mechanism for providing feedback between those responsible for their care and the counselors should be developed. Backup referral sources for individual therapy also need to be identified.

In my community experience, two male and two female clients and male and female coleaders comprised a group. The first session began with the negotiation of a contract. The coleaders told the group what their obligations to the group were and helped the counselees identify their responsibilities as group members. Since vid-

eotapes were to be used during the sessions, each client was required to sign a consent form. During a first session, one woman cried because she had never before been privileged to sign her name to a legal document even though she was not under guardianship.

With the initial group, it soon became evident that the planned curriculum had to be discarded. Greater needs than information giving became apparent. The former institutional pattern of living had promoted conformity, regimentation, group controls, and group discipline. The members were unable to make individual, responsible, and self-satisfying decisions about how they wanted to express themselves sexually. They needed a great deal of assistance in analyzing the factors involved in the various means of sexual expression so that they could made decisions based on an awareness of the possible contingencies of their actions. Among the areas discussed were masturbation, sexual fantasies, pornography, casual pickups, effects of alcohol on behavior, approximations to intercourse, intercourse, short-term heterosexual and homosexual relationships, prostitution, venereal disease, contraception, long-term relationships, marriage, abortion, sterilization, and child rearing. In addition, knowledge regarding sexual organs, characteristics, and functioning was clarified. The process of examining consequences before acting led the group members to apply the same process in making satisfactory and responsible decisions regarding other aspects of their life-style and total life program. Such decisions included selling personal real estate, continuing in school, changing jobs, and voting on the abortion reform issue in Michigan.

Another major task identified was to help the counselees develop a valid self-concept. They had strong negative feelings about the label of mental retardation. They had heard the words used in relationship to themselves and had experienced negative consequences throughout their lives. It became necessary to assist them to accept the reality that retardation was one of their human qualities, but not the only one. This acceptance required a great deal of discussion and exploration regarding what "retardation" is and what it is not. The counselors explored the various characteristics that fall under the label, and the counselees identified which of those characteristics applied to themselves. Other human qualities such as talents, likes, dislikes, feelings about self, and all the other characteristics that make up any individual personality were explored. Again the clients differentiated among these and picked those that applied to themselves. Through this process, the clients came to recognize that each had a multitude of components in their personhood that had little or no relationship with the condition of retardation. Mental retardation as it applied to themselves was put into appropriate perspective as their awareness of individual qualities developed.

During the session, real and current situations were discussed. Some deep-seated problems were revealed that required individual therapy. One young lady had never had anyone help her deal with a very traumatic life experience. She had had a baby in the institution 3 years before reentry into the community. The infant was placed for adoption, gone before she had even seen it. She was then sterilized without having the opportunity to decide about the operation. She felt that her inability to have children would prevent anyone from wanting to marry her. The group members assured her of her attractiveness but also understood her feelings of anger, rejection, and humiliation. These were subsequently dealt with in individual therapy.

The need for explicit rules was apparent, particularly before the clients had developed appropriate strategies for making choices. One young woman barely missed being involved in a possible tragedy. She had accepted the offer of a stranger in a bus station to go with him to Detroit where he would set her up in an apartment and give her $20.00. Fortunately, this conscientious young lady told the stranger that it was a rule that the house managers were to be notified whenever a resident changed prearranged plans. Over his protests, she made the telephone call and was told to come home because of the dangers inherent in the situation. The stranger had disappeared when she went to make the telephone call. She was so confused and frightened by the experience that the house managers spent a great deal of time helping her resolve these feelings.

Since decisions regarding expression of sexuality have significant social implications, the understanding of personal and others' feelings and the ability to verbalize regarding these are of primary importance. The use of role play and discussion of feelings, as portrayed in such photographs as those in the *Family of Man*,[19] are helpful. Role play can be videotaped and played back for analysis by the group in a subsequent session.

The need for clear communication within the total counseling and support systems is clearly apparent. Counseling without this is not only unwise but dangerous and can result in painful consequences for the client.

Counselor issues

Counseling regarding sexuality, whether with parents or directly with their adolescents and adults, requires specific qualifications and knowledge. Nurses who assume the role of sex educator and counselor must be knowledgeable and comfortable with their own sexuality and that of others.

The most important question nurses need to ask themselves is how sexually secure they themselves are. Their attitudes and how these affect their behavior in counseling cannot be overemphasized. Over a lifetime, people develop attitudes regarding sexuality; how they feel as females or males, how comfortable they are with their own sexual situations and the reasons for these states, and the degree of comfort they experience in dealing with disparities between sexual behaviors that one permits for oneself and accepts in others. A thoughtful examination of various forms of sexual expression and of where one is, both intellectually and emotionally, is necessary. These are basic to a nonjudgmental acceptance of a wide range of behaviors. Acceptance of people where they are, wherever that may be, is necessary for the client to experience trust and to wish to continue. No needed changes can occur unless this happens and unless the counselor is an astute and empathetic listener. For example, when a couple who is homosexually expressive is counseled it should be ascertained if both partners are comfortable with the current practice. Is there a need for intervention? Just because they are involved does not mean that this particular activity is truly desired by both partners. A man may be involved in homosexual behavior because that is what he learned when he was in an institution and had no opportunity for alternative types of relationships. He may be continuing it in the community out of fear of the consequences of changing. These could include fears of physical reprisal from his partner or anxieties about approaching women.

Knowledge of a wide variety of sexual topics is necessary. Nurse counselors may have to deal with a wide range of sexual behaviors: masturbation, premarital intercourse, unprotected intercourse, incest, bestiality, pedophilia, homosexuality between consenting partners, homosexual rape, and many others. Behaviors such as these occur within nonretarded populations, also, and are presented here only as examples to stimulate thinking.

Counseling in the area of sexual expression requires that the counselor be comfortable in hearing and using "street" terminology. Use of the client's terms when eliciting knowledge or responding to the questions or concerns of both adolescents and adults communicates acceptance of the counselee, or client, through the use of the same vocabulary. When a counselor proceeds too quickly to correct the terminology used, an opportunity is lost for dealing with the client concerning some important issue within the client's reality situation. When lessons in semantics are substituted for dealing with issues, individuals are left with no alterna-

tive but to turn to peers, pornographic literature, or other sources for information that might misinform while doing nothing to facilitate the resolution of painful feelings. The lesson regarding appropriate terms can come later.

Knowledge of crisis intervention and conflict management is also needed. Problems of sexuality, when not prevented, can produce both conflict and crisis, as the various examples used throughout this chapter have illustrated. Comfortable nurse counselors apply knowledge using the skills they have. But what of the nurses who wish to become involved, who have skills and knowledge, but do not know how they feel about practices that are not permitted for themselves? Desensitization workshops might be helpful. Their proliferation may speak to the large number of people who are in conflict about the new sexuality and its promise of enhanced personal fulfillment. Would-be counselors benefit most when they are able to discuss their feelings in a nonjudgmental situation. Some are able to do this in groups, whereas others need privacy. Films depicting various forms of sexual practices are shown in theaters. These should be viewed with someone the nurse feels comfortable with and who accepts personal reactions without judgment.

The nurse who has never counseled people who are handicapped will benefit from viewing films about intimate sexual activities in which the actors are people who have a disability. Some feelings about disability itself can be surfaced in this way. These films are available for preview from many university and school district film libraries. The nurse could also talk with someone in the field about the kinds of issues that are brought to counselors. Many questions could be asked that would elicit feelings. How do you feel about contraceptive use for unmarried adolescents? Would you be able to facilitate a young woman's purchase of a safe dildo, especially if she were using an unsafe object, such as a bottle, for the same purpose? What information will you want to have from parents and their daughters when the parents want their daughters to have a hysterectomy so that they can be rid of a recurring monthly "problem" and ensure sterility? What will you discuss when a parent asks you if an adult son or daughter should marry or live together on a trial basis? How do you react to the use of "street" sexual terms? These are but a few of the questions that will elicit feelings. If readers experience discomfort in dealing with any area, they should try discussing these issues and using the language that communicates the client's reality with colleagues with whom they feel safe.

There are people in nursing and in other disciplines who would be willing to help these nurses practice dealing with problems and the feelings they arouse. Experience helps to increase counselor comfort. Comfort is of paramount importance not only to promoting acceptance of people where they are but also because the nurse counselor will be role modeling in counseling with people who are retarded and their parents. It is acceptable to say, "I really don't know enough to help you with that concern, but I can get in touch with someone who can help me." Perhaps the nurse will want to decide that direct consultation should be arranged. In any case, personal feelings or a lack of knowledge should not be permitted to interfere with helping.

SUMMARY

This chapter discusses major needs in the development of sexuality of adolescents and adults who are retarded. One major need is related to lack of experience in making informed choices or responsible decisions, expressing and appropriately handling feelings, and being comfortable with their own bodies. Suggestions have been presented regarding ways to provide for the development of these positive functions early in the lifetime of the child, as precursor experiences, so that problems commonly encountered in pubertal and adult counseling would be reduced.

The paucity of case descriptions regarding assessment and counseling guidelines for individual or group work with the retarded has been recognized. Examples of assessments and of group and individual methods have been presented to serve as possible resources to nurses who are engaged in this valuable and much needed service.

REFERENCES

1. Andry, A. C., and Schepp, S.: How babies are made, Alexandria, Va., 1968, Time-Life Books.
2. Bakwin, H., Renshaw, C., and Elkind, D.: Erotic feelings in infants and young children and commentaries, Medical Aspects of Human Sexuality **8:** 200, 1974.
3. Baran, S. J.: TV and social learning in the institutionalized M.R., Ment. Retard. **11:**36, 1973.
4. Baran, S. J., and Meyer, T. P.: Retarded children's perceptions of favorite television characters as behavior models, Ment. Retard. **13:**28, 1975.
5. Fischer, H. J., Krajicek, M. J., and Borthick, W. A.: Teaching concepts of sexual development to the developmentally disabled; a guide for parents, teachers, and professionals, Denver, 1973, J. F. K. Development Center.
6. Gellert, E.: Children's conception of the content and function of the human body, Genet. Psychol. Monogr. **65:**293, 1962.
7. Grunewald, K.: The mentally retarded in Sweden, Kyköping, 1974, Länstrycheriet.
8. Hall, J. E.: Sexuality in mental retardation. In Green, R., editor: Human sexuality, a health practitioner's text, Baltimore, 1975, The Williams & Wilkins Co., pp. 185-189.
9. Hillsman, G. M., and O'Grady, D. J.: Helping adolescents with mental retardation, Child. Today **10:**2, 1972.
10. Katz, G.: Sexuality and subnormality; a Swedish view, London, 1970, The Millbrook Press, Ltd.
11. Kempton, W., Bass, M. A., and Gordon, S.: Love, sex, and birth control for the mentally retarded, revised edition, Philadelphia, 1972, Planned Parenthood Association of Southeastern Pennsylvania.
12. Lief, H. I.: Introduction to sexuality. In Sadock, B. J., Kaplan, H. I., and Freedman, A. M., editors: The sexual experience, Baltimore, 1976, The Williams & Wilkins Co.
13. Mattinson, J.: Marriage and mental handicap; a study of subnormality in marriage, Pittsburgh, 1970, University of Pittsburgh Press.
14. Morganstern, M.: The psychological development of the retarded. In De La Cruz, F. F., and LaVeck, G. D., editors: Human sexuality and the mentally retarded, New York, 1973, Brunner/Mazel, Inc.
15. Murdock, C. W.: A constitutional perspective upon sterilization as a family planning technique for retarded. In Rowitz, L., and Meyer, R., editors: Out of the maze; family life education for vulnerable populations, Chicago, 1974, Division of Health

Services in Region V, U.S. Department of Health, Education, and Welfare.

16. Pattullo, A.: The socio-sexual development of the handicapped child; a preventive care approach, Nurs. Clin. North Am. **10:**361, 1975.

17. Perske, R.: About sexual development; an attempt to be human with the mentally retarded, Ment. Retard. **11:**6, 1973.

18. Perske, R.: New directions for parents of persons who are retarded, Nashville, Tenn., 1973, Abingdon Press.

19. Steichen, E.: The family of man, New York, 1955, The Museum of Modern Art, New York.

20. Wilbur, C., and Aug, R.: Sex education, Am. J. Nurs. **73:**88, 1973.

CHAPTER 19

An alternative to institutionalization for severely involved newborns

MARY SCAHILL CHALLELA

When a severely handicapped child is born, parents are often advised to place the infant in an institution for "the child's own good and the sake of the family." The infant as a person is dismissed as having no chance for a normal life and as having a particularly devastating effect on the rest of the family because of the demand, time, and expense involved in care. Although such advice may be given with good intentions to parents, it does not deal with the immediate crisis of the birth of a defective child.

Placing a child at birth does not allow parents an opportunity to make this difficult decision after careful consideration of other alternatives. In fact, they are often led to believe there are no other alternatives. Parents need time to recover from the fact of the birth itself: to ask questions, to deal with their feelings of grief and anger, and to mobilize their strengths. "It is during this early period that parents are groping for help," one father stated.[11] "However . . . help and information [are] rarely found and very often whatever information is obtained is erroneous and misleading."[11]

This chapter focuses on the question of whether home care of a severely mentally handicapped newborn is an acceptable alternative to immediate institutionalization. The answer is considered from the viewpoint of dealing with the crisis of birth of a mentally retarded infant and its significance to parenthood. One program of early nursing intervention is discussed as a model to demonstrate how nurses might deal with the problem.

MEANING OF PARENTHOOD

LeMasters states that parenthood itself is a crisis.[8] Parents who have organized their lives and feelings around circumstances that did not include an infant face a period of disorganization and stress. The family as a social unit must now incorporate another individual into its structure. New roles and relationships will need to be learned and old roles relinquished or modified. As each child is added to the family, roles and relationships become increasingly complex as time, effort, and responsibilities are realigned.[16] When a normal child is born, parents are not expected to make immediate decisions about the future, such as what the child will be like in 1, 5, or 10 years hence. Yet, if a child is abnormal and the advice is to institutionalize at birth, parents are required to make such a decision.

This chapter was supported in part by the Maternal and Child Health Services, Project No. 906, U.S. Department of Health, Education, and Welfare.

In our society, the family is the social unit in which children are desired and nurtured. Having a baby is a time for celebration and joy. A defective child means added social, economic, and emotional burdens for the family. The emotional component must be dealt with before other aspects can be approached.

(Parents make a great emotional and material investment in preparing for the birth of an infant who embodies their hopes and ideals for the future as well as their immortality.)The mother is often confused about her ability to care for the infant because she is caught up in feelings of dependency immediately postpartum and in societal demands that she be a competent mother. However, she transfers love to her infant as she provides needed care; in return, she feels loved when the child responds to her care. For the father, a new infant may be a symbol of success. Furthermore, the ability to produce a normal child is culturally and psychologically an affirmation of one's personal adequacy.

Consider the contrast when a defective child is born. The joy and fulfillment of the anticipated healthy infant are gone. Instead, there is an atmosphere of sadness and grief. How can parents love this person who is imperfect? How can they be proud of their accomplishment?

DEFECTIVE CHILD AS CRISIS

Much has been written about parents' reactions to the birth of a defective infant within the framework of grief and mourning. Freud conceptualized mourning as a reaction to the loss of a love object.[7] Solnit and Stark have utilized Freud's psychoanalytic theory in stating that the birth of a defective child may be seen as the sudden loss of the expected healthy child.[18] The mother cannot complete the normal mourning process relative to the loss of the "fantasy" child of her pregnancy before she is forced to invest herself with the handicapped infant as a love child. Having prepared herself to nurture and be satisfied with the child during pregnancy, she has failed to create what she intended and feels damaged by the "new child"—the defective one. Her adaptive skills have been exhausted. However, there is no turning back, and the mother feels trapped.

According to crisis theory, the way in which crises are resolved affects one's ability to deal with subsequent crises. Therefore, when help is given, the objective is to enter "the life situation of the individual, family, or group to alleviate the impact of a crisis."[13] This is done by alleviating the stress and helping the person(s) affected to problem solve and bring their feelings into focus, thereby strengthening themselves for future experiences.[15]

As individuals strive for emotional equilibrium, they utilize a series of adaptive mechanisms that are facets of the equilibrating process. Adaptive techniques may cause other imbalances that need to be resolved and incorporated into existing behavior patterns. General modes of adaptation are partly determined by the individual's past behavior, sociocultural experiences, and the present situation.[10] Thus, the parent of an abnormal infant may need to learn some special techniques of caring for the child and will have to cope with attitudes of family and friends.

Lindemann in his study of bereavement found that there was a definite sequence of events with both psychological and somatic symptomatology: somatic distress, somewhat altered sensorium, preoccupation with feelings of guilt, feelings of hostility toward other people, and a formalized manner of social interaction.[9] Mastery or failure of the grief process is determined in part by the individual's facing or avoiding the associated physical distress and the necessary emotional reaction to the situation.

Although the individual's ability to cope with a crisis is determined in part by previous handling of other stressful events, a person can learn new patterns of resolving conflicts during the disorganization period that accompanies each new crisis. The outcome is governed by the kind of interaction that takes place between the individual and the key figures in the environment.[13] It is also influenced by the amount of physical and psychological energy available to the person.

If it is accepted that the birth of an abnormal child is followed by a period of mourning and stages that must be experienced for a healthy adaptation to the stress, then energy is needed by the parents for this process. Therefore, it seems reasonable to conclude that there is little, if any, energy left to cope with making other decisions of a crisis nature. This is especially true if the decision involves separation of a part of oneself, namely, the child. Time is the important element that must be considered—time to question, be angry, deny, and finally to reach an accommodation with the reality of the child's existence; time to be relieved of the ego-shattering feelings of guilt and blame; and time to make rational decisions based on many factors. Institutionalization may be the final decision, but it should be made after feelings and attitudes have been dealt with and other possibilities explored.

Given other alternatives, placement at birth is often influenced by such factors as the child's appearance, potential for life, financial and educational status of the family, support systems available, and the amount of care required by the infant. Fackler's study of parents following institutionalization revealed other factors that influenced their decision: feelings and attitudes of neighbors and professionals, their own feelings of adequacy, their ignorance of resources, and misconceptions about mental retardation.[5]

CHANGING ATTITUDES

At the present time in our society, attitudes toward defective infants and institutionalization are changing.[6] Institutionalization often includes dehumanization either for the "protection" of society, as with the mentally ill or legal offenders, or for the "good of the individual," as with the handicapped or mentally retarded. As a result of these changing attitudes, deinstitutionalization of those who are men-

tally ill or mentally retarded is being stressed and implemented. Since Bowlby's[4] study of children in institutions and Robertson's[14] study of hospitalized children, child care experts have recognized that institutionalization or confinement usually has a detrimental effect on child development. Children reared in such settings usually lack the warm, affectionate, intimate contact with a loving and giving adult that is necessary for healthy personality and physical development.[4] There is also clear evidence that abnormal children cared for at home do better physically and emotionally than institutionalized children and that isolation of mothers from their newborns can be damaging.[2] Parents deprived of the parenting experience may have more guilt and uncertainty about their ability to care for an infant. "At least we tried," the young parents told the nurse when their severely damaged child was institutionalized at 3½ years of age. "We miss him and he will always be our son; we will never forget him." One year later the mother stated, "We worry about him as if he were normal."

The concept of normalization, as stated by Bank-Mikkelsen, emphasizes the need for mentally retarded persons to have an everyday life as similar to that of their normal peers as possible.[19] Although Bank-Mikkelson was primarily concerned with implications for living facilities for the retarded, the normalization concept has been applied to other life situations. Therefore, it is reasonable to apply this concept to the abnormal infant. If the usual pattern of care for an infant is with parents and siblings in the home, then this is the best place for infants in the majority of instances. Likewise, the normal pattern of parenthood is for the child to live at home. Parents should have the time and the necessary information to decide for themselves what they wish to do.

NURSING INTERVENTION

One program that focuses on early intervention with parents of abnormal infants is conducted by the nursing department in the Eunice Kennedy Shriver Center at the Walter E. Fernald State School.[17] The early nursing intervention program was established in 1970 to provide immediate assistance to parents at the time of birth of a defective infant. Crisis theory is utilized in this program of intervention. A concern of the nursing staff was the need to counter advice given most parents to institutionalize the child immediately. Such advice is in direct conflict with the psychological needs of parents following delivery. It also does not deal with the fact that there is a dearth of immediately available placement facilities. If available, such institutions are usually too expensive for most parents. Immediate placement also completely denies the infant the opportunity for life in a normal environment. The early nursing intervention program was designed to offer parents information about alternatives, guidance and assistance in home care of the child, counseling and emotional support, and assistance in accomplishing institutionalization, if necessary, using crisis intervention techniques and theory.

It is not enough to merely help parents work through their feelings and establish a new equilibrium as they progress through the crisis, as described by Caplan.[13] Of equal importance is the need to provide guidance and assistance in caring for the child at home.[1, 15, 18] In many instances, this means reinforcing the mother's skills in child care, encouraging her to pick up, feed, and bathe the infant as she would a normal baby. If the infant has feeding problems, as many do, the nurse helps the mother find solutions, such as holding the infant away from the body if the baby does not like to be held or advising the mother to use a soft nipple and showing her how to keep the infant's lips together to stimulate sucking if the infant has difficulty sucking or has tongue thrust. The following case study serves as further illustration:

Amy was a severely damaged newborn whose survival was not threatened but who took a long time to feed. She had profuse amounts of mucous and required frequent suctioning. Her mother wanted to take her home but was afraid she could not manage. The nurse from the Center visited frequently to follow up on the suction technique taught in the hospital. She helped the mother manage the tube feedings and, later, bottle feedings. She gave her information regarding the infant's problem of microcephaly and helped both parents deal with their feelings of guilt and hopelessness. She recommended genetic counseling, after which she reinforced the information given by the geneticist.

Many parents have little factual information about their infant's condition and practically none about available resources for the present or future. Many have little understanding about the child's potential for development or the degree of handicap. Some think the child will never progress beyond the newborn stage, whereas others think the child will have a slow start but will be just a few years behind normal siblings. In some situations, professionals have given parents information, but they were either unable to comprehend or simply did not hear it. A great deal of the nurse's time is spent reviewing factual information and gradually imparting new information as the child matures and as the parents are more able to listen.

Beck has identified some needs that apply to parents of retarded children. These include understanding: (1) the meaning of "retarded," (2) the degree of handicap, (3) the child's assets and needs, (4) the effect of the child's presence on family life, (5) the fact that behavior can be influenced, and (6) knowledge of community services.[3] It is most helpful for nurses to keep these basic needs in mind as they offer services to parents of mentally retarded infants and children.

In some instances, a newborn may be so neurologically damaged that care at home may be impossible. Placement might be the most appropriate course. Even so, placement takes time due to the lack of facilities and expense involved. It may be necessary for the infant to remain in an acute care hospital for immediate care. During this time, the nurse may visit the parents at home or in the hospital, thereby assuring them of the nurse's availability for supportive counseling and assistance in finding a suitable placement. Occasionally, the institution may be able to take the infant immediately. More often, a pediatric nursing home may provide the answer. Parents of infants who are placed need much support as they deal with the crisis of birth plus the need to separate from a child they have never really known. They are also sometimes confronted with the angry feelings of staff if they do not visit their child, as in the following case study:

Timmy was born with a major chromosomal defect. He was immediately transferred to a medical center in a city several miles away from his parents. No one knew whether or not he would survive. The parents were very young, and the mother did not visit Timmy, making the nursing staff angry. When the social worker called, the nurse made plans to visit the family immediately. The young mother stated that Timmy was their child and responsibility and that they were prepared to care for him at home if necessary. Having delivered by cesarean section, she had been advised not to travel for a week. She had also been advised by her pediatrician and her parents not to visit him at all. During the nurse's visit, she expressed a longing to know what Timmy looked like. "If he dies, I'll never know." The nurse suggested that a picture be taken in the hospital, a common practice in all newborn nurseries. The mother confided to the nurse that her husband was very hurt and cried at night. He had visited the child once, and she would like to see him, too. The nurse offered to accompany her within a few days. When the nurse conveyed this information to the social worker, arrangements were made to have a picture taken and to alert the staff of the parents' interest, concern, and impending visit. Unfortunately, the child died before the visit occurred, but a friend who had seen Timmy talked to the mother and described his appearance. The nurse visited the parents several more times, providing emotional support. The mother was experiencing a second period of grief.

In all situations, the nurse should be available to the parents by telephone or in person. Some parents may be angry about the lack of resources, and others because they do not feel it is their responsibility to care for the child. These are the parents who need the empathetic understanding or presence of a supportive person. In many instances, they are fully aware of the child's condition and potential. They are afraid of becoming attached and believe the child will have an adverse effect on other children in the home.

Sometimes it is possible to help parents look at their feelings and gain some insight into the dynamics involved. Reassurance of the nurse's interest and availability as well as the existence of community resources as the child grows older often helps parents make the decision to take the child home. Some parents are vehement about their feelings and unwillingness to try home care. For any intervention program to be successful, it is essential that the parents make the decision regarding institutionalization, that the nurse helps them live with their decision, and that the nurse accepts the decision as well.

A follow-up study of the early nursing intervention program at the E. K. Shriver Center was conducted from March to May of 1975, by a nurse who was not involved with any of the families who had received this service. The purpose of the study was to assess the effectiveness of this program by obtaining parents' feelings about the agency's response to their request for help and the parents' evaluation of the nurse's assistance in terms of function and effectiveness.

Nineteen families who were referred to the Shriver Center nursing department between 1969 and 1973 for early intervention were contacted for the follow-up study. Thirteen of these families had requested residential placement, and six had requested a home program. Within this group of families, nine infants had died during the first year; all infants were severely impaired. Although the majority of the mothers in this group stated that the Shriver Center was their only source of help, those mothers whose infants were beyond the newborn period at the time that intervention was initiated stated that no help was available. This finding certainly emphasizes the need for referral of families at the time of birth or diagnosis of mental retardation to an agency able to deal with this problem.

In evaluating the nurse's function and effectiveness, four mothers indicated that the nurse did not provide information about the child's condition or other available resources for care. One mother felt that the nurse was ineffectual in securing institutional placement, and another mother felt that the nurse did not help her relationship with her infant. On the other hand, one mother reported that the nurse was the only professional who helped her, and another reported that the nurse was instrumental in obtaining respite, or temporary care. Another mother was impressed that the nurse visited her in the hospital shortly after delivery of her child and felt that the nurse was the only person who "really cared." After her child was placed in an institution, this mother remarked that she had not felt pressured in making the decision. Although these results indicate many positive feelings about the nurse's function and effectiveness, some work remains in order to continue to improve the feelings of parents about nursing intervention with severely impaired children.

Although the early nursing intervention program has been ongoing since 1970, the problems with professional staff in the hospital are unchanged. Institutionalization is still advised by this staff in spite of the increase in public awareness of and response to the needs of handicapped children. Mental retardation is still considered by many staff members to be a hopeless situation as well as a stigma. Even when the parents' needs are recognized and efforts initiated in the hospital, this effort ceases when the child is discharged. As one mother described her feelings, she felt awed and embittered by the indifference of professionals with whom she and her husband met. She was also frustrated by bureaucratic red tape in placing her child and the lack of resources available in the community.

One way of counteracting problems with the attitude of professional staff is to provide conferences and workshops for nurses who work in newborn and intensive care nurseries. Educational sessions provide nurses the chance to learn skills needed in order to give appropriate intervention at the time of

birth of a handicapped infant. Nurses are then more likely to become a referral source for agencies able to provide assistance to the parents. However, nurses must be aware of their own feelings and attitudes about mental retardation.

In providing intervention, nurses should be aware that parents have moments of despair and sorrow, even after they have made an apparent adjustment to having a mentally retarded child. This phenomenon is termed chronic sorrow and is described by Olshansky.[12] Although parents of retarded children experience chronic sorrow, it does not prevent them from deriving comfort and satisfaction from even modest achievements of their children. As one father so aptly expressed it, "Do not feel sorry for handicapped children. They need acceptance and encouragement, not sympathy. They are capable of leading happy and rewarding lives; for leading a happy and rewarding life is not at all dependent on one's degree of intelligence."

Early contact with a nurse who can offer assistance in daily care in addition to supportive counseling provides parents an opportunity to explore their feelings about the crisis of having a mentally retarded child. It can also help parents make realistic plans for the continued care of the infant and to help them make decisions about the future, reflecting their needs as well as those of the child.

SUMMARY

The importance of helping families cope with the crisis of the birth of an abnormal child has been presented. The needs of these parents have been compared with the needs of parents of normal newborns. Parenthood as a period of adjustment and coping has been explored. Finally, one program of early nursing intervention with parents of abnormal infants has been discussed and analyzed. It is hoped that nurses will utilize crisis intervention theory and techniques, as well as sound nursing practice, in assisting parents of mentally retarded children.

REFERENCES

1. Aguilera, D., and others: Crisis intervention; theory and methodology, St. Louis, 1970, The C. V. Mosby Co.
2. Barnett, C., and others: Neonatal separation; the maternal side of interactional deprivation, Pediatrics **45:**197, 1970.
3. Beck, H. L.: Counseling parents of retarded children, Children **6:**225, 1959.
4. Bowlby, J.: Maternal care and mental health, New York, 1966, Shocker Books.
5. Fackler, E.: The crisis of institutionalization of a retarded child, Am. J. Nurs. **68:**1508, 1968.
6. Fletcher, J.: Attitudes toward defective newborns, Hastings Center Rep. **2:**21, 1974.
7. Freud, S.: Mourning and melancholia, collected papers, vol. I-V, New York, 1924-1956, Riviere, J., translator, Jones, E., editor: **4:**143, Basic Books, Inc., Publishers.
8. LeMasters, E. E.: Parenthood as crisis. In Parad, H. J., editor: Crisis intervention; selected readings, New York, 1965, Family Service Association of America.
9. Lindemann, E.: Symptomatology and management of acute grief. In Hardy, M., editor: Theoretical components of nursing, New York, 1973, MSS Information Corporation.
10. Martin, H., and Prang, A.: Human adaptation. In Hardy, M., editor: Theoretical components of nursing, New York, 1973, MSS Information Corporation.
11. Nazareth, G. R.: On being a parent of a retarded child, 1973, Providence, R.I., unpublished paper.
12. Olshansky, S.: Chronic sorrow; a response to having a mentally defective child, Soc. Casework **436:**190, 1962.
13. Parad, H. J., and Caplan, G.: A framework for studying families in crisis. In Parad, H. J., editor: Crisis intervention; selected readings, New York, 1965, Family Service Association of America.
14. Robertson, J.: Young children in hospitals, New York, 1958, Basic Books, Inc., Publishers.
15. Robischon, P.: The challenge of crisis theory for nursing, Nurs. Outlook **15:**28, 1967.
16. Rowe, G.: Development of a conceptual family framework in study of the family. In Nye, F. I., and Berardo, F., editors: Emerging conceptual framework in family analysis, New York, 1966, Macmillan Inc.
17. Scahill, M.: A program of nursing intervention with abnormal newborns and their families, 1974, Waltham, Mass., unpublished paper.
18. Solnit, A., and Stark, M.: Mourning and birth of a defective child, Psychoanal. Study Child **16:**523, 1961.
19. Wolfensberger, W.: The principle of normalization in human services, Toronto, 1972, National Institute on Mental Retardation.

ADDITIONAL READINGS

Caplan, G.: An approach to community mental health, New York, 1961. Grune & Stratton, Inc.

Deutsch, H.: Motherhood, psychology of women, vol. 2, New York, 1945, Grune & Stratton, Inc.

Kennedy, J. F.: Maternal reactions to the birth of a defective baby, Soc. Casework, **51:**410, 1970.

Rykeman, D., and Henderson, R.: The meaning of a retarded child for his parents; a focus for counselors, Ment. Retard. **3:**4, 1965.

CHAPTER 20

Use of play in an institution

BARBARA NEWCOMER McLAUGHLIN

PLAY FACILITATES DEVELOPMENT

Play is an important medium for facilitating the development of normal children. There are four basic premises that warrant special consideration when play is viewed as promoting growth. First, play is a natural medium that children will seek on their own to practice developmental tasks if the opportunity to do so is made available. Second, in order to promote play as a facilitator of development, play materials and toys appropriate to the child's developmental level must be made available. Third, play is more likely to facilitate children's development if they receive some encouragement and interaction during play from significant adults in their environment. Fourth, new skills are frequently learned as a child begins to imitate peers, which reinforces the value of group play as stimulating growth and development.

The development of play follows a sequential pattern that is a predictable progression from simple to complex levels. Between the ages of 1 month and 1 year, an infant learns through play. The time spent playing is used to practice motor skills, acquire control of the body, and gain general coordination of movements. Play is especially important to help an infant gain limited control over body movements and develop ability to make sounds. Initially, an infant's play centers around

the development of eye-hand coordination and motor play for exercise. A few simple toys, such as rattles, mobiles, and cradle gyms, are especially important. The motor activity of play remains an infant's chief source of developing sitting, crawling, and pulling to stand. Many things are explored with the mouth, and a variety of multi-textured, multicolored objects are important. A variety of sounds are also stimulating, such as bells, noise-making toys, and music. Infant play consists primarily of sensory-motor stimulation of all types, such as colors, texture, sounds, activity, physical contact, and verbal communication.

Play develops during the toddler period and is based not only on motor skills but also on social and emotional development. A toddler is very active, moving freely from place to place. The toddler enjoys solitary as well as parallel play, and imitative behavior is prevalent. Toddlers have gained control of the finer muscles in their bodies and particularly enjoy manipulating toys and materials. Constructive play, such as modeling with clay, making mud pies, and digging in the sand, begins to be expressed by a toddler. The selection of toys for toddlers should include their individual likes and dislikes, though usually they like push-pull toys and toys that open and close. Toddlers need plenty of space in which to play and a permissive atmosphere that is controlled by a loving adult.

In the preschool stage, many changes are seen in personality development, ability to deal with reality, and control of feelings. The child has made a shift from solitary play in infancy and parallel play as a toddler to cooperative play as a loosely organized play group emerges. The child begins self-expression more with words and less with actions. Active games are increasingly important, but the child also enjoys quiet activities as an increase in constructive use and manipulation of materials is seen. The preschool child needs to develop a sense of initiative, needs to play in groups that include slightly older and younger children, and needs increasing amounts of independence.

The school-age child is primarily interested in the immediate environment and the immediate present. Opportunity to express feelings and find acceptance is important. The play of a school-age child is a spread of scope and movement. Again, very active play is apparent in addition to times of quiet play. Children enjoy group activity: loosely formed clubs, sports, rules, and collections of items in terms of quantity, not quality. The school-age child's needs center around developing a sense of industry, and a more serious aspect of play is seen. An increasing degree of intellectual stimulation in games and projects is noticed. The socializing aspect of play is extremely important because almost all group play means working in close cooperation with others.

Play is an important medium for facilitating development as it follows a predictable, sequential pattern while the child grows and develops. Play is a natural medium that normal children will develop on their own to meet appropriate developmental tasks, if given the opportunity to do so along with encouragement from the significant adults in the environment.

PLAY FOR MENTALLY RETARDED CHILDREN

Play is an important medium for facilitating the development of children. This is no less true for children with mental retardation than for normal children.[3, 4, 10, 12-14] A survey of the published literature has shown that there have been few well-designed and effectively completed experimental studies concerned with play and those who are mentally retarded. Studies of play in this field have been primarily concerned with the refutation or demonstration of change in the areas of personality adjustment or intellectual performance. However, in the few case reports[15] and in the available research reports,[6, 11-13, 16] investigators have shown that children who are mentally retarded do change their behavioral and intellectual functioning as a result of play therapy or play treatment programs.

Despite the fact that play is an important medium for facilitating a child's development, several aspects are often overlooked when play and mentally retarded children are considered. Many play materials that are designed for nonretarded children are unsuited for a retarded child of the same chronological age. When mentally retarded children are able to negotiate such play materials, they are usually chronologically older and much stronger than the nonretarded child for whom the materials were designed. Play materials that are safe for a nonretarded child are frequently dangerous when used by a retarded child of comparable mental age.[3, 4]

A retarded child also will have special deficiencies that make play difficult, such as learning slowly, requiring much repetition, depending on examples rather than words, and attending to things rather than ideas.[4, 13] Games that normally would be suited for a retarded child's developmental age are likely to be considered "too easy," yet the games intended for the chronological age are too complicated.[3] Therefore, games and play activities for a retarded child must be simply structured and concrete and must demand little thinking or language facility.[13]

Benoit found that despite the importance of play for development, children who are mentally retarded usually do not receive sufficient play opportunity.[4] This is especially true for retarded children who live in institutions or training schools. Benoit states that it is primarily through group play that a retarded child can obtain beneficial stimulation necessary for optimal development; therefore, solitary play is seldom successful. Benoit found that play activity during a child's early years did exert measurable effects on the child's growth in social competence, muscle coordination, and motivation.[3] However, he found that much of the material written on group play did not apply to the retarded due to a failure to consider the conditions of overcrowding in institutions and training schools, as well as the need to safeguard play equipment that is easily destroyed.[3]

Play therapy

Play therapy is frequently viewed as an inappropriate treatment modality for those who are mentally retarded. Mentally retarded children have special deficiencies that make play difficult; they exhibit characteristic behaviors, respond for a shorter time duration, and respond with less intensity than do nonretarded children. Play therapy is usually associated with the ability to utilize cognitive function and language in an abstract fashion.

However, the little research that has been done in this area has yielded some important results that conflict with this opinion. Probably the most extensive research in the area of play therapy with mentally retarded children has been done by Leland and Smith.[10] One of their objectives of play therapy states that it is particularly important to emphasize the positive sides of the development by emphasizing ways in which the child is similar to others rather than constantly emphasizing differences. Second, helping the retarded child to increase mastery of motor skills, to increase language ability, and to achieve social gain through development of new interaction patterns are techniques presented by Leland and Smith.[10] Improving the mentally retarded child's developmental skills in the language and social areas will in

turn improve the interaction with other children, again emphasizing ways the child is similar to others.

Play for institutionalized mentally retarded children should include both directive and nondirective play. Play opportunities that encompass a variety of cognitive and social development, including gross motor, fine motor-adaptive, language, and personal-social skills, are extremely important.

Directive play consists of the adult assuming the responsibility for guiding the play, initiating activity with play materials, and entering into the play with the child or children. Activities need to be planned in advance, and play sessions should be organized to include activities that will stimulate cognitive and social functioning. A wide base of play experiences needs to be provided; however, caution must be exercised to plan only one or two different activities per play session.

Nondirective play consists of the adult leaving the responsibility and direction to the child or children. The adult presents play materials and then allows the child to use the materials or toys as desired. The adult presents the necessary materials to complete one or two activities, again including materials that stimulate a variety of cognitive and social skills. The adult allows the child to choose which materials, if any, are wanted. With nondirective play, the adult intrudes in the play only when the child asks or when it is necessary to protect the child's safety or prevent destruction of play materials.[1, 10]

Research indicates that another important aspect of play therapy with mentally retarded children is facilitation of more rapid progress in learning new developmental skills. Newcomer and Morrison found that following three ten-session blocks of play therapy (first and third blocks were directive therapy; the second was nondirective), children in both individual and group play therapy increased their functional levels in gross motor, fine motor-adaptive, language, and personal-social skill categories when compared with children in a no-treatment group.[13] However, in this study no differences were found between children receiving group therapy and children receiving individual therapy.

Another study was completed to determine the effects of directive versus nondirective play therapy with institutionalized mentally retarded children.[12] All children received the play therapy on an individual basis. The DDST was administered before and after the play therapy sessions, and the resultant data supported the hypothesis that play therapy was effective in increasing developmental level.[9] The data did not reflect that directive therapy was more effective than nondirective therapy.

Play opportunities for mentally retarded children

It is extremely important when play opportunities for mentally retarded children are planned to consider the developmental level of the particular children involved. An initial developmental assessment of the child's developmental level (such as the DDST) is needed so that activities that are appropriate to each child's particular level of functioning can be planned.

Play opportunities for those who are mentally retarded must include a variety of activities that will stimulate cognitive and social development. Activities that stimulate gross motor, fine motor-adaptive, language, and personal-social development must be included. The same activities, skills, and toys need to be available for both directive and nondirective play, as well as for group and individual situations. In directive play settings with more than one child, all the children should be asked to do the same activities together. In nondirective play, children should be allowed to play together or separately as they wish. Play groups need to be selected carefully to ensure that children with similar developmental levels are grouped together. It is well to group children of some slightly advanced developmental levels with others less well advanced.

Gross motor activities are those that develop the use and coordination of the gross motor muscles. Initially, the child will progress from rolling over, sitting, crawling, and pulling to stand to walking. Gross motor activities may include playing with large blocks, push-pull toys, slides, or wagons. Coordination is increased through practice in balancing, throwing, hopping, jumping, or running.

Skills within the fine motor-adaptive area deal primarily with eye-hand coordination and perceptual-motor ability. The young child learns to grasp, reach, transfer, and coordinate a neat pincer grasp. Activities may include thumb-finger coordination, peg boards, puzzles, drawing, painting, or cutting.

Language skills include developing speech, improving vocabulary, comprehending words, and following directions. The child learns to vocalize, babble, imitate sounds, develop words, and combine words to form sentences. Specific activities that may enhance language development include imitating speech sounds, identifying pictures in books, talking on a telephone, and naming body parts.

Personal-social development consists primarily of learning the activities of daily living. Children learn social behavior, self-feeding, dressing, and interaction responses in their own environment. Activities that may be used for development of these skills include feeding, washing and drying hands, dressing, performing simple household tasks, and playing interactive games.

Play within an institution

Although play for institutionalized mentally retarded children should include both directive and nondirective play and both individual and group play, some observed differences are worth mentioning.[13] There are benefits of directive, individual play by virtue of the fact that the play is directive in nature and on a one-to-one basis. Directive play with an individual child is probably most organized due to the one-to-one relationship with an adult. Usually one activity, skill, or toy is introduced at a time, and the adult directs the child in the proper use. The environment is organized to a maximal level, and children appear to use a structured environment or organize their play efforts.

Nondirective play for both individual and group situations is unstructured. The interaction with the adult is left to the discretion of the children, and the adult intrudes only within the realm of safety factors. Since play activities usually provide new experiences, particularly for those who are institutionalized, mentally retarded children are frequently content to spend extended periods of time investigating equipment and toys by themselves. One disadvantage of nondirected play is that children appear to have a low ability to organize an unstructured play environment, either as individuals or within a group situation.

Nondirective play for groups of retarded children provides the least structure. In a nondirective play situation with an individual, the child has a one-to-one relationship with an adult, which is an advantage in the child's ability to play. With directive play in a group situation, children are also provided structure, though contact with the adult is less than one-to-one. Mentally retarded children in directive group play usually interact in groups of two and three as opposed to groups of larger size.

Case study. The following case study illustrates the technique and procedure utilized for a play therapy treatment program. The child discussed is part of a larger study described elsewhere.[12]

T.D. was a 9-year-old girl who was institutionalized in a large state training school for those who are mentally retarded. Testing revealed an intellectual level of 4, a mental age of 3.1, and an adaptive behavior level of 4.[8] The DDST was used to measure developmental level before the initiation of play treatment.[9] This test includes items arranged in developmental sequence that measure four categories of abilities: (1) gross motor, (2) fine motor-adaptive, (3) language, and (4) personal-social. Items were administered to the child in each category within an area between the point where

the child passed all of the items and the point where she failed all the items. Developmental scores were determined for T.D. Within each of the four categories, she was assigned one point for each skill passed according to the criteria defined in the test manual. Developmental scores were determined only for the purposes of this project, and it must be emphasized that the DDST in its original form is not designed to derive a developmental or mental age or an IQ score.

T.D. received the following points for skills accomplished before the play project intervention:

	Pretest scores	Maximum potential scores
Gross motor	17	31
Fine motor-adaptive	11	30
Language	5	20
Personal-social	11	22

A directive play program was initiated for T.D. on a one-to-one basis with an adult. The play was guided by the adult initiating activities with predetermined materials. Activities were planned to include one or two activities within each of the four skill categories during each session. The sessions extended for 45 minutes per day and were continued over a 3-week time period. The child was seen in the same playroom for each session, and the playroom was equipped with standard materials, such as balls, crayons, paint, clay, blocks, and furniture.

T.D.'s pretest and posttest scores on the DDST scales are as follows:

	Pretest scores	Posttest scores
Gross motor (31)	17	22
Fine motor (30)	11	21
Language (20)	5	5
Personal-social (22)	11	15

New skills accomplished by T.D. following the directive play program include the following:

Gross motor
  Regards face
  Smiles responsively

  Plays peek-a-boo
  Helps in simple house tasks
Fine motor adaptive
  Follows past midline
  Follows 180°
  Sits and looks for yarn
  Passes cube hand to hand
  Bangs two cubes held in hands
  Tower of two cubes
  Dumps raisin from bottle
  Tower of four cubes
  Tower of eight cubes
  Imitates vertical line within 30°
Language
  None
Personal-social
  Walks up steps
  Pedals tricycle
  Balances on one foot 5 seconds
  Balances on one foot 10 seconds

The case example has shown that the directive play program was effective in increasing T.D.'s developmental level. The directive play was extremely organized due to the one-to-one relationship. One activity, skill, or toy was introduced at a time, and she was directed in the proper use. The play efforts were directed toward activities that were appropriate to her functional level. The environment was organized to a maximal level, and T.D. appeared to use the structured environment to organize play efforts.

Summary. Several questions must be raised regarding the total picture of play treatment to increase the developmental level of institutionalized mentally retarded children. First, it is important to consider the effects due to the children's institutionalization. Zigler and his associates[2, 5, 17-19] studied the socially depriving effects of institutionalization and the relationship between social deprivation and desire for adult reinforcement. Balla and Zigler found that certain tendencies toward psychological growth in evidence after 3 years of institutionalization were still in evidence after 6 years of institutional living.[2] Impressions are that the relationship between social deprivation and increased motivation for adult social reinforcement depends in part on the level of social deprivation before

institutionalization. Institutionalized children are usually considered to be highly socially deprived, and the children in play programs quickly become attached to the adult and to the playroom. The nurse or other adult has the potential to be highly socially reinforcing to the child while responding to play activities.

The increase in developmental level seen in children following play treatment needs further investigation to determine whether similar changes would occur in noninstitutionalized mentally retarded children. With regard to the level of social deprivation, certain differences warrant attention when play therapy for retarded children who are not institutionalized is considered. Nurses could teach parents to develop play programs incorporating the concepts of play therapy. Parents need to know that play opportunities for mentally retarded children must include a variety of activities that will stimulate cognitive and social development. Activities that need to be included are ones that promote gross motor, fine motor-adaptive, language, and personal-social development in both directive and nondirective fashion and individual and group situations. Parents providing such intervention should be aware of basic concepts of growth and development and that all efforts should be directed to the child's particular functional level.

In addition to parents providing intervention for noninstitutionalized retarded children, nurses could offer such intervention to a child in the home environment. Preschool and special education programs for the mentally retarded could be designed to incorporate the basic principles of play therapy intervention to facilitate growth and increase developmental level.

A second question relates to whether changes in the DDST scores are stable over a period of time. Follow-up data should be collected to determine whether ongoing play treatment is necessary to maintain the developmental level increases.

A third question is whether a play program does indeed constitute "play therapy.'' The adult (therapist) in the case study presented was trained in the principles of nondirective therapy as enunciated by Axline[1] and in the principles of therapy with retarded children as described by Leland and Smith.[10] There appear to be two basic objectives for play therapy with mentally retarded children, both of which seem equally significant. Improving a mentally retarded child's emotional health and self-concept, as well as facilitating cognitive growth by increasing developmental skill level, requires special intervention. Although an increase in mentally retarded children's developmental levels has been observed,[12, 13] evidence is not conclusive that specific training or therapeutic principles are necessarily factors in producing the change.

A fourth consideration is Erikson's premise that children use play to work through each developmental crisis. Erikson's guide offers insight into both the sickness and wellness of human personality. The following four stages represent areas of crisis that must be met with satisfactory solution to promote good emotional health.

1. Basic trust versus basic mistrust (first year of life)
2. Autonomy versus shame and doubt (second and third years of life)
3. Initiative versus guilt (third and fourth years of life)
4. Industry versus inferiority (fifth year to adolescent years)[7]

Erikson believes that play facilitates personality growth by allowing a safe arena for children to try out and work through new developmental challenges.[7] Institutionalized mentally retarded children appear more susceptible to the negative pole of each developmental crisis; thus, play therapy could be used as a preventive measure.

The final question relates to whether or not relatively untrained personnel, such as volunteers and foster grandparents, could have produced the same results, given the same amount of time spent with a child on a one-to-one basis. If this hypothesis could be supported, it would have major implications for institutionalized mentally retarded children. An increase in a child's developmental level could be expected to occur with slight alteration or modification of the child's usual activities of daily living.

Before the initiation of a program that would incorporate relatively untrained personnel, it would be mandatory for the responsible professionals, usually nurses, to develop a staff learning program for attendants and volunteers in the basic techniques of play therapy intervention. Concepts of growth and development, along with a basic understanding of activities appropriate to a child's functional level, must be taught.

Overcrowding, understaffing, use of expensive equipment, and lack of understanding of the value of play are all concerns to be considered. Institutions are currently becoming less crowded, and the staff-resident ratio is improving. Equipment need not be expensive, and much play stimulation could occur during the course of daily activity if attendants and volunteers were knowledgeable of appropriate techniques and principles. Hopefully, the social interaction involved in play would facilitate development and serve as a means of counteracting the decline in developmental level relative to age that has been demonstrated with institutionalized mentally retarded children.[12, 13, 19]

REFERENCES

1. Axline, V.: Play therapy, New York, 1947, Houghton Mifflin Co.
2. Balla, D. A., and Zigler, E.: Preinstitutional social deprivation, responsiveness to social reinforcement and IQ changes in institutionalized retarded individuals, Am. J. Ment. Defic. **80:**228, 1975.
3. Benoit, E. P.: More fun for institutionalized retarded children, Am. J. Ment. Defic. **58:**93, 1953.
4. Benoit, E. P.: The play problem of retarded children, Am. J. Ment. Defic. **60:**41, 1955.
5. Butterfield, E. C., and Zigler, E.: The influence of differing social climates on the effectiveness of social reinforcement in the mentally retarded, Am. J. Ment. Defic. **70:**48, 1965.
6. Chess, S.: Psychiatric treatment of the mentally retarded child with behavior problems, Am. J. Orthopsychiatry **32:**863, 1962.
7. Erikson, E. H.: Childhood and society, New York, 1963, W. W. Norton Co., Inc.

8. Fogelman, C. J., editor: AAMD adaptive behavior scale manual, Washington, D.C., 1974, American Association on Mental Deficiency.

9. Frankenburg, W. K., and others: Denver developmental screening test manual, Denver, 1970, The University of Colorado Medical Center.

10. Leland, H., and Smith, D. E.: Play therapy with mentally subnormal children, New York, 1965, Grune & Stratton, Inc.

11. Leland, H., Walker, J., and Taboada, A.: Group play therapy with a group of post-nursery male retardates, Am. J. Ment. Defic. **63:**848, 1959.

12. Morrison, T. L., and Newcomer, B. L.: Effects of directive versus nondirective play therapy with institutionalized mentally retarded children, Am. J. Ment. Defic. **79:**666, 1975.

13. Newcomer, B. L., and Morrison, T. L.: Play therapy with institutionalized mentally retarded children, Am. J. Ment. Defic. **78:**727, 1974.

14. Piers, M. W., editor: Play and development, New York, 1972, W. W. Norton & Co., Inc.

15. Sarason, S. B., and Doris, J.: Psychological problems in mental deficiency, ed. 4, New York, 1969, Harper & Row, Publishers, Inc.

16. Schachter, R. F., Meyer, L. R., and Loomis, E. A.: Childhood schizophrenia and mental retardation; differential diagnosis before and after one year of psychotherapy, Am. J. Orthopsychiatry **32:**584, 1962.

17. Zigler, E.: Mental retardation; current issues and approaches. In Hoffman, L. W., and Hoffman, M. L., editors: Review of child development research, vol. 1, New York, 1966, Russell Sage Foundation.

18. Zigler, E., Butterfield, E. C., and Capobianco, F.: Institutionalization and the effectiveness of social reinforcement; a five and eight year follow-up study, Dev. Psychol. **3:**255, 1970.

19. Zigler, E., and Williams, J.: Institutionalization and effectiveness of social reinforcement; a three-year follow-up study, J. Abnorm. Psychol. **66:**197, 1963.

ADDITIONAL READINGS

Barnard, K. E., and Erickson, M. P.: Teaching children with developmental problems, ed. 2, St. Louis, 1976, The C. V. Mosby Co.

Biggar, J.: Psychotherapy and child development, London, 1966, Fairstock Publications.

Ginott, H. C.: Group psychotherapy with children, New York, 1961, McGraw-Hill, Inc.

Haworth, M. R., editor: Child psychotherapy; theory and practice, New York, 1964, Basic Books, Inc., Publishers.

Kessler, J.: Psychopathology of childhood, Englewood Cliffs, N.J., 1966, Prentice-Hall, Inc.

McCandless, B. R.: Relation of environmental factors to intellectual functioning. In Heber, R., and Stevens, H., editors: Review of research in mental retardation, Chicago, 1964, University of Chicago Press.

Marlow, D. R.: Textbook of pediatric nursing, Philadelphia, 1977, W. B. Saunders Co.

O'Neil, S. M., McLaughlin, B. N., and Knapp, M. B.: Behavioral approaches to children with developmental delay, St. Louis, 1977, The C. V. Mosby Co.

Smart, M. S., and Smart, R. C.: Children; development and relationships, New York, 1972, Macmillan, Inc.

CHAPTER 21

The transition from institution to community living

JUDITH BICKLEY CURRY

In recent years, many overcrowded institutions have begun efforts to return retarded residents to the community. Some adults with severe physical disabilities or nursing care needs have been placed in nursing home settings. Many adults who need sheltered living or work environments have been placed in community facilities, such as halfway houses, where some degree of supervision is available. The goal for most of the adults who have minimal or moderate handicaps is to enable them to become self-sufficient members of a community. In some instances, however, adults have been discharged from institutions with very little educational, vocational, sexual, or social preparation. Their adjustment to community living has been more difficult due to the lack of a support system during this transition period.

In the past, nurses have not been involved to a great extent in this support system. Traditionally, nurses employed in institutional facilities have limited their responsibilities to providing physical care to the residents and teaching and supervising aides who assist in the routine, daily care. Community health nurses have focused their responsibilities on children and families who already reside in the community. There has

been little effort to coordinate care for those individuals who are preparing to move from institutions into community living arrangements.

The purpose of this chapter is to identify some of the problems and issues involved in the retarded individual's transition from the institution to a more self-sufficient community life. The roles and responsibilities of nurses in alleviating or preventing some of the problems associated with the transition are discussed.

INFLUENCES ON THE TRANSITION FROM INSTITUTION TO COMMUNITY

A number of factors have influenced recent efforts toward deinstitutionalization. In the late 1960s and early 1970s, overcrowding was a major problem in most public institutions. Even though overcrowding existed, institutions had long lists of individuals waiting to be admitted. Administrators of large institutions, recognizing the problems of overcrowding, understaffing, and increasing financial constraints, began looking for alternatives to residential care.

At the same time, the need for improvements in residential care and services was recognized. Policy statements for use as guidelines in improving services were published in 1968 by NARC[5] and in 1970 by the President's Committee on Mental Retardation.[6] The formation of the Accreditation Council for Facilities for the Mentally Retarded within the Joint Commission on Accreditation of Hospitals resulted in the publication in 1971 of standards for residential services.[8] These standards were consistent with the policy recommendations of NARC and the President's Committee on Mental Retardation. They also incorporated: (1) the concept of normalization, (2) a philosophy of individualized programming for the development of maximum potential, (3) consideration for the quality of services rendered, (4) a humanizing environment, (5) coordination efforts with community agencies to provide a full range of comprehensive services, and (6) consideration of the rights of retarded individuals.

Another impact on residential services was the initiation of right-to-treatment court cases. The first case, *Wyatt vs Stickney,* was filed in September, 1970, in Alabama. It resulted in the determination that a resident has a constitutional right to treatment, and it established standards by which adequate habilitation could be evaluated.[3] Similar cases have been filed in other states. Most of them are still in the long process of appeal. However, these suits have been responsible for upgrading care in many residential facilities and for bringing legal services to institutionalized individuals.

During this period of service reform in institutions, community services for retarded individuals were expanding. Halfway houses and group homes were developed. Client programs, such as citizen advocacy and protective services, were initiated by many state agencies. In order to alleviate the need for institutional admission, respite care facilities were developed. With the expansion of a variety of community service agencies for children and adults, the need for permanent residential care for many individuals was lessened.

One of the major influences of this period was the federal Developmental Disabilities Act* (PL 91-517), which went into effect in October, 1970. The Act authorized formula grants to states for[2]:

1. Developing and implementing a comprehensive and continuing plan.
2. Providing services to the developmentally disabled.
3. Constructing facilities for the housing of services.
4. Training specialized personnel for services and research.
5. Developing or demonstrating new or improved techniques of services.
6. Constructing university-affiliated facilities to house the interdisciplinary training of professional personnel.
7. Administering and operating demonstration and training facilities.

A major reason for the trend toward community care is the belief that retarded individuals belong in the community and not in specialized, isolated residential facilities. The outcome of expanded community services will be that more retarded individuals will remain in the community and be provided services by already existing resources. At present, however, the reentry into the community of a large number of previously institutionalized individuals is of primary concern.

ISSUES AND PROBLEMS IN THE TRANSITION
Readiness of the client, community, and professional

In the effort to discharge residents from institutions as rapidly as possible, numerous problems have occurred. Some residents have been placed in community nursing or group care homes, which in turn have become smaller institutions with little improvement in services or quality of care. Many staff members of these homes, including nurses, have not been prepared for working with retarded persons. Many residents have been discharged into the community

---

*Developmental disability is defined as a condition attributable to mental retardation, cerebral palsy, epilepsy, or other neurological handicapping condition closely related to mental retardation.

without adequate preparation, adjustment periods, and support systems. Many retarded individuals have not been ready for community life, and many communities have not been ready to accept retarded persons.

The lack of preparation and necessary adjustments has been exhibited in some communities by resistance to requests for zoning approval for group homes and living arrangements. Many of those who resisted group homes in their own neighborhoods were professionals who worked in fields closely related to mental retardation. Public attitudes toward retarded persons have changed in recent years. However, the general population, including professionals in service fields, has a long way to go in achieving community acceptance of individuals with disabilities. Before attempting to educate lay people about the mentally retarded individual's rights as a citizen, nurses and other professionals must examine their own attitudes and become more accepting of others' disabilities.

Socioeconomic issues and the work ethic

In most instances, a retarded adult's success in adjusting to community living has been equated with an ability to be employed as a wage earner. This may be an unrealistic expectation for some individuals, especially those who have spent a number of their adult years as unemployed residents of an institution. Zipperlen points out that competitive work is basically selfish and that many retarded persons are more interested in the result of their work than in earning money for themselves.[9] Retarded individuals cannot be expected to easily adjust to financially supporting themselves through competitive employment when the institution has previously provided for all material needs. Professionals should recognize and accept that there will be retarded individuals in the community, with or without families, who will need financial support from social service agencies.

Retarded persons who have been able to handle competitive employment are usually in low-paying, manual work situations. Because of their low-income levels, most retarded adults who have achieved some degree of self-sufficiency in the community have moved into low-income housing areas. Unfortunately, some professionals do not feel comfortable working with low-income families. If these professionals find themselves working in such situations and do not admit their discomfort, the provision of services will be inadequate.

Agency objectives versus client needs

All too often, the objectives of programs and care for retarded individuals have been those that benefit the agency or professionals involved rather than those that benefit the clients.

After discharge from an institution, Mr. S. was to receive assistance from a state vocational training agency. The worker assigned to the case decided that Mr. S.'s physical appearance detracted from his training and employment potential. Before the training would begin, Mr. S. was advised to show up at the worker's office clean shaven and well groomed every morning for a week. When Mr. S. was unable to meet this unrealistic demand, he was terminated by the agency as a failure. No consideration was given to Mr. S.'s needs or why he was unable to achieve this task, and no referral was made to other agencies for assistance.

Working with individual needs is time-consuming and requires participation of the client or family in determining goals and objectives. Many agencies, with the objectives of turning out a certain number of successful cases, have not been willing or able to spend the necessary time to begin their efforts at the same level as that of the retarded individual or family.

Dependency to independency

Most residents of institutions have been conditioned for years to be dependent on the institutional staff for all needs. Very little independent activity has been encouraged or even tolerated. Some initial dependency on community professionals or agencies can be expected from retarded adults who are discharged from institutions.

Mrs. B., an expresident of an institution, was married, lived in the community, and was the mother of two preschool children. She had received threats from several agencies to remove her children. In attempting to establish a trusting, helping relationship with a new agency, the nurse encouraged Mrs. B. to call anytime she needed assistance. After several months, the nurse realized that Mrs. B. was calling almost daily—sometimes for information, and other times for favors.

One day the nurse refused a request from Mrs. B. to drive her to a well-baby clinic for routine care. She was advised to see if a neighbor could take her for the appointment and informed that the nurse would call her later. Feeling guilty about refusing this request, the nurse sought counsel from a social worker who also knew the family. Both agreed that the family could handle this situation because they had done so in the past. It was also decided that the family needed to become more independent.

On the follow-up call to Mrs. B., she had received assistance from a neighbor for transportation to the clinic. The nurse praised Mrs. B. for handling this situation on her own. After several more months of selectively refusing requests that Mrs. B. had demonstrated she could handle, her telephone calls came less often and were more appropriate.

In cases where retarded individuals have had negative experiences with agencies or professionals or when the person is new to community life, some initial dependency may be encouraged. However, professionals should be aware of what is happening and know when to begin working toward independency as a long-term objective in treatment plans.

Neighbors can be significant resources in the community support system for retarded adults. In many communities, retarded adults are easily accepted by the other families in the neighborhood and provide each other with needed support, such as sharing transportation, baby-sitting, shopping, and emergency services.

Health education needs

Retarded adolescents and adults have the same needs for health education services as do all persons. If retarded persons have as-

sociated medical problems, they may need more intensive nursing services. Most individuals will need a greater amount of time and help in adjusting to the community health care system, since most institutions have previously been the sole provider of all the medical and dental services for residents.

Health education needs of retarded individuals in the community include:

1. Understanding of illness and disease, including communicable diseases, such as venereal disease.
2. Prevention of illness and daily health regimens.
3. Knowledge of community resources and how and when to use them (medical, dental, nutritional, and mental health).
4. Knowledge of human sexuality, family life, family planning, and alternative life-styles.
5. Information about medications and drugs.
6. Recreation, exercise, and leisure-time activities.
7. Safety factors and accident prevention.

Health education services should be initiated in the institutional setting. Most institutions, however, have not provided adequate educational services for residents. Therefore, the need is greater for nurses and other professionals to provide for health education needs after the retarded person returns to the community.

The right to have a family life, to marry, and to have children

The rights of retarded individuals to have a family life, to marry, and to have children have been expressed by the International League of Societies for the Mentally Handicapped[1] and by AAMD.[7] In 1975, however, forty-one states still carried statutes that prohibited marriage for persons with mental disabilities or who had been confined in institutions. In forty-one states, the permission of retarded parents was not needed in order to remove children for adoption.[4]

Despite outmoded state statutes, many mentally retarded adults are marrying and raising children in the community. Few studies have been done concerning the success or failure of these marriages and families. Marriage and the right to have children are still controversial issues among both professionals and the general population. One marital failure or success of a retarded individual should not be generalized to all retarded persons. Each situation should be considered on an individual basis with respect for the person's rights, desires, and capabilities.

When a retarded mother announced that she was expecting her third child, professionals in the agency that coordinated services for the family blamed the case coordinator, a nurse, for the lack of "successful" teaching about birth control. Before the pregnancy, however, both parents had decided that they wanted a third child. They had also decided that the mother would have a tubal ligation after delivery because they felt they could not support more children. The nurse felt that education and counseling had been successful because the parents had made their own decisions about their family.

More positive attitudes are developing toward marriage of retarded individuals who live in the community, particularly for those without children. Acceptance has seemed to be more related to the need for marriage in order to combine incomes and for companionship rather than related to the fact that marriage is a normalizing societal experience. Institutions have not adequately prepared their residents in sexual, marital, and family life needs. Educational programs and more normal experiences throughout childhood and adolescence in institutions and community facilities should be made available in order to prepare young adults for informed decision making about their lives.

Documentation and reporting

The issues of documentation and reporting are important to the deinstitutionalization efforts. Many residents have lengthy records that cover a long period of years. When they move into a community, the entire record, or portions of it, may be transferred to other agencies. In many instances, data in a client's record may be outdated, such as IQ scores that are 10 years old. Data may also be subjective and even erroneous.

Often, records and referral information precede the client's personal contacts with agencies. These reports can influence the attitudes of professionals toward the client.

In one agency, the case worker received a report stating that a retarded couple was living together but not legally married. Since there were children in the home, the case worker immediately began investigating the legal aspects of child guardianship. If the case worker had waited until after meeting the couple, many hours of investigative work could have been saved. The couple had a marriage license, which they proudly displayed.

Professionals working with retarded clients should not prejudge the individuals based on referral information and reports. Nurses should use such material selectively and discriminatively. In written reports, care should be exercised to record only pertinent, factual, and objective data. Verbal reporting and passing of information are equally important and can be as helpful or as damaging to the client as written information.

Interagency coordination

Some retarded individuals may not be known by service agencies in their community. Many individuals, however, are known by one or more agencies. Some may have had contacts with and services from numerous agencies. Unless one professional or agency has taken responsibility for coordinating all services for one retarded individual or family, very limited contacts have existed among agencies.

Coordination of care should begin before discharge from the institution. Interagency conferences should be held routinely to assist in coordination efforts. For the client, the advantages would be to eliminate confusion, ease transition from one agency to another, and provide a central contact person or agency for assistance. The advantages for agencies include better utilization of manpower, elimination of duplication of services, and a better service delivery system.

ROLES AND RESPONSIBILITIES OF NURSES IN INSTITUTIONS

Nurses who work in residential facilities have been expanding their roles and responsibilities. Many institutions are changing from a medical model to a developmental approach to care and services. In many of these facilities, nurses are moving into programming and administrative positions within the organizational structure. Nurses are increasingly evident in positions such as unit managers or program directors, with responsibilities that extend beyond traditional bedside nursing care to total programming for residents.

With these expanded functions, nurses in residential settings can greatly influence the types and quality of programs, activities, and services for their clients. They can also provide positive contributions to policies and decision making at the administrative level. In facilities where it is still difficult to have an impact on the philosophy and objectives for the benefit of all residents, nurses can influence the quality of services on an individual, one-to-one basis.

The standards for residential facilities developed by the AC/FMR should be used as a resource by nurses in institutions to plan, administer, and evaluate nursing care services.[8] These standards require that nursing personnel be involved in the provision of comprehensive services to clients, beginning with preadmission planning through discharge and referral to appropriate community resources.

To assist in the adjustment problems related to transition from institution to community, nurses in residential settings should be involved in the provision of the following services.

1. The resident should be prepared for discharge. This should begin at the time of admission to the institution. No admission should be considered permanent. If the ultimate goal for all residents is to be returned to the community, programming and ser-

vices should be developed to meet that goal.

2. Provision should be made for normalizing living conditions and experiences. Some of the ways in which this can be achieved are through (a) allowances for privacy and personal effects, (b) flexibility in schedules for activities of daily living, (c) coeducational activities and living arrangements, (d) frequent trips and outings in the community, and (e) encouragement of heterosexual relationships and opportunities for dating.

3. Clients should receive encouragement and provision for their participation in decision making. Too often all responsibility for decision making is taken away from the client at the time of admission. All decisions for the individual, including what clothes to wear, are then made by the residential staff. To as great an extent as is possible, all clients should be allowed to participate in making decisions about their care, activities, interests, and programming needs.

4. Clients should be educated and counseled about health concerns. These services should be constantly available and should include health needs, personal hygiene, sexuality, family life and alternative lifestyles, family planning, prevention of illness, and recreational and leisure pursuits. Services may be provided in group settings or on an individual basis. If a nurse does not feel comfortable discussing some of these areas, other nurses or other professionals interested in these topics should be utilized as resources.

5. Family participation in residential care and treatment should be encouraged. Many families relinquish responsibility for care of a retarded person on the admission of that individual to an institution. For many families, institutionalization is the greatest crisis with which they have to deal. Support for families to assist them with the separation anxiety, financial burden, and guilt surrounding the placement decision can be provided by nurses, both in the institution and in the community. If plans for the client include a future return to the family, ongoing involvement by the family is mandatory. The longer retarded persons remain in an institu-

tion, the more difficult it is for their families to take them back into the home. Nurses should allow, encourage, and welcome family participation in daily care such as feeding, therapy programs, and other activities.

ROLES AND RESPONSIBILITIES OF NURSES IN COMMUNITY FACILITIES

Nurses in community health practice may be employed in a variety of service agencies, including local health departments. Most community health nurses have not had specialized education and experiences in mental retardation. However, community nurses have responsibilities in areas with which nurses in institutions have not been primarily involved, such as coordination of care for individuals and families among a number of health service agencies.

In the future community nurses will come in contact with increasing numbers of mentally retarded individuals and their families. At present, however, these nurses can make a great contribution toward improving the adjustment problems of retarded persons in the community through the provision of the following services.

1. They can coordinate services provided by the support system in the community. The nurse can be the liaison between the retarded person and the community agencies that are involved in providing services for that individual. The retarded person may need assistance with making agency contacts and discriminating among appropriate service resources. Nurses can help by making initial contacts, advising about appropriate services based on needs, and teaching the retarded person how to use the system.

2. They can serve as advocates for the needs and rights of clients and families. Community nurses should be knowledgeable about the trends in services for mentally retarded persons. Nurses have a responsibility to educate other professionals and the general public about changing services. They also can serve as an advocate for appropriate care and treatment based on individual needs and legal rights. On some occa-

sions, nurses have to remind other professionals of unfulfilled promises of services to clients and families. Community nurses can be of further assistance by serving on committees and task forces in order to influence services and legislation that protect the rights of retarded persons.

3. They can encourage client independency and participation in decision making. Community nurses, other members of the team, and retarded adults should work together in planning short-term and long-term goals toward self-sufficiency of the client. Some professionals may have difficulty decreasing or terminating relationships with clients due to their own dependency needs. If the retarded person is able to function appropriately in a community, nurses should encourage that independency by positive reinforcement. Retarded individuals should be allowed some reasonable risk taking in making informed decisions about their lives.

COORDINATION BETWEEN INSTITUTION AND COMMUNITY

In order to improve the deinstitutionalization effort, better communication and coordination must take place between institutions and communities. Nurses in both settings should initiate relationships in order to establish the roles and responsibilities to be carried out by each. As institutions become less isolated and are utilized as another resource within a continuum of community service providers, nurses will have a greater responsibility for contributing to the continuity of care. As an example, a community nurse might go into the institution to assist in the preparation for discharge and to establish a relationship with the resident. In another situation, the nurse from an institution might make a home visit to a family to discuss the care and services provided by the residential facility. The continuity of care, alleviation of adjustment problems, and maintainance of family involvement should be the major concerns of nurses in institutions and community agencies.

OUTCOMES OF INTERVENTION

Through improved and expanded nursing services and better coordination of efforts between agencies, many objectives may be realized. One of these might be to avoid the duplication and fragmentation of services to clients and families. Improved coordination will assist retarded individuals and families to cope with the adjustment surrounding admissions to, and discharges from, institutional facilities.

In addition to improving the quality of services, better utilization of nursing manpower can be realized. Knowledge and resources can be shared among those nurses working with an individual client or family. Nurses in both settings will have greater opportunities for updating knowledge and improving skills in working with retarded individuals through team efforts. Finally, nursing services provided through teamwork should lead to increased levels of independent functioning by retarded persons and their families. This outcome should be the major goal of all nursing services and should be the indicator of the effectiveness and success of service delivery.

SUMMARY

This chapter has focused on the recent developments in deinstitutionalization and some of the issues and problems related to readjustment of retarded individuals in the community. Nurses in institutions and community settings have major roles in alleviating some of these problems and influencing the issues. Some of the ways in

which nurses can assist in these efforts have been discussed. Innovative practice in this area is encouraged. The primary goal for nurses helping in the transition process is to increase the level of independent functioning of retarded individuals and their families.

REFERENCES

1. Declaration of general and special rights of the mentally retarded, Oct. 1968, The International League of Societies for the Mentally Handicapped.
2. The developmental disabilities act; a view and review, U.S. Department of Health, Education, and Welfare, Social and Rehabilitation Service, Rehabilitation Services Administration (SRS) 74.25080.
3. Friedman, P.: Legal aspects of institutionalization of mentally retarded citizens, presented at the Legal Planning and Legal Rights for Mentally Retarded and Developmentally Disabled Ohioans, Columbus, Ohio, 1973.
4. Hobbs, N.: The futures of children; categories, labels, and their consequences, Report of the Project on Classification of Exceptional Children, San Francisco, 1975, Jossey-Bass, Inc.
5. Policy statements on residential care, adopted by the Board of Directors of the National Association for Retarded Children, Oct. 1968.
6. The President's Committee on Mental Retardation: Residential services for the mentally retarded; an action policy proposal, Washington , D.C., 1970, U.S. Government Printing Office.
7. Rights of mentally retarded persons, official statement of the American Association on Mental Deficiency, Ment. Retard. **2:**56, 1973.
8. Standards for residential facilities for the mentally retarded, Accreditation Council for Facilities for the Mentally Retarded, Joint Commission on Accreditation of Hospitals, Chicago, 1971.
9. Zipperlen, H. R.: Normalization. In Wortis, J., editor: Mental retardation and developmental disabilities, an annual review, vol. VII, New York, 1975, Brunner/Mazel, Inc.